"Pretty Ugly" is a fascinating tale that takes us from Kansas City to Washington, D.C. and on to Ireland – a genuine tour de force from a global journalist turned global novelist. It's a fast-moving triumph from a writer who really knows his way around human relationships, especially those involving politicians, editors, doctors and even strangers lurking in the mysterious fogs of Éire!" (STEPHEN FARNSWORTH is a political science professor and founder of the Center for Leadership and Media Studies, University of Mary Washington. Multi-book author, Fulbright scholar and national commentator, including The Washington Post, Reuters, The Chicago Tribune and MSNBC.)

"Start with a natural raconteur who is at home in Romania as Kansas City. Add a shot of old-school newspapering, a sinister dose of big medicine and the right mix of Irish humor and moral indignation, and you get a novel as bracing as a shot of Jameson." (MIKE WEATHERFORD is Arts & Entertainment Reporter and Columnist for the 'Las Vegas Review-Journal' newspaper and author of 'Cult Vegas.')

"Seasoned journalist and writer John Sean Hillen has filed a story that's as entertaining as it is timely. "Pretty Ugly" is a richly written novel that is both journalistic procedural and cautionary tale about the cosmetics industry, politics, and corporate journalism. When they collide, it can be pretty ugly." (JOHN DEDAKIS is a novelist, writing coach, former CBN White House correspondent and senior copy editor for CNN's 'The Situation Room with Wolf Blitzer.' Adjunct journalism faculty member at University of Maryland-College Park.)

"Rich in detail, this is a novel by an astute observer. Sean Hillen is a curious and peripatetic writer and he gives his readers a remarkable sense of place and time in this elaborate story of political, journalistic and medical intrigue. From a midwestern newsroom to the halls of Congress to the 'brown-black turf bogs beyond Cnoc Fola,' Hillen not only takes us on a narrative journey, he places us there." (JIM KUHNHENN, newspaper bureau chief, editor and Congressional and White House correspondent, past president of the Washington Press Club Foundation and former member of the Congressional Standing Committee of Correspondents.)

D1530019

Pretty Ugly

a novel by

Sean Hillen

ISBN-10: 1523361158
ISBN-13: 978-1523361151

seanhillenauthor.com

Dedication

'Pretty Ugly' is published in memory of the late Massachusetts Senator Edward Moore 'Ted' Kennedy, known as 'The Lion of the Senate.' who spent a great part of his exemplary political life supporting varied consumer health issues and was particularly active in attempting to better regulate the cosmetics industry. May his name be writ higher than the Washington Monument itself.

I also dedicate 'Pretty Ugly' to a pre-eminent medical practitioner and teacher, now sadly gone from us, who encouraged me both as a health correspondent and in my first faltering footsteps into authordom. 'Doctor Gray' in 'Pretty Ugly' is a fictional character named to honor Doctor E. Grey Dimond, cardiologist and founder of the University of Missouri-Kansas City (UMKC) School of Medicine and the international Diastole Scholars' Center, now under the direction of its president, Nancy Hill.

With the agonizing decline in investigative reporting in all but the bravest and strongest of newspapers, it would be remiss of me not to mention one shining example in the field that I had the privilege and honor of calling friend. A gentle, soft-spoken man and fierce reporter – sadly departed, long before he should have left us – he not only possessed the determination and stamina to run multiple marathons but also to track down and reveal corruption at the highest levels of society, from the Midwest to the East coast, from Kansas and Missouri to New Jersey. Pulitzer Prize winning, Dunstan 'Dusty' McNichol, meet Colm Heaney.

Acknowledgements

Thanking all those people who helped me in this literary endeavor might well end up being longer than the book itself. My deepest gratitude, however, go to a host of people in various countries, in diverse fields, who contributed their expertise to help me avoid inane inaccuracies in several domains including health, media, cosmetics and politics, not to mention the native Irish language, Gaeilge. Any mistakes remaining are entirely of my own (un)doing. Blame for this lies primarily at the feet of unbridled imagination, born of a Celtic DNA.

First and foremost of those whose support proved invaluable is my Transylvanian wife, Columbia. May Mother Nature lavish its bounties eternally upon her for her infinite patience. As my anam cara ('soul mate' in Irish), my editor, my designer, my marketing director, my brand manager… one of my favorite poets, W. H. Auden, put it best,

> "*my North, my South, my East and West,*
> *My working week and my Sunday rest,*
> *My noon, my midnight, my talk, my song;*"

But even that's not enough.

Then I dance a dizzy waltz from tiny rocky islands off the northwest coast of Ireland to the metropolises of Belfast, Galway, Dublin, London, Zurich, Kansas City, Las Vegas, Tucson, Washington and New York to round-up all those whose literary footprint lies within the pages of 'Pretty Ugly.'

Not in alphabetical order nor necessarily in order of importance, they include:

Word lovers Mark and Tina Gregory in Belfast and Connie Ward in Switzerland who waded through 'Pretty Ugly' wearing microscope editing lenses.

Sandra Katz, book lover, skilled ophthalmologist and incurable world traveler who with long-time friend, Diane Stephenson, considers Paris and Havana equally intriguing in so many different ways.

For scientific help in better understanding the power and potential of nanoparticles, my deepest gratitude goes to Professor Terry Tetley, researcher and professor at the Faculty of Medicine, National Heart & Lung Institute, Imperial College London who initiated the college's strategy on 'Nanoparticles and Health' as well as to Doctor Olwyn McWeeney and barrister-cum-medical writer, Paul McGinn, for their advice.

I would be amiss not to mention Dr. Felix Sabates founder of the University of Missouri-Kansas City School of Medicine's Department of Ophthalmology half a century ago, of the original founders of the Missouri Ophthalmologic Society and the 'Sabates Eye Centers.' As health correspondent for 'The Kansas City Times,' interviewing him increased my knowledge exponentially about the human eye, our body's most complex organ. It's amazing something so small can have so many working parts.

I also wish to acknowledge the important research and consumer activism of Stacy Malkan, author of 'Not Just A Pretty Face' and co-founder with Janet Nudelman of 'The Campaign for Safe Cosmetics,' a coalition project with founding members including Friends of the Earth, the Breast Cancer Fund, Commonweal, the National Black Environmental Justice Network, Alliance for a Healthy Tomorrow, Women's Voices for the Earth, National Environmental Trust, Clean Water Fund, Massachusetts Breast Cancer Coalition, the Environmental Working Group, as well as Health Care Without Harm, a worldwide organization of health professionals, environmental groups and governments to promote safe practices and products in healthcare. The American Medical Women's Association and the Society for Women's Health Research are also lobbying for safer cosmetics.

Aside from former Senator Edward Kennedy, credit also goes to a succession of other leading politicians, including former Missouri Senator Thomas F. Eagleton, who have tried to regulate the cosmetics industry. As this book goes to print, Senators Dianne Feinstein of California and Susan Collins of Maine have proposed a new Personal Care Products Safety Act which is being discussed in the Health, Education, Labor and Pensions (HELP) Committee.

My knowledge of Irish islands is due in great part to helpful 'Sabba' Curran, captain and operator of ferry boat, 'The Cricket,' to Donegal's Gola Island and Pól Ó Muireasáin, Brussels-based linguist extraordinaire 'as Gaeilge' and self-styled sea-forager.

On the esoteric subject of entomology, biologist Mircea Ciuhrii deserves strong praise for his development of skin creams using insect proteins whom I interviewed at his Bucharest lab. Ciuhrii sadly passed away earlier this year.

As for close journalism colleagues in both print and broadcast, I deeply apologize for tying you to a railing and making you read this manuscript, thank you:

Stephen Farnsworth, who has parlayed his extensive media acumen into academic excellence as professor of political science and international affairs at the University of Mary Washington, Fredericksburg, Virginia.

John DeDakis, CNN editor for 25 years and former senior copy editor for 'The Situation Room with Wolf Blitzer' and now creative writing coach and author of four suspense novels.

Jim Kuhnhenn, who spent much of his illustrious journalism career in Washington as newspaper bureau chief, editor and Congressional and White House correspondent, and who is as insightful an analyst of a football game as he is of intrigue on the 'Hill.'

Mike Weatherford, long-time reporter and columnist for the 'Las Vegas Review-Journal,' who may yet, one hopes, with his brilliant script-writing skills, turn 'Pretty Ugly' into a much-loved, Oscar-winning movie, starring…

To you all I say a huge thank-you (as Gaeilge: Go raibh maith agat). With your help and encouragement, 'Pretty Ugly' has gone from thoughts in my mind to words on a page.

Chapter one

Kate Moss. Naomi Campbell. Heidi Klum. Elle McPherson. Sienna Miller. The crème de la crème of fashion and style. A gathering of elites. Giants of stage and screen, stars from the intoxicating world of scent and sparkle. The most delectable of eye-candy parading their wares.

She approached, knowing the routine. No turning of heads. Unforgivable in such heady company. Pretense was the watchword. Overt displays of interest avoided at all costs. Furtive, nonchalant, all-encompassing glances best advised. She could almost hear the hum of electrical impulses racing from optic nerve to brain. Analysis of every contour.

Downward thrust of her hips, the drop of her arms, the fullness of her breasts, the angle between head and neck. She knew the telltale signs they were looking for. Thickness in the ankles. Tiny blue threads behind the calves. The ghost of stretch marks along the lower thigh. A bulge of flab lurking beneath armpits. Why? A potential rival? Her? Hardly. Not now. Not anymore. Remembering the preying eyes, the unspoken slights and stares, she controlled the urge to hurry on. She imagined – though harsh reality meant imagination was hardly necessary – their air of superiority etched with regal-like arrogance. The prerogatives of rare species - the rich, the famous, the supremely, stunningly, sublimely beautiful.

She drew in a deep breath, slowly, softly. With the power of instant observation, a primordial trait peculiarly inherent to womankind and particularly adept when applied to other members of the gender, she noted their trademark expressions, their fixed public faces. Some wore porcelain smiles; some as solemn as stone; others mocking and playful; still others devilishly wayward.

And the make-up. A state-of-the-art science in all its wondrous glory. No lumpy powders or scratchy pencils. Acetate reds to glaze lips. Lurex

1

golds to highlight cheeks. Mink browns to accentuate eyes. An artisan's well-honed skill applied with excruciating patience. Forcing wrinkles to surrender their ill-gotten gains and skin immune from crack and ripple under the relentless glare of smoldering studio lights. Delicate dusting, broad brushstrokes almost imperceptible in their lightness, faithfully following the natural contours of the faces they caressed so lovingly. Perfectly applied they might be, but to the knowing eye the imperfections remained glaringly obvious. Veneer that failed to vanquish vanity. It took so little to show so much. A cocktail too many. A sleepless night. Cross-Atlantic long-hauls in pressurized cabins. Free radicals, nasty little molecules, potent toxins with a lifespan of a millionth of a second, that poked holes in skin fibers, attacked collagen, weakened support structure.

The result: catastrophic collapse. A crack below a pouting mouth. A discolored crease in the cleft of the chin. Hyper pigmentation. Under-eye circles. A solitary spot where a spot simply shouldn't be. Standing, staring, she knew the effects of oxidative damage only too well. No better person to notice them. After all, hadn't she been one of them. Queen of the product junkies? Hadn't that led her to this?

Seeing the parade of faces before her, she remembered, and her shaky self-esteem shook a little bit more, for she wore no face powder, not even a swipe of foundation. And for reasons she dare not think about, not a single stroke of concealer. Her face felt like plastic, her hair nylon wire. Glancing down, things got worse. No satin, no silk, no leather no lace. Plain, worn sneakers. Jeans threaded at the bottom, a faint star-shaped shadow of soil clutching obstinately below the knee. Was a disguise really necessary? She wasn't even herself – yet.

The resolve she'd built up on the journey here slowly unraveled, unhinging carefully-crafted determination, sending shivers of discomfort through what she now felt was an utterly ill-dressed, ill-kept, ill-fitting body. She had been warned certain situations might bring this on. That she needed to stay strong, ignore the inner voices. She thought she was prepared. She was wrong. Whatever semblance of self-belief she had set out with swayed like the proverbial reed in the wind. Confused, naked, vulnerable. Caught unaware and, lacking decent heels - so comical if it were not so serious - firmly flat-footed. She sensed the swift spinning downward spiral begin again, bringing with it the fear, the self-flagellation. How could she not control simple emotions in a situation as simple as this, among cardboard cutout women whose company she'd shared often? Remembering the breathing techniques, she tried to calm her racing heart. There's nothing to be ashamed of, she repeated mantra-like under her breath, reminding herself of her familiarity with the faces before her, recalling specific places, occasions. Canapés, carpets, catwalks; clinking glasses at glamorous galas.

For goodness sake, she'd sat half-naked with them in frenetic pre-show dressing rooms, with urban sexy-chic bras scattered about; skimpy, alluring panties draped over chairs, colorful French corsets dangling from hangers. They'd exchanged dirty jokes and raucous laughter and snide remarks lightly cloaked in humor. They'd gossiped like old hags dressed in the finest of haute couture.

So why should she feel any different now, she wondered, scolding herself for her cowardice. The answer, more than obvious. This wasn't a carefully controlled, closed-doors circumstance, with primping, pampering publicists with a prancing menagerie. She stood in the middle of an uncontrolled, most public of public places, a shopping mall for goodness sake. She glanced nervously around. No extended lenses, no whirring monitors. No blinding flashes. No prodding microphones. No peering, peeping paparazzi. Safe. For now at least. How long could she go on like this? When would the nightmare end?

Patricia paused, a rollercoaster of emotions sweeping over her. Confused, bemused, amused. Not knowing whether to laugh or cry. Then, awkward about doing it, but realizing it was the perfect time, she adopted the pose she'd been shown. A matador before a kill, she lifted her chin high, stuck out her chest, stared directly into the eyes staring directly at her. If anyone saw me, recognized who I was, they'd believe I'd gone crazy. Feeling better, she glanced at her watch. She'd better rush. Couldn't be late for her appointment. Turning, she traced an uneven line on her neck gingerly. Then pulled her hand away quickly.

Behind her, faces on the multi-colored billboards outside the store window remained immobile, their piercing eyes unblinking.

Outside, traffic roared by. Life went on.

Chapter two

Slippery, shiny, slimy, they sucked silently, succulently, on the shifting soft skin of a sickly soul. Of course it would never get past the copy desk but teasing out the tongue-twister tickled him no end. And it helped while away the time as he cruised well beyond the speed limit along the wide swathe of Interstate 70, past endless fields of Kansas corn undulating either side of him.

Images of the little creatures had filled him with a rising sense of expectancy, presenting him with the hope of a perfect start to a languid, Midwest summer morning and a welcome respite from newsroom troubles.

He pictured them advancing slowly, purposefully, over ever-so-slight ridges of human skin, bone and muscle. Like snow trekkers seen from high above, they'd leave little trails of glistening silver, then burrow assuredly into wrinkles where blood had gathered like miniscule droplets of dark stagnant water in tiny furrows. Their detection and drilling skills exquisite, a true miracle of nature. No effort wasted. No time lost. Quiet, utter efficiency. Bio-mimicry. If oil companies could genetically reproduce them in giant form and harness their innate search-and-find talent, they'd save billions worldwide in wasted bore holes, he mused, smiling at the absurdity of the notion.

He imagined these diaphanous, marshmallow-like creatures in the flesh, hearing their soft moans of pleasure as they curled and swelled with every mouthful like mini-sausages pulsating slowly on a sizzling barbeque. Their voracious appetites, their meticulous, unerring motion, their precise in-built sense of location as they searched for nutritious life-giving liquid mere millimeters beneath a leathery wrinkled cheek, these were things that made his professional pulse quicken.

Art ops were bountiful. With a decent photo – sensitive enough not to make readers throw-up into their cornflakes - it could make a page one lead with a difference. But considering he was in the conservative Land of Oz and that the President was still battling baddies abroad, he knew it would more likely be earmarked for the metropolitan page mélange wrapped around federal court, education board and city hall coverage. At least it might 'put some crab in the crab soup,' as his neighbor on the desk next to him liked to say, as well as escape 'the horrible huddle' normally associated with front-page offers. Too many self-important editors, like bees drawn to honey – or, more apt, hungry hyenas feasting on a still beating heart - offering endless suggestions, making countless changes, leading inevitably to stories so disjointed they read as if the sentences suffered from rickets. Yes, losing the front page was always a disappointment but avoiding the ritual mauling was fair compensation.

The main reason Colm was feeling in an ebullient mood matching the cloudless sky above, was that at last he had something to write about. Hot days in the dead of summer were a reporter's nightmare. "Tedious, monotonous, 'n as slow moven as a crocordaihle on a suhn-baked mud flaht," was how his flustered southern colleague put it, his inimical nasal West Texas twang causing bouts of laughter to echo around the newsroom.

The press release had arrived late yesterday, too late for the final edition, its slick design a singular illustration of American medicine as the sophisticated, publicity-driven multi-billion dollar marketing machine it had become. It was neatly printed on quality letterhead, the logo of the medical center embossed along the top. Well written, too, the five 'Ws prominent in the opening paragraphs reflecting the undeniable talents of an ex-hack's hand at work, journalistic skills used in the pursuit of public relations' goals, high salary, bonuses and generous benefits.

Short, succinct, with punch, the first word faithfully adhered to the golden rule of intros: neither 'the' or 'a.' It struck a fine balance – informative with a catchy opening and the medical center mentioned from the off. Its quirky, tantalizing news lead was a red flag to a bullish reporter. That's why Colm re-read it. That's why it didn't end up spiked and in the trash as had the osteoporosis update from the Dairy Farmers of America and the monthly list of free pre-natal clinics at Baptist Health Clinic and the University of Kansas Medical Center.

Ancient remedy aids patient
Returning to the days of our medieval ancestors, doctors at the

University of Kansas Medical Center are using leeches - those flabby, bloodthirsty little creatures - to help treat certain skin disorders. And in a particularly remarkable case, special leeches flown in from California will be used to help a middle-aged woman from Olathe, Kansas avoid a major infection that could leave her face severely scarred for life following a surgical incision that failed to heal properly.

A tingling feeling crept over him, the kind he felt when a tantalizing story jumped out at him. That's why he was heading to work early. He wanted a head start. Other papers would be on to it and he'd be embarrassed if left behind at the starting line. The thought made him push down harder on the accelerator.

After all, he had a job to do. Not to mention dealing with Pratt, a troublesome managing editor who'd use any excuse to make his life a misery.

Chapter three

Robbed of everything but hope
GALVESTON, TEXAS - When human skin meets fire it doesn't flame – it burns, darkening until it blisters and peels. To survive, the victim must undergo debridement; an excruciatingly painful process to cut away contaminated skin.

Six-year-old David DaBell of Odessa, Mo., has had to endure that and other treatments at the Shriners Burn Hospital for Crippled Children here after a fire at his parents' home burned skin over 70 per cent of his body.

David is motionless and speechless, communicating only with his eyes as he lies on a special bed of silicon beads, his charred body wrapped in bandages.

Doctors' main concern is that David will succumb to infection. The flames destroyed his nerve endings and the lack of protective skin allowed bacteria to run rampant. Six square yards of cadaver skin have been applied to cover the wounds, while any remnants of good skin have been stripped off for harvesting.

By the time an eight-hour surgery was over, David's body was a patchwork of new and old skin. He was iridescent with layers of silver sulfadiazine and sulfamylon antibiotic solution.

"He was almost dead for 48 hours," said Doctor David Herndon, medical director of the burn unit. "He lost a catastrophic amount of fluid. He was bloated, his arms severely swollen as capillaries leaked fluid…"

Doctor Gray leaned back from his computer with a sigh. It might just work. He seemed the kind of reporter he needed. Of course there were risks but at this stage there were no other options. For the nth time, he wondered. Was he making the right decision? The thought sent him back to the fateful day a few weeks before when he'd got the call.

***

"Jack, I'm so glad to hear from you. Any news?"

"Of course, Gray, aren't I the best ophthalmologist you know?"

"You might well be. But that'll depend very much on what you've got to tell me."

"My, my, you are piling on the pressure. I've not seen you this jittery since your fainting frolics that day in Mass Gen."

Gray smiled with nostalgia. His old friend was right. It wasn't often he was this nervous. Not since that forgettable afternoon as an enthusiastic young medical student when he'd collapsed watching emergency treatment of a chemical skin peel gone wrong. Jack was there. Had caught him as he fell. Said as he lifted him that he'd saved his career from literally 'crashing to the floor' and a lifetime's supply of fine wines was but fair reward. The mistake he'd made, however, was not specifying the exact amount, so Gray had escaped penury through his residency years by sending a single bottle of vintage red once a year.

"OK, I've got the file here in front of me," Jack resumed. "Arrival at the hospital after the crash is probably the best starting point, though we can't ignore the report by the lead paramedic at the accident scene. He said, and I quote, 'the subject seemed dizzy, rubbing her eyes constantly complaining of pain and severe itching.'

Gray jotted the words, 'initial complaints - dizziness, itchiness' in a notebook.

"A doctor wrote on the admission form, wrongly as it turned out, 'severe posterior blepharitis in the left eye'," Jack continued. "I'm afraid, Gray, medical training isn't what it used to be, eh?"

Getting no reply, he continued, "Initial examination showed chronic inflammation of the right eyelid but no signs of chalazions."

Gray started writing again, 'initial misdiagnosis.'

"Closer examination by attending physician showed cornea also affected. Gentamicin was instilled and eye was patched. Patient kept for further treatment and observation. Next day ophthalmologic consultation documented impaired vision and a corneal abscess in patient's eye. Gram stain of corneal scrapings revealed gram-negative rods. Culture of the corneal scrapings presented pseudomonas aeruginosa with identical antibiotic susceptibility patterns. Following inpatient therapy, including subconjunctival gentamicin, infection eased. Upon discharge from hospital, however, dense inflammatory corneal infiltrate and subsequently, diffuse neovascularization of the cornea developed."

"Could it have simply been glass fragments from the car's smashed windscreen?" Gray ventured.

"Negative. No evidence of that. No foreign bodies detected in tissue samples."

"What other avenues did you explore?"

"We checked for keratitis."

"Amoebic?"

"She doesn't wear contact lenses so hardly likely. No presence of acanthamoeba in corneal culture."

"Bacterial?"

"Negative both for staphylococcus aureus and pseudomonas aeruginosa."

"What about viral? Herpes simplex?"

"No dendritic ulcers."

"I suppose onchocerciasis is out of the question?"

"River blindness? We considered it. An interesting possibility. Probably would have been the most celebrated case ever recorded. Considering what she does for a living, she could have been the tragic, modern-day Nefertiti, Queen of the Pyramids."

"What the heck? You've lost me."

"Our lady travels to exotic places. In fact, she was in Egypt recently on what they call in the business, 'a shoot.' But that's where the remote possibility of river blindness becomes even more remote. Her customary lodgings during such soirées could hardly be described as mud and wattle huts in a mosquito-infested village along the Nile. She stayed in a seven- hundred-dollar-a-night luxury suite in the Four Seasons Cairo. That financial information comes from a reliable source for I'm too much of a gentleman to ask her directly. Head of cardiac surgery here told me he enjoyed such grave hardship at a conference on gene therapy last year. Obviously Gray, we have chosen the wrong specialty."

"That, my dear friend, is a discussion for another day."

"Indeed," Jack went on jauntily. "So, the chance of blackflies leaving nematode larvae on our patient's pillow instead of mini-mint chocolates is close to zilch."

"I see."

"By the way, she was there for Vogue. A special swimsuit issue she told me. But riverside bathing wasn't part of the itinerary. In fact, strictly forbidden. She wasn't allowed to take a single swim the entire time she was there, not as much as a quick sit-down in the Jacuzzi. Bizarre eh! How can you promote a swimsuit without taking a swim? "

Knowing how little it took for his friend to wander from the subject at hand, Gray didn't respond. His silence, however, didn't stop him doing so.

"The answer is - and I quote our good lady on this – '*chlorine has an oxidizing effect on human skin. It splits hydrogen from water, causing the release of nascent oxygen and hydrogen chloride. Highly corrosive, it attacks the epidermis, removes protective oils and proteins and leaves skin dry and cracked, eventually leading to premature wrinkles.*'"

"Impressive."

"Indeed. I kid you not, Gray, this lady may know more about skin than you and I put together. If she ever considers a career change - which unfortunately for her, with what has just happened, may be right about now - I'd advise you to get her on your staff pronto. Beautiful, and - surprise, surprise, considering the general IQ level of those doing what she does – as bright as a button. Just what you need to freshen up that dowdy research facility of yours there among the corn fields."

"My dear esteemed colleague," Gray put in, sensing the need to rein in his friend's musings. "Beauty, as we are very well aware, is in the eye of the beholder – and that goes for this fine lady, my fine lab and this piece of fine land on which it is located. Now can we please get back to discussion of the eye and leave philosophical ramblings on the nature of beauty for another time?"

"Of course, my equally esteemed colleague, as you wish. Let me read on."

Gray waited anxiously.

"Ok, says here, 'no sign of bites or worms around the eye tissue, so onchocerciasis definitely ruled out."

"Tumors?"

"We checked for choroidal melanoma. Did I say checked? Quadruple checked. Using every examination modality we could muster. Ophthalmoscope to MRI. No sign of abnormal pigmentation or dilated vessels. Vascular layers beneath the retina clear. Doesn't smoke so no obvious carcinogen links. No family history either."

"Floaters?"

"Plenty. And often. Said they sparkled like diamonds. We thought the floaters might be due to chronic, long-term stress from the intense glare of camera lights and flashbulbs. An everyday vocational hazard, I'd guess. But no. She said no major problems before. Only recently. Nothing severe. Nothing like that night."

"So that's it?"

10

"Not quite. Getting back to that old Egyptian dowager Nefertiti."

"Must we?" Gray's sigh of protest went unnoticed.

"During this time, I happened to be indulging in my favorite pornographic magazine,, 'Analytical Chemistry,' and therein I found a fascinating article about how our ancient ancestors, including the great Queen herself, used a lead-based substance in their cosmetics, especially for eye makeup."

"To avoid a lesson in classical history, are you saying Patricia used something like that?"

"Be patient my friend. Hear me out. During their research, scientists analyzed samples from ancient Egyptian makeup containers that had been preserved in the Louvre in Paris. They identified four different lead-based substances all of which produced nitric oxide in cultured human skin cells. As we know, nitric oxide is a key signaling agent in the body, revving-up the immune system to keep out invaders, particularly nasty little viruses from the dirty Nile river waters."

"So you're saying the ancient Egyptians may have deliberately used lead-based cosmetics to prevent eye disease? While fascinating medical anthropological research, I still don't see the remotest connection to this case."

"Not to worry. Just another example of my superior intellect. Bear with me a moment, all will be revealed forthwith. Move the clock forward several thousand years from Nefertiti's day. No longer is there lead in cosmetics. It's too risky. Instead, the beauty industry uses other substances. Things that even our nitric oxide triggers may not help detect. Things that slip past the guards right into the bloodstream, maybe even across the blood-brain barrier and cause all sorts of problems.... are you with me?"

"I quite certainly am not, but I'm certainly listening."

"As we know, with the help of nitric oxide, the inner blood retina barrier contains tight junctions that prevent diffusion of damaging materials from the blood into the retina and vice-versa."

"Yes." Doctor Gray mumbled, trying to work out where Jack was going.

"Now what if a substance was created that caused the system to loosen these junctions just enough to let small molecules pass through? A bit like sneaking past the velvet rope at a gala party to where all the action is."

"What?"

"Never mind. Anyhow, the key to getting in - to the retina, not some post-Oscar party - is claudin-5, an important component of these junctions. Without it, they aren't so tight. By blocking the cells in and around the eyes from making claudin-5 at the blood-retina barrier, you tweak the system so that it allows molecules of a certain size in."

"Okay, but why would you do that?"

"To deliver."

"Deliver? Deliver what?"

"Think, my old friend. Put that famed, fearless intrepid mind of yours to work."

"Low molecular weight drugs into the retina to tackle conditions like macular degeneration and diabetic retinopathy?"

"Ah, a lovely idea and one that might work well one day. May even be your ticket to Oslo to pick up the big prize one day. But my dear Gray, while your selflessness and generosity of spirit make you an invaluable member of the national medical consumer movement, your commercial innocence sometimes astounds me."

Gray remained deep in thought, trying to unravel his friend's verbal poetry.

"You are, of course, absolutely right, but looking in the wrong place for the answer," was the reply to his silence. "America is in the midst of a billion dollar research frenzy but unfortunately it doesn't focus on the efficacy of precise administration of therapeutic drugs. In fact, the lucrative product research I speak of is part of the reason why people like you and I are so apprehensive. This, my friend, is our call to arms. Think toxic cosmetics."

Gray's eyes shot open as realization dawned. The word burst from his lips.

"Buckyballs."

Chapter four

The gleaming silver and chrome doors swung round silently with the slightest of touches. A blackberry Chesterfield sofa and a Gemelli coffee table stood in the center of the lobby. Glossy magazines - Glamour, Marie Claire, Elle, Cosmopolitan – carefully arranged on top, emanated a sense of hominess, an invitation to cozy up, relax, unwind, be a friend of the family.

Nearby, an elongated column of empty space rose dizzyingly up through the central spine of the 30-story building, reminding Larry of a private visit his father had arranged for him once to the NASA launch pad when he'd looked up in awe with a child's eyes into a huge empty space that seemed to stretch forever. Such was the dramatic effect this lobby had, he'd often watched with amusement as first-time visitors, like tourists to New York, craned their necks to stare into the void, puzzling over what esoteric Law of Nature kept the sides of the column from peeling apart like the skin of a giant banana.

Already late, he made a beeline for the elegant reception desk and a young woman with a beguiling smile. He gave her the name of his contact and waited while she announced his arrival.

"Mr. Jackson said the meeting's taking place in the ground floor conference room," the woman said, putting the phone down. "He'll be with you in a moment."

Larry turned without a word. The three-hour drive south through 'Indian country' as he called it - Amagansett, Sagaponack, Shinnecock Hills, Patchogue - and the slow traffic on 495 had left him in need of a good stretch. After the urgent message he'd received, he now regretted his decision to prolong weekend's frolics out at Montauk. Cloudless skies had made it difficult to resist staying another day. Even harder to resist was the provocative Charlene as she padded naked across the thick carpet of his beachside condo. All thoughts of Monday morning traffic and a client strategy meeting dissipated in a tangle of silk.

But even his high-level connection might not be able to save him if he screwed up this plum account. Reputational damage didn't even begin to describe the possible outcome if things went belly-up. Then where would he be?

To make his morning worries complete, the newsreader on WYNC had given valuable airtime to the man causing the trouble, his least favorite politician speaking on one of his most favorite subjects. His annoyance had grown so much he'd banged loudly on the car horn, noting with a certain degree of relish the nervous starts he caused among passersby. That's when the idea came to him. The oldest trick in the book. Scare tactics. It was the only way. His mind went into overdrive, an array of options opening up. It was just a matter of deciding which one to try first, and on whom. Where minutes before he felt reluctant to face the demanding top executive of Bellus, now he felt a throbbing pulse of excitement. Suddenly, he was impatient to be in the conference room, to move into action, to borrow some of the bullying techniques he'd grown accustomed to down through the years over the dinner table at home.

He ambled along the wall that ran around the ground floor, admiring the line of full-color photographs affixed there. Though he had looked at them a hundred times, he never failed to derive pleasure from seeing them over again, recalling almost word for word the short explanatory texts printed below each in bold Times New Roman font on laminated white boards.

Unlike the usual photographs in corporate offices, these were not solemn head-and-shoulder portraits of company past presidents or 'royal' members of the family dynasty. Instead, dressed in open-necked shirts, workaday pants and simple skirts and blouses, the people captured here in celluloid were more plebian than regal. Young and old, male and female, black, Asian, Hispanic, white, they gazed out, a look of innocent puzzlement on their faces unaccustomed as they were to being the center of attention.

Stopping at the photograph of an old woman, her leathery, wrinkled hands wrapped around a tiger-striped cat ensconced in her lap, Larry smiled with satisfaction. It had taken a helluva lot of persuasion to get Betty to pose, but well worth the wait. That photo, he remembered, had been his breakthrough, a dream start to a consultant-client relationship. It all started when word leaked out about the treatment of animals in the cosmetic testing labs. Like many companies in the industry, Bellus had been caught totally unprepared by the strength of feeling on the issue. Placards baring the words 'Animal killers' outside the front gates every morning startled both staff and management. Television footage of passionate protesters - not long-haired hippies leftover from the '60s but gray-haired retirees in their '60s - brandishing images of deformed rabbits, mice and guinea pigs - led to a slump in morale and in sales. Overnight, the humdrum phrase 'eye irritation test' took on a more menacing meaning. Crisis management became the hot game in town and in a knee-jerk reaction, companies in the cosmetics world bolstered their staff with outside advisers - particularly those with the right connections.

"That's how I went from foul-smelling glue to sweet-smelling perfume," was how he liked to describe his change of fortune, conveniently omitting to mention the key role of his well-placed supporter.

"It's a no-lose situation," he'd been told by the one man who boasted he'd never missed an opportunity. "You've worked in public relations for how many years now? Getting only hand-me downs, barebones clients. You've pushed pennies in a slot machine long enough, peddling paints. Time for the major leagues. A high-paying consultant position that'll make you big bucks. Then a cushy executive number with a big mahogany desk and your own leggy secretary."

Larry didn't protest even though he knew the debt would never be forgotten. Truth was, he was plain tired of adhesives. Just thinking about 'em gave him a headache. Working with 'em gave him an even bigger one. So many warehouses, so many factories, always getting the wrong kind of high.

While he was more than ready for change, the speed of transformation took his breath away. During the five years prior, he'd risen less than majestically from marketing associate to marketing executive at McCann & McKenzie Image Makers, from 35k to 39k plus company car – an off-red utilitarian Ford Mondeo hatchback, plenty of space for cans in the trunk. Then bingo, he'd celebrated the start of each of the last five with a new set of wheels, swinging from classic to sports as the notion took him. Not to mention the purchase of a Manhattan loft apartment with views over the Museum of Natural History and a Long Island beach-house with an outdoor terrace shaped from the smoothest of cedar beams; a Jacuzzi out back and - as he liked to say to bar buddies at the 'Touchdown' – "that other all-important prerequisite for personal happiness - a bevy of beautiful babes."

Larry knew the move meant mothballing his pride but he contented himself with the thought that while the door might have been shown to him, it was he who'd walked through. If truth be known, he didn't have to knock. Or at least not very loudly.

At first, the utter simplicity of the idea seemed to have no merit but he couldn't shake it. Now it was almost legendary. How 'Betty No Name' had captured the media's attention, a household catchphrase on the streets of New York. No picture editor could ignore the raw emotional appeal of the 'Queen of the Homeless,' the vivid before/after images when she'd been cleaned up by Bellus, 'the friendly corporation,' and put in a hostel. The Post and The Daily News ran regular updates on her 'road to transformation,' as they penned it, each article ratcheting up Larry's reputation a notch more. That's when it dawned on him that he was a natural-born troubleshooter, with flair, innate charisma and what he liked to term, *a predator's instinct for the kill.* 'I gave the makeup industry a fresh make-over,' was the phrase he used to impress.

"Saying hello to an old friend?" the sound of a familiar voice behind him shook him out of his reverie. "Best hundred dollars we've ever spent."

"That much?" Larry replied sarcastically, turning with outstretched hand to greet Jackson, Bellus's business development manager.

"Almost."

They laughed, backslapping each other.

"She's back home," Jackson added. "I saw her in the park the other day. Seems more content than ever. As does Tabby."

"I'm fine with that," he replied, leaning closer, whispering conspiratorially. "Just as long as the media don't find out."

"I hope that's the only thing they don't find out."

"That bad?" Larry asked, sensing his colleague's concern.

"There's market rumors. Competitors tossing garbage. Delays. Research flaws. The usual. Investors are edgy. Been fielding calls all week from big fund managers."

"Maybe just routine pre-roadshow nerves."

"Under normal circumstances, I'd agree, but these aren't normal circumstances, are they? That stupid model and now this snoopy Midwest doctor. I didn't want to spoil your love-in weekend but the big guy on the top floor is worried. We've only one chance to get this right. It could be the biggest birthday bash in the history of the company.... or the last."

"And what about the Scent on the Hill event?"

"Window dressing as usual. Fluff. Cathy's in charge."

Larry rolled his eyes.

"Forget her," said Jackson, noting his friend's reaction. "Focus on the other thing, that's what's important. A helluva lot of money's gone into this baby, we've gotta make sure the little bundle of joy is delivered healthy and rosy."

"It will, don't worry."

"Easy to say, harder to do. The crisis over eye irritation tests will seem like kindergarten play if this goes belly-up."

Larry stared hard into the face of the other man.

"I have an idea," he blurted out.

"Great, he'll want to hear it, we'll all want to hear it."

"Maybe not."

A momentary silence passed between them.

"I smell something nasty," Jackson said.

"Let's deal with one smell at a time, shall we?"

Chapter five

A large clock with oversized black numbers high on a white pillar showed 8.45.

Below it, Michelle, the tall, thin, pencil-shaped news secretary, was dressed in a short pink skirt showing a generous length of leg strapped to dainty patent high-heels. Bending over what resembled a large canvas laundry basket on wheels, she dipped her head into it to appear a few seconds later with a handful of letters. She repeated the movement, reminding Colm of a hungry flamingo pecking greedily in shallow water for wayward fish.

Reluctantly, Colm turned away, making a beeline for the cluster of reporters' desks at the far end of the large L-shaped room. Once seated, he lifted a press release from a stack of documents. Scanning it quickly, he grabbed the phone and dialed the number along the top.

"Good morning, this is Allison, may I help you?" a cheery voice answered.

"Hello, Allison, Colm Heaney from The Kansas City Guardian. I just received your intriguing release on the skin treatment. If it's okay, I'd like to come by with a photographer to see the procedure."

"Yes, of course, we'd be delighted." The enthusiasm in the woman's voice showed her delight that the medical writer of the city's leading paper was interested. With more than 20 hospitals and clinics in the metropolitan area, Colm was well aware of the promotion power he wielded.

"Allison, if another paper prints the story before us, we can't..."

"Don't worry," the voice said, hastily interrupting. "Dr. Gray was particularly insistent we send the release to you first. He'll be very happy. I'm sure we can even arrange for you to come this afternoon if you like."

"That'd be great."

"I'll call you back in a few minutes. Will you need anything special?"

"I'm sure the shooter will want to get pics of the leeches being put onto the patient's face."

"Of course."

"Could you also send me any background you have on these delightful little fellas. We'll also need a photo release form signed by the patient. The images may be a bit sensitive." He paused. "As for the leeches, I'll leave that up to your persuasive powers to get them to sign." A momentary silence greeted his words, his effort at levity a failure. Then the voice on the other end burst into chuckles of laughter.

"I'll do my best but everybody knows their legal rights these days. They might sue for invasion of privacy."

Colm smiled, satisfied. Charm had worked. It could mean advance story tips. Allison sounded young, intelligent, maybe even pretty. The day had just gotten even better.

Putting down the phone, he glanced up at a square table opposite strewn with documents and newspapers. This was the sacred territory of the four assistant editors – *'masters of the news universe'* as they liked to call themselves. Between the table and his desk, a narrow corridor stretched the length of the room, linking the reporting, copy-editing and photo departments in a maze of desks and chairs. Waiting for the call back, Colm watched the daily routine of the newsroom unfold, realizing more than ever how the cacophony of sounds from *'the orchestral news-pit'* made him feel part of something important. A global information crossroads right here in a single room.

To his ears, the music began as sporadic low humming sounds – cursory, monotone *'Good morning'* greetings muttered as staff stumbled dull-eyed through the doors. Then the soft tread of footsteps on carpet and tile as a procession of people, like spiritual pilgrims, lined up to pay homage to the revered Buddha in the corner – *'Almighty Giver of Life'* as one wit had scribbled on a note attached to the coffee-maker.

Hearing a squeaking sound, Colm turned quickly to see Joe the Flow, the paper boy, sweep round the corner from the sports department as if rushing desperately to catch a departing train. A thick stack of newspapers tucked under his arm, he scampered round the room, tossing one off at each chair he passed, his body leaning at an acute angle with the weight of them, but righting itself gradually as his burden reduced.

As Colm's copy landed with a thud on his desk, Joe winked cheekily at him then careened on by. It was only a matter of time before the Flow would meet his destiny, probably some wintry morning after trampled snow had melted treacherously on the tiled newsroom floor. He imagined the Flow sliding helplessly, toppling head over heels, his precious newspapers scattering everywhere. Bets were already being placed as to when that fateful day might be.

Meanwhile, the papers that had just been delivered snapped open in the air in unison like regimental flags on a ceremonial parade ground. Faces disappeared behind pages as reporters and editors familiarized themselves with yesterday's world. A subdued hush fell upon the scene, a stillness interrupted only by the crinkling of paper, a batch of chicken eggs hatching around the room.

Within minutes, comments emerged like spiders under stones.

"The president looks like he has a severe headache in the lead photo."

"He does. It's called the American economy."

"Take a look at page six. I'm sure the new Iraqi Defense Minister is wearing a toupee. With all the overseas development money you'd think they could buy him a better one than that."

"The federal procurement agency wouldn't notice."

"Are you kiddin'? If they give one to every member of the entire Iraqi army it still wouldn't notice."

Colm likened this part of the morning to the orchestral strings section. Simple, unadorned notes, isolated comments, soft snatches of conversation lightly played out, twirling round each other like random, floating feathers of thought. Then the brass and wind sections began - telephones buzzing sharply, voices rushing down mouthpieces, batting out questions – times? places? people? – a barrage of heavy, jarring sounds rising higher and higher, shattering the earlier atmosphere of quiet gentility. The crescendo would rise further as shouts reared up across the room, editors and reporters exchanging quick-fire views on story ideas, angles, sources to be contacted, column inches needed, art possibilities discussed.

"Give me a killer lead."

"Keep the headline tight. Twenty point."

"Thirty inches, ok?"

"The Second Coming wouldn't get you that. Fifteen. Space is as tight as a duck's ass."

Within an hour, the newsroom would be a walking, talking wave of reporters, photographers, editors and secretaries with the four editors the central focus of a lively buzz of activity. With up to six reporters each under their control, they were news traffic cops operating amidst a constant blur of chattering sound as the world unfolded its wings for another day's flight, from the narrow varnished oak benches of the Jackson County Courthouse to the barbed wire borders along the Gaza Strip.

Snatches of half-sentences floated upwards... *double homicide, verdict today... behind home-base... move closer... get some sweat... teacher cut-backs... react... parents... council members... call the school super...*

Though it was still some time before the day's first editorial meeting, jockeying for space had already begun. It would reach its finale mid-afternoon in the glass-paneled office at the other end of the newsroom where lively gesticulations indicated which stories might get top billing and which got canned. Sometimes reporters would gather in knots to watch the animated goings-on. With falling circulation and recent talk of staff changes, more people than usual came to observe matters. A raised hand, a raised voice, silence – all became fuel for the raging rumor mill. Colm no longer watched the ritual. His last invitation to the glass-house was not one to savor. Sight of Edward Pratt, the managing director, padding his portly, self-important self around the newsroom made the hairs on the back of his neck stand up. Their recent confrontation over an investigative story Colm had worked on for weeks was still raw. Pratt had spiked it, mainly because it centered on an old college buddy of his.

Shaking off the memory, he glanced over at Kevin McCarthy, his editor, sitting behind a computer, the top of his head, round, bald and shiny, bobbing up and down like an apple in a basin of water. A phone squeezed between ear and shoulder, he spoke in short, rapid bursts, his index fingers weaving an intricate tapestry back and forth across his keyboard. Realizing this was not his calmest of moments, Colm turned to the second man he needed to talk to.

Head down, deep in concentration, his wire-rimmed glasses balanced precariously on the bridge of his nose, George Whitsmith sat staring open-mouthed at a screen filled with page designs as if it was a crystal ball foretelling his future. Colm knew what he was doing. A dedicated, single-minded mission to persuade the news desk to publish more pictures by presenting them with his early mock-up pages based on story proposals and advance ad bookings.

"Good news, George," Colm called out confidently over the clatter of conversation.

The man glanced up, his eyes lost in pixels and column inches.

"I've a medical story that screams photo. Should get good play."

George gazed over, blankly at first, his fogged mind slow to emerge from what Colm coined his '*Hypotenuse dream world.*' Then his hands shot high in the air and he started waving them back and forth, his eyes blinking wildly like an exuberant fan at a rock concert.

"At last, at last, not a head and shoulders of our beloved mayor babbling on about parking meter charges and garbage collection," he said, taking hold of his belt-loop and rotating his drooping pants as if screwing them up over his generously protruding belly. Waddling over to a small, square table nearby, he swept up a photo request sheet from a narrow ledge, then bounced his way over to Colm as if his feet were made of sponge-ball. Leaning down he placed his elbows firmly on Colm's desk, his face close to his. "Thank you, dear magnificent, merciful, munificent, medical maestro," he whispered conspiratorially. "Your meaningful news makes me feel marvelous. Your tender act of kindness towards us writhing souls is beyond words. Even if you do nothing else today to show you've walked through God's sweet pastures, you've already gained a righteous path to Heaven. We will capture the moment in all its glorious splendor."

Colm tried not to laugh but it proved difficult. George's proclivity for melodrama was legendary – a natural element of his sexual proclivity. Only the most hard-hearted could resist his boyish charms.

"My all-conquering Alexander, Prince of Fortune, Savior of Sanity," George continued, batting his eyes flirtatiously. "Kindly write the exact time and place on this piece of parchment and I will be eternally indebted. As will Margaret, the poor cutesy teensy-weensy little kitten. I had to send her to some horrid, nasty place to take pics of that fatuous chief of police, he of the hairy armpits and beetroot face who's receiving yet another nebulous award for saving Mankind from imminent disaster. Please write down as many details as possible so the little dear will not lose herself. These hospitals are such a maze old people spend months in them. Not because they're sick but because the poor souls wander around and around trying to find their way out."

Colm nodded in agreement, remembering how he'd often got lost, confused by the bewildering array of interconnecting wings, corridors and elevators and the complex lettering, numbering and coloring system.

George placed the photo sheet in front of him.

"I owe you a large cold one, or rather, a hot one," he said, winking suggestively, touching Colm delicately on the shoulder with his pinkie. "The silly summer season has well and truly begun. Nothing's happenin'.

My guys are getting claustrophobic in the studio taking still-lifes of sizzling T-bones for the shopping supplement. And worse, some of them are vegetarians."

Just then, Colm's phone rang. Time to go.

Chapter six

An hour later, leaving his black Fiero on the second level in the medical center car park and remembering for the umpteenth time to replace the cracked wing-mirror, Colm walked along a connecting bridge over the street towards the main building. Repeated renovations and extensions had given the complex the look of a giant concrete octopus, the central dome the head and tentacle-like corridors spreading out in all directions.

The glass sliding doors to the lobby, their thin rubber edges frayed with use, whooshed open as he walked through. Inside, a ceiling fan feathered his hair. He glanced up as a middle-aged man pushing a wheelchair moved towards him. An elderly woman sat in it, wrapped tightly in a Paisley blanket. She was tiny and pale-faced like a ceramic doll and appeared to be in a deep sleep, her cheek resting on the metal rim. Colm stopped as the man moved across his path. Caught in their own worlds, neither noticed him.

He watched momentarily as the woman was wheeled across the large lobby. Mopped and buffed, the floor gave off a lustrous sheen that made his eyes glaze over. He looked up at the clock above the reception desk. He was fifteen minutes early. Standing there, unsure how best to pass the time, a strong sweet scent wafted through his nostrils. A man carrying armfuls of flowers tied in bunches, was walking into a nearby gift store. Colm wandered over. Inside, soft cuddly toys lined display shelves. Miniature dinosaurs with big, bright eyes and the words 'I Miss You' emblazoned on their pot-bellies and soft pink pussy cats with silky black whiskers and the message 'Get Well Soon. I Wanna Curl Up Together' on their backs. One corner of the store was festooned with colorful balloons. Ahead of him, the man placed the flowers, a mixture of daffodils, tulips and roses, in plastic pots of water. To the right of the entrance, a wooden stand held an assortment of music CDs.

Curious, Colm wandered over and started to read the labels: '*Mother Nature presents Beethoven, gentle sounds of the evening blending with the great composer's most famous symphonies;*' '*Best of Johann Strauss, the Waltz King featuring the Wiener Philharmoniker;*' '*Journeys in the Light, Musical Meditations.*' Reading them reminded him of his father's efforts years before to open his mind to the delights of the piano, paying a blind woman to come to his home each week to teach him. He remembered not getting much further than E,G,B,D,F and F,A,C,E, which he dutifully scrawled on the keys in pencil. The opening notes of 'Rudolf the Red-nosed Reindeer' and 'I Was Born Under a Wandering Star,' a Lee Marvin hit at the time, represented the dizzying heights of musicianship he reached. He remembered walking the blind woman home, her hand lightly on his arm, and he afraid of her sightless eyes. Dark swirling ringlets of hair made her seem witch-like and when she'd stop and stare into his face every few minutes, he'd think he was about to be turned into a toad or a swamp creature of some kind as punishment for his woeful musical efforts.

Maybe that's why his attention was captured by the intriguing artwork on one of the CDs on the rack. A swirling image depicting what seemed to be a thick fog sweeping around the base of some mountains with a sweep of frothy sea in the background. The more he looked, however, the more this image receded, making way for another very different one, one that seemed the vague outline of two figures emerging from the fog. At first, he thought it a trick of the bright ceiling light above him but the more he looked, the clearer the image became, as if the sketch was being revealed to him in slowly changing stages like one of those trick three dimensional prints. He still could not make out if the figures were human or animal, male or female, but as he raised the CD closer the shapes became less blurred, taking on more recognizable form until he realized he was gazing at an elegant woman, with a dreamy, sad, faraway look in her eyes, and a man, slim but muscular, a determined expression on his face.

Colm was shocked at how he could not have recognized the two figures immediately, entrancing and unsettling as they were. While their faces, heads and shoulders became more discernible, the rest of their bodies remained wraith-like, woven into the thick fabric of fog sweeping around them, disappearing in a mass of circular, feather-like shapes trailing off and merging into their surroundings. Both figures were the epicenter of the fog itself, emerging naturally from it and disappearing just as naturally back into it, their bodies almost shapeless. Amorphous as they seemed, it was almost as if they stood on the threshold of parallel worlds, the past and the present, yet didn't belong fully to either.

Inexplicably, Colm was left perturbed by what he saw. Why, he had no idea. A rush of emotions shook him accompanied by a keen sense of loss. The rush of feelings left his senses shaken. Strangely, there was no title on the CD cover to give him a clue as to its contents. Nothing but the haunting image of two people, entangled, trapped even, inside the thick, enveloping fog. Colm turned the CD over. It was completely black, devoid of explanation. Then he noticed it – in one corner, tiny lettering, scribbled as if by hand and in a shade of black deeper than the background, making it hard to see. With an effort, he made out the words: 'Niamh's Lament for Tír Na nÓg.'

Tír Na nÓg, he remembered, the ancient Irish legend about the fabled 'Land of the Ever-Young.' He was trying to recall who Niamh was, or her lament, when his name rang out loudly on the public address system overhead.

"Would Mr. Colm Heaney please come to the reception desk. Paging Mr. Colm Heaney. Hospital personnel are waiting for you at the main reception desk."

He reluctantly replaced the CD back on the shelf. Maybe he'd drop by on his way out and buy it. He stepped into the lobby. An exceptionally pretty woman with shapely legs, standing alone in the middle of the tiled floor, caught his attention. She was staring, a hint of sadness in her eyes, into the far distance. Colm followed her gaze. The wizened woman was alone in the wheelchair beside the elevators, her companion momentarily gone from sight. Frail as she was, she seemed to have diminished even more. It was as if gravity itself was literally squeezing the life out of her. He half expected her to disappear like a wisp of smoke into the very fabric of the Paisley blanket that covered her. The idea haunted him. The thought she could go into an elevator unwell and not come out and that so few people in the entire building might even be aware she'd gone. How could life pass so quickly, he thought, in a place where things moved so slowly?

Just then, her companion returned and pushed the button. The elevator doors slid open and the wheelchair moved out of view. As the doors closed, Colm waited, watching until the master console lit up 7. His senses filled with a mix of relief and guilt. Relief it wasn't himself on the way to oncology. Guilt that he had come here hungry for a front-page splash on the back of someone else's suffering. He wished such situations were rare. Unfortunately, they weren't. The greater the suffering the better the story was the norm. And he, a magician with a pen for a wand, turned pain into prose.

He turned, his mood falling to the floor like a lead weight. The brunette dressed in a matching charcoal-colored two-piece suit remained motionless, staring. Realizing her role wasn't much different to his own, he wondered if she felt similar emotions. Should he ask? Probably best not to. He walked towards her, his approaching footsteps causing her to snap out of her reverie and turn quickly. Seeing him, her frown transformed instantly to a broad smile. He vaguely remembered meeting her before, but couldn't recall where.

"Allison?"

"Yes. Colm?"

She stepped toward him, extending her hand in greeting. Placing his hand in hers, he felt its smooth softness, its smallness caressing his own, a letter slipped in an envelope.

"It's nice to meet you again," she said, then seeing the quizzical look on his face, added, "You came once to do a story on Alzheimer's. About Timmy who kept his slippers in the refrigerator and walked the streets in his pyjamas looking for his dog who had died thirty years before."

Colm remembered. The man couldn't recognize his wife anymore, thought she was a thief breaking into his home to steal his Labrador, Faithful. That was more than a year ago. The woman in front of him had been a junior in training, he recalled, nervous, awkward, unappealing in her shyness, fading into the furniture as she shadowed a senior communications staffer. The zest, poise and confidence she showed now were reasons why Colm hadn't recognized her.

"Actually," she continued, beginning to blush at the attention she was receiving. "I meant to ask earlier if it would be okay to use your story as part of our lobbying effort to the state legislature for more research support."

"Of course, I'd be honored," Colm said without thinking, his mind still digesting the change in her. "I hope it'll help."

"Great. And thanks again for coming. They're excited, all waiting for you in the treatment room. Your photographer is already there."

They started to make their way along the nearest corridor. The walk was long, past groups of interconnecting corridors, their walls painted in greens, purples and yellows to identify them.

Allison told him about some of the other research work being carried out, her tone indicating if he was interested, he should just tell her and she'd arrange everything. As they turned a corner, past a sign that read

D 12, she slowed her pace as she approached a room immediately ahead. A whiff of disinfectant tickled his nose.

A red-haired woman, boyish in tight-fitting jeans and plaid shirt, sat busily wiping a camera lens with a white tissue. A white lab coat was folded on her lap. Hearing their footsteps, she glanced up and raised a hand in recognition. He returned the gesture, reassured to see Margaret McDowell. Her penchant for capturing images thick with emotion, whether at home plate or in a hospital bed, was well regarded.

A middle-aged woman with ferret brown eyes amid a tangle of blonde hair, popped up from behind a reception desk.

"Hi Allison. Hello, Mr. Heaney, I'm Helen," she said jauntily, shooting out her hand. "Welcome to KU. Everything's ready to go. If you could both just put these on, we can go right on through."

She took two white lab coats from behind her desk.

"Doctor Gray has gone in to talk to the patient. He's waiting for you just inside."

As Allison took off her stylish jacket and slipped it off her shoulders, Colm noticed how the tightness of her crème-colored silk blouse outlined the contours of her breasts, the hollow of her stomach. Regular workouts, he guessed. He also noticed her left hand devoid of a ring. His rising notions of romance were interrupted as Helen ushered them past a heavy door marked Suite B. They walked in solemnly one by one. Inside was silence. He felt as if he was entering a Requiem Mass.

The first thing he saw was a metal table in the middle of the room. Instruments were lined up on it in neat rows - scalpels, scissors, forceps, rolls of bandages and thin squares of gauze on a plate soaked in a thick unctuous brown liquid. A small oblong box, its top covered with a dark cloth, stood beside them. Hearing a sound, Colm turned, a gurney stood against a wall. His gaze fell directly upon a bare foot sticking out from one end of a crisp, white sheet. At the other end was a heavily wrinkled parchment of face, as ashen a color as he had ever seen.

Chapter seven

The tall, silver-haired doctor led Colm along a corridor to a heavy wooden door. Standing aside, he ushered him with a mock ceremonial wave of his hand, guiding him towards two comfy mahogany armchairs of burgundy leather.

"Now that you have all you need for your leech story, let's enjoy that wonderful tradition you have across the pond," he said, with almost childlike delight, walking towards a small cupboard at the far end of the room. "Afternoon tea and scones smeared with generous dollops of jam and cream. When I go to conferences in London, it's an anachronistic occasion I enjoy immensely. And, of course, old-fashioned fish and chips in a wrapper. But please don't tell my wife. For my nutritional sins, she threatens to have me bound and gagged, cut into dainty parts and preserved in a jar of formaldehyde. She teaches dietetics, you see, and says she'll use my various bits and pieces to illustrate the ill effects of poor nutrition. Rather unladylike and most unbefitting a highly-educated professional such as she."

Chuckling at his own humor, he lifted several scones from a plate inside the cupboard.

Colm shifted himself into a comfortable position in the armchair, the fabric giving a soft sssshh sound as he sank into it. Glancing to his side, his eyes popped open in shock. He jerked back involuntarily. Not three feet from him, perched on a small table, two haunting eyes gazed with what seemed ferocious animosity directly into his. Or rather two eye-sockets. In a shiny, smooth patina of bare skull. Staring accusingly from their eerie, ivory-colored hollows.

"Ah, I see you've met Georgiana," Doctor Gray said, turning upon hearing the sudden movement and seeing Colm's blanched face. "A gift from morbid colleagues upon my seventieth year in this human

29

envelope. Or perhaps a subtle hint it's time for me to move on to the next world and let someone else take over." His smile broadened, "But just to be ornery, I think I'll have them wait a few more years. By then I should have the entire skeleton."

Colm smiled, sitting back up and feeling a little more relaxed. He liked this congenial man with his deprecating sense of humor.

The table beside him was piled high with materials and an impressive collection of objects in no particular order, clumps of pens, scalpels, pencils, scissors, erasers, felt-tipped markers, two stethoscopes, a fan-shaped collection of newspaper and magazine clippings, and a single set of forceps. Thick stacks of documents either side maintaining a precarious balance to the whole, preventing the table from tumbling over and scattering its diverse contents across the floor. A copy of *Natural Health Magazine*, with its front-page strapline, '*Complementary Therapies for Mind, Body & Soul*' lay open, impressing Colm. Midwest doctors, conservative by nature - Kansas was among the last states even to permit chiropractic - the doctor's reading displayed an openness perhaps not shared by many of his colleagues. Curious, he glanced up at the tall mahogany bookcases lining the walls. Through glass panels, he could make out the titles of magazines – *Dermatology Review, New England Journal of Medicine, JAMA, American Medical News*. A smaller open cupboard nearby revealed a display of vintage laboratory instruments, including an archaic copper-colored microscope.

Setting down a tray with scones, a teapot and two delicate porcelain cups on the table, the doctor cleared his throat. "Do you mind if our conversation here stays strictly confidential?" Colm glanced up, surprised at his abruptness.

Seeing his reaction, the doctor continued. "Your visit comes at a most opportune time but what I might say is sensitive. I'm throwing caution to the wind and placing trust in intuition. To use journalistic parlance, I'd like our conversation to remain off-the-record though I promise. You'll be the first to know when the time is right."

He hesitated momentarily. "Is this agreeable?"

Colm disliked off-the-record conversations, double-edged swords often providing explosive information but information he couldn't use. And if he'd a dollar for every time a source had said, 'you'll be the first to know,' he'd be a rich man. However, his interest was piqued by the doctor's hint of secrecy and his journalistic instinct told him better to have something off-the-record than nothing at all. Also, he hadn't enjoyed a good cup of tea with scones, jam and cream since emigrating.

A wave of nostalgia rushed over him.

"You have me where you want me, doctor," he said, accepting a pro-offered scone. "I'm all ears."

"Excellent. I hoped you'd understand." The doctor let out a deep breath. "I'm involved in something that could have far-reaching consequences. But it's still hush-hush. Nothing's been released yet, in specific medical journals or the general media."

He pulled one of the stacks of documents closer to him, tapping on it with his index finger.

"Like most of our work here, our research focuses on innovative skin rejuvenation treatments," he began. "We've been conducting experiments using natural substances - those things Mother Nature creates so abundantly all around us – plant fiber, fruits, herbs, leaves, berries, marine plants, even tree bark and sap."

Colm's eyebrows arched with interest.

"If I slip into jargon, don't hesitate to stick up your hand up and utter the magic phrase, 'I surrender.' My students say I talk too fast but I tell them I have less time left than they so I have to speak quickly to fit everything in."

Smiling, Colm took a pen from his pocket and pointed questioningly to his notebook. "Background only," he said reassuringly.

"Mmmm." The doctor seemed unsure. Then, reluctantly nodding, he stood up suddenly and began pacing slowly around the room as if shifting into lecture mode.

"As skin plays such an important role in our very survival, never mind how we feel and look, you can imagine how much investigation has gone into uncovering its make-up and what affects it," he began. "Billions of dollars have been poured into skin research in sophisticated research centers worldwide and these are neatly divided into two camps. The purely medical, inevitably - and unenviably – the limited-budget kind, the more intellectual, as my colleagues and I like to think. And the unapologetically commercial, the cosmetic one with vast, endless budgets."

Doctor Gray stopped pacing and sat down.

"On the medical side, finding new ways to rejuvenate damaged skin is invaluable in so many treatments. The list would take hours to go through. Instead, let's just take the one that first brought you to our attention here."

Colm glanced up. Our attention? Whose attention? He was about to ask but it was answered for him.

"Burns. Like your friend David."

At first, the name meant nothing. Then he remembered. The boy badly injured in the house fire. The rush to Galveston, the marathon operations. The code blues.

"Most of those kinds of skin traumas are caused by these, whether from severe heat, cold, chemicals or electricity," the doctor continued, shaking Colm out of his reverie. "As you probably know from your own articles on David, we've come a long way dealing with even the worst of them. But we're still searching for ways to rejuvenate damaged skin so scarring doesn't occur. That's the medical side. Now the cosmetics. Over the years, with Hollywood, red-carpet events, celebrity websites and gossip magazines, 'the perfect look' has become an ever more popular catchphrase. Looking young, having unblemished skin, is a national fixation, some saying it's the number one criteria cited today for success and happiness..."

An abrupt silence fell upon the room. Colm glanced up quickly. The doctor's back was half-turned to him. He was gazing at a framed photograph on his desk. When he turned around again, his face bore a wistful expression. Seeing Colm staring at him, he tried to regain his composure. But it took effort. That much was obvious. Whatever the cause, the sudden change of demeanor seemed more personal than professional. He reverted back to lecture mode.

"Every year, an estimated fifty billion dollars is spent in America trying to maintain that youthful look. The unofficial motto of this immensely profitable industry is, '*Preservation at all cost.*' Not surprisingly, with such lucrative returns, some cosmetic companies have become the nation's industry blue-chip giants with huge research budgets and state-of-the-art high-tech laboratories that make public health research facilities seem as sophisticated as a child's chemistry set."

Colm was becoming puzzled. And annoyed. At himself. He prided himself on grasping a news angle early in an interview, maybe even have a thirty-five-word intro in mind, but here he was plain confused. Was this a hard news story about an experimental skin technique? A feature article on the pros and cons of non-profit medical versus for-profit skin research? Or something else altogether? Like something hidden behind a shower curtain, it was blurred but it was there. Discomfited as he felt, the doctor didn't seem to notice. He was off again.

"Realizing that valuable independent skin research is being conducted but that it receives poor public funding, the cosmetic industry cleverly began offering generous amounts of money in return for experimental data they could use to formulate and refine their own commercial products and stay ahead of their competition," he continued. "Such funding is usually in the form of science fellowships, equipment or a new center named after a distinguished, long-serving professor. Many research labs accept the deal. Sometimes, it's the only way to avoid shutting their doors. We've been close to that here. But this little lady keeps me honest."

He stretched over, lifting the skull from the table.

"She's my confessor, my conscience, my constant in an ever-changing constellation of maybes and what-ifs until I shuffle off this mortal coil. Georgiana here would eat my scones, and probably my briefcase as well, if I lowered my standards."

His eyes twinkled with mirth.

"Ethical problems sometimes arise when test results don't match the expectations of managers of cosmetic companies. That's when they decide what information is released and what is withheld. Such decisions can often run counter to the public good."

He paused and started flipping through pages of the document stack on the table. Transparent pockets, individually labeled, with scribbled notes clipped to glossy color photographs. Colm couldn't make out what they showed, but the doctor slipped some from their pockets and handed them to him.

The image in the first one was a blur to Colm. As if the camera was out of focus. Then he recognized what it was and winced. The contorted face of a small animal, the red rims of its swollen eyes filled with yellow-pus. The other photographs were equally dramatic. All of animals, some missing large irregular chunks of hair as if shaved with an old razor. In others, bare skin covered with open, runny sores, thin films of blood splotched across them, parts of which had hardened into long narrow brown ridges, like dry crusts of bread.

"Syrian golden hamsters, rats, mice, rabbits, experimental subjects," explained Doctor Gray.

"They look awful, what caused this?"

"Cosmetics."

"You must be kidding."

"Unfortunately I'm not. It's the sad price we pay for protecting the public. Believe me, humane conditions were applied. Pain was kept to a minimum. I've had a border collie for fourteen years and a tiger-striped tabby so I know full well the love and companionship four-legged creatures offer. Unfortunately, this is the only way we can find out what detrimental effects toxic ingredients in cosmetics could have on people."

Colm stared again at the photos, unable to believe simple cosmetics could cause such horrors.

"It's one of the main reasons we started looking more closely in Mother Nature's pantry," the doctor continued. "To see if she offered anything we could use to treat skin without scarring or major side effects."

Just then a shrill sound interrupted the silence. Getting up quickly, the doctor went to his desk, lifted the phone and began speaking. Not wanting to look at the photos, Colm gazed idly around him, his eye falling upon the opened file on the table. He could just make out the title at the top of the page, 'Profiles: Natural Healing Properties Applied to Skin Rejuvenation Techniques.' Curious, he drew it closer and began reading. The first pages were clinical notes written in small tight lettering with a maze of statistics and charts in various color codes.

Making no sense of them, he skipped on, stopping at two glossy photos taken of the same scene but from different angles. They were simply labeled, in thick capital letters, 'PATRICIA ROBERTS, WESTON, MISSOURI.' The first showed a group of doctors and nurses dressed in green and white gowns gathered around a metal-rimmed bed all focusing on someone lying prostrate there. A woman, her long strands of auburn hair sprayed out from under her head on the pillow. In the first photo, her eyes were closed, as if she was asleep. In the other, lying in a similar position, they were wide open, as if she was listening closely to what someone was saying. Her face was smooth, oval-shaped with high cheekbones, her eyes the color and shape of almonds. A cloth covered part of her cheek and neck but as Colm leaned closer, he thought he could make out what looked like a series of sharp, uneven ridges. It was as if something or someone had grabbed the skin and pulled it out of shape as if it was plasticine. A man was gazing intently down at her and though a mask covered his mouth, Colm recognized him instantly. The same shallow bend of the back; the silver wisps of hair; the tall, slim gait. It was Doctor Gray.

Lost in concentration, Colm didn't hear the voice at first.

"I'm afraid we live in a litigious society but I'll excuse this as a journalist's inveterate curiosity and pretend your eyes were closed," it said.

Colm eyes shot up. Doctor Gray stood over him.

"I'm sorry," Colm blurted out, flustered.

"It's okay, maybe even inevitable. The poor woman's had more media attention than a person would ever wish for. Or want."

The statement made Colm recover his poise quickly. "Media attention? For what?"

"Well now, Colm, let's not go into that right now. Even in an off-the-record interview, you know very well I can't divulge patient information."

Embarrassed at just been caught in flagrante delicto, Colm felt he was in no position to persist. He'd bide his time to see what else he could learn. Also, there was something in the doctor's calm expression that set him wondering. It was as if Colm finding the photographs came as no surprise to him, as if the doctor fully expected it. As if....but that wasn't possible. Was it? Why?

"Now, where was I?" the doctor said sitting down again, swiftly changing the subject. "Ah, yes, Mother Nature's talent for healing. We experimented with a wide range of plants, herbs and seeds, both temperate and tropical. Ones with strong liposome content and keratinous proteins for rejuvenation of skin structure. You name it, we investigated it – camelina, passionflower, evening primrose. We made potions for drinking, poultices for the skin."

The thought struck Colm that the doctor might begin to rhyme off a hundred and one cures for warts using dandelions, nettles and buttercups. Thankfully that didn't happen.

"Results were promising, but not overwhelming," the doctor said, ambling across the room. "We needed something new, something non-toxic that had never been used before. That's when I met the Insect Man. That's when he showed me this."

He lifted a dark object from under the table, holding it high in the air, almost triumphantly as if it was a hard-won sports trophy.

"If my memory serves me right, I think 'oul Sod' is the term you Irish give it."

For a few seconds, all Colm could make out was a solid irregular object the size of his hand, then the full realization dawned on him. It was a simple lump of turf. He stared at it, dumbfounded. Either the man before him was some sort of creative genius or a scientific mind gone sadly astray. He wasn't sure which, but he was sure willing to find out.

Chapter eight

Colm was mulling over his meeting with Doctor Gray as the hospital exit door opened propelling a wave of hot, humid air at him, clinging to his face like melted plastic.

He stopped suddenly. There was something he'd forgotten. But what? The sliding door closed, then opened, then closed again as if impatient for him to decide whether he was coming or going. Then he remembered. The CD, the one with the intriguing title and the mysterious cover. Won't take but a few seconds to buy. Spinning on his heels, he re-traced his steps through the lobby.

As he approached the store, he could see several people standing at shelves lined with cuddly toys and candies. As he headed for the music section, he stopped momentarily, grabbing bottled water from the refrigerator. Oven-like temperatures outside meant he'd need it. Glancing down the CD titles, he noticed the one he was after wasn't where he'd left it. He looked more closely, a vague sense of disorientation falling over him. The others were there. *'Beethoven in the Evening,' 'Best of Johann Strauss,' 'Journeys in the Light.'* Just where he had seen them, but not, what was its full title again, ah yes, *'Niamh's Lament for Tír Na nÓg.'* In fact, there was none on Celtic music at all. And no covers remotely resembling the one that had intrigued him earlier. His concentration was interrupted by a light cough. The young salesgirl stood beside him, bright-eyed, ready to please.

"Can I help in any way?" she said, her voice lively.

"Hi, it's me again," Colm replied. "Yes, I'm looking for a CD. Of Celtic music. Had a strange cover on it, two figures in a swirling fog. It was here when I came in earlier."

"Oh, yes, I remember it. I'm real sorry but you're just too late. Someone bought it a few minutes ago."

"Ah," he said, his face registering disappointment. "Just my luck." Then as an afterthought, "Got any more in stock?"

"Might have," she chirruped good-naturedly. "I'll go have a look. Will only take a second."

Turning, she walked quickly to the customer desk and began searching in a computer. To pass time, Colm glanced nonchalantly around the store. Behind him, a balding, middle-aged man held a fluffy toy in each hand as if unsure which to choose. A plump woman beside him, his wife perhaps, was offering her advice. In the far corner, another woman, her back to him, stood swirling a spoon slowly around in a coffee cup, seemingly lost in a dream world. She wore a long coat and a scarf was wrapped around her neck. Strange clothes to be wearing on a scorching day like this, he thought. As if she was trying to hide herself among layers. She seemed pensive. Maybe medical test results or an upcoming operation. She reminded him of someone but he couldn't think whom.

"I'm really sorry, I've looked several times." It was the salesgirl. "Can't even find any record of the one we had. It's as if it never existed."

"Ah, well, thanks for looking," replied Colm. "It seemed interesting. I'd never seen anything like it before."

But the girl wasn't paying attention to him. Her gaze had wandered to a point over his shoulder. Suddenly she leaned closer, a hint of a smile on her face.

"You could always ask if she'd sell it to you," she whispered conspiratorially.

Colm was taken aback. "What?" he said, nonplussed.

"No harm in asking, right?"

Colm gazed at her, completely lost.

She tilted her head sideways as if indicating something. He turned slowly, his eyes following hers, catching a sideways glimpse of the woman in the scarf and baggy coat moving quickly out of the store and turning into the crowded lobby. Why did he think she looked familiar?

"No, that's okay," he said, unable to shake off the thought he'd seen her somewhere before. "She got there first."

"Suit yourself. Your call." The girl's tone was one of disappointment, as if she'd just been robbed of a touch of romantic intrigue that could have brightened up her day. "Anything else then?"

"Nope, that's it. Just this water."

"Okay, let's go ring it up."

She turned towards the cash desk, Colm following.

"That'll be a dollar fifteen."

Still wondering what it was about the woman that baffled him, he fished in his pocket for change, pulling out a clump of coins, his car keys nestled among them. Setting the keys on the counter, he began counting. That's when it hit him. An instant realization.

He spun away from the counter, sending coins spilling from his hand, falling to the ground before the shocked salesgirl had a chance to grab them. Mumbling an apology, he began gathering them up but he knew he'd never catch her if he didn't move fast.

"I'll just be a second," he mumbled. Then he was gone.

How could he not have recognized her? The contrast between in-the-flesh reality and a two-dimensional photo? The circumstance? Her on a bed in a surgical room surrounded by doctors versus her sipping coffee alone in a gift store. Paper-thin hospital gown versus full-length coat and scarf. But it was the face that was unmistakable. High-cheek bones, skin as smooth as alabaster. And eyes. Sensual, full of …he didn't know what exactly but it caused a stirring within him. The combination of beauty and vulnerability that had captivated him then, did so again now with even greater force. He ran out of the store into the open lobby, his eyes sweeping around the large open space. With visiting hours about to start, it had become crowded. Knots of people blocked his view. He tilted his head to see past them, but couldn't. Like a child looking for its favorite toy, he stood on tiptoes but that didn't help much either. He still couldn't see her. She couldn't have just disappeared. His gaze swung across to a bank of telephones against the wall. She wasn't there either. Nor was she at the central reception desk.

Then he caught sight of her. Or at least a part of her. The scarf, its edges trailing behind her as it vanished out the exit door. Though it was only a few seconds, he felt as if a physical part of him had been ripped away, leaving him less than he was before; a fragmented person losing the part that made him whole. It was a ridiculous thought, he knew, but the power of it sent him headlong through the lobby, zigzagging this way and that, bumping into people as he went.

Outside the sliding doors he was met by a maelstrom of cars and people. He looked frantically up and down the street, glare from the blinding sun making it hard to focus. No sign of her. Maybe she'd taken the outside elevator to the upper levels of the parking lot. He headed there. Then spied her. Or at least thought he did. The transformation left him momentarily unsure. She was different. She was taking off the scarf and getting into the driving seat of a red Mondeo, her thick auburn hair cascading around her shoulders. There was something not right about her but he couldn't put his finger on it nor did he have time to think more about it for she had already switched on the ignition, the engine beginning to hum smoothly. He tried to run along the sidewalk, shouting, waving his hands in the air, but there were too many people blocking his way. Sweat began trickling down the back of his shirt. He stepped on to the road, started yelling, "Stop!" but his call was lost in all the commotion, the sound of car engines, the general chatter of conversation. He could swear he saw her head angle slightly as if she'd caught a brief glimpse of him in the rear-view mirror and as he drew closer, the rhythm of the engine changed, flattening out, sending a flood of relief through him. He slowed down, expecting it to fall silent. Instead, the sound suddenly rose higher, the car pulled away from the kerb with a screech. He started running again but it was too late. The distance between him and the Mondeo widened. It surged up the hill. Then disappeared out of sight on to Rainbow Boulevard.

He stopped, exhausted, an emptiness clawing at his stomach as if he hadn't eaten for days. He was sure she had noticed him, shouting, waving his hands in the air. So why rush off? Fear? Of what? Him? *More media attention than a person would ever wish for. Or want,* the doctor had said. But she couldn't possibly have known he was a journalist. They'd never even met. Or had they? He stood perplexed. The feeling he'd had in Doctor Gray's office when he'd been caught looking at the photographs returned, this time more forcefully. Had it been meant for him to see her? Something strange was going on. Something tantalizing lay below the surface, beyond his understanding, for now, like a mysterious box just out of reach on a high shelf. While unsure what was going on, he was damn sure of one thing. There were no coincidences in life. He had to get to the bottom of this and there was only one clear way to do that.

Chapter nine

Thin shafts of sunlight filtered down over a gray downtown Manhattan. Even the multitude of neons seemed colorless and uninviting in the approaching dawn.

Glancing up from his newspaper, Richard Browne gazed out of the car's tainted window towards 42nd Street and Broadway and wondered – not for the first time - how on earth a single advertisement up there on 1 Times Square Building could be worth more than a quarter of a million a month.

Word on Mad Ave was that Colgate-Palmolive, Kraft, Johnson & Johnson, Kia and L'Oréal were all paying this. Electronics giant LG was paying over a hundred and sixty grand for the corner wrapping above Planet Hollywood and the Mountain Dew sign below it had gone for close to two hundred. The six-story, three-dimensional display of a giant beanstalk topped by a castle probably cost Washington Mutual even more.

Browne made a quick count of the ads and multiplied by the average rate. He didn't need a calculator. He had been so long in the business he could work up numbers minus commissions on the back of a postage stamp. It was all in the zeros. The pulsing lights looming up ahead were worth the princely sum of sixty-nine million dollars a year, he concluded, give or take a few hundred grand. Not to mention the millions that went into creating the customized, weatherproof, high-definition LED signs. Browne shook his head, partly in disbelief, partly in anger. Talk about a prime piece of property. An outdoor owner's wet dream. A few bricks in this wall could run a good chunk of my media empire, he thought, and if print media continued its slide, it would soon run it all. The jungle of colors blinking taunted him with a single word that had become his, and every other newspaper editor's nemesis - digital. Here, staring at him from above and below, with The New York Times opened on his lap, was old versus new media.

He returned his gaze to the newspaper and the article he had been reading a half-hour before.

'Reader's Digest Association, the venerable staple of doctors' waiting rooms and middle-class bedside tables, has announced plans for voluntary bankruptcy as it became the latest victim of the advertising recession.

Equity investors led by Ripplehood Holdings, which announced the $2.4 billion acquisition in November 2006, will lose their entire $600 million investment.

Reader's Digest, launched by a husband and wife in a backroom in New York in 1921, began as a mail order collection of condensed articles from other magazines and evolved into a direct mail pioneer and one of the world's largest publishers.'

Browne rubbed his tired eyes and shook his head in resignation. On Monday, the *Tribune Company*, owners of the *Chicago Tribune* and the Los Angeles Times, had filed for bankruptcy. The New York Times Company followed saying it might mortgage its Renzo Piano-designed headquarters building by Times Square to reduce debt.

The recession had turned the long, slow decline of newspapers into a brisk fall and his own company was no exception. At this rate, they'd all be lucky to make it to the weekend. His eyelids felt heavy. Lost sleep clawed at him for attention. He couldn't remember the last time he'd had five hours, never mind seven or eight.

Not for the first time, he cursed the Internet. The list of electronic usurpers was getting longer by the day. Readers had become too used to free information on the web to pay for newspaper subscriptions. And Craig's List, Monster.com, Realtor.com were the reasons why his sales managers walked around with funereal faces. Once generous clients had become less kind with their budgets. Financial body blows were raining in thick and fast and like a prizefighter past his prime, titan newspapers everywhere stumbled blindly around on their feet, bracing themselves for the knockout blow.

The equation was simple. Media, like all business, was a game of numbers. In the case of newspapers, it was the number of eyeballs. Towering above him, Times Square attracted more than forty million of them. With saturated television coverage, that shot to two hundred million when the midnight ball dropped. Sadly, with subscriptions and revenues declining, newspapers couldn't even begin to imagine such numbers - even in their heyday.

Browne wondered for the umpteenth time where it was all heading. America, the cradle of democracy, without newspapers? Unthinkable. Wasn't it? He stopped mid-thought. What was he doing? He had spent the entire weekend at his Hamptons' beach house doing the very same thing, turning down offers of tennis foursomes, poolside cocktails and succulent barbeques, to pour over P&L figures, HR reports and industry analyses until his sinuses had flared. Now, Monday morning with a board meeting less than two hours away, he needed a break.

As usual, traffic choked the broad sweep of 7th Ave., the grinding of brakes and screeching of horns heralding the mass morning exodus from home to work, the street becoming one long narrow strip of ceaseless ear-splitting sound with high-rises either side creating a natural amphitheater. Steam poured out of vents and gratings, as if a bubbling cauldron of boiling liquid flowed beneath.

The sleek green Lexus SC430 slowed near Shubert Alley, stopping smoothly under a green overhead canopy in front of an imposing building.

"Ave a goodun, Gov'noh." George tipped his cap in deference as he pulled open the car door. "Ah'll talk to Martha later 'bout pick-up time."

Browne nodded appreciatively, bemused how his long-time chauffeur had managed to maintain such a strong English accent after almost a lifetime across the pond. Of all places, he concluded, there was no real benefit in developing an American accent here. In Manhattan, the modern-day Babylon, home of the exile, his lyrical tones found a natural resonance in the vast linguistic sea.

As he got out of the car, the acrid stench of gas fumes filled his nostrils, causing his eyes to smart. Countless mornings imbibing the heady stuff had yet to make him immune. His tear ducts exploded and he took out a handkerchief to stem the flow. At times like this, with the smell and the noise all but suffocating his senses, his wife's words besieged him with strong logic, 'you don't need the salary, darling, less so the stress. You should ease off the pedal. That's what wise men in their 60s do. We'll be putting you into a coffin with banknotes as a shroud.' An avid gardener and lover of the sea, she missed no opportunity to try to woo him away from his executive's chair with the smell of fresh fruit, flowers and floppy beach-chairs. His response: 'Doris, I'd probably suffocate sooner outside beside the sea than inside a stuffy boardroom.'

Glancing up along the façade of the 10-storey building, the view imbued him with a keen sense of pride, sending the years rolling back in an instant. From cub reporter to corporate rider. Not bad for a local boy from the *'burbs with no high falutin'* education at an Ivy League School or rich parents footing the bills. He surveyed the building's smooth Hummelstown brownstone facing, remembering the day he'd carried the vote on it as the company's new headquarters. Not an exact replica of the Barbour County Courthouse in West Virginia that had first taken his fancy, but close enough – encapsulating a heightened sense of power and prestige. A broad band of plate glass curved around the top floor resembling a huge transparent polo collar. It was a quaint architectural addition he had personally requested and worth every cent, permitting him a panoramic view over the Upper West Side, past Central Park and on to the George Washington Bridge. The seven hundred thousand had been a relatively modest indulgence considering the elevating circumstances of the time - the company's stock soaring and he with the moniker *'publisher of profit,'* the blue-eyed media boy of the Street. Ebullient board members were in no mood to say no to anything he suggested then. It seemed such a long time ago. How fast fortunes change, how fickle the financial marketplace, he mused.

Bright lights flickered in the glasshouse. He imagined a petite porcelain cup packed with pungent aroma, offering him a moment's respite from the monetary madness. He hoped his traditional morning espresso would raise him to the requisite level of intensity he intended to introduce at the meeting.

Climbing the marble steps, he passed the polished brass nameplate, Leland Newspapers, Inc. unaware of the uniformed doorman's greeting. His mind wrestled with the conundrum before him. Initially, it had seemed quite straightforward – a simple *'surplus to requirements'* situation, one he had faced many times before – removing a longtime executive who had lost his verve and replace him with someone with more fire in their belly.

Then - to avoid fall-out among other top echelon figures fearing they'd be the next to go - convince them it was an unavoidable, one-off action to save their own jobs. A generous severance package and a formal award for long-time service at an expensive dinner with remaining managers usually settled the matter. The exiting executive would retire to a life of golf and vacations, dinner parties and perhaps a few well-paid speaking engagements, and his natural successor would slip effortlessly into the chair.

In this case, however, there was no natural successor. Cronyism has become a tick-borne disease, with both commander and his closely-knit crew suffering from it. Comforted by overly thick expense accounts and plump sofas, they had slipped nonchalantly into cruise control when print media had ruled the roost. Now, with things less rosy, none of them seemed inclined to shift into higher gear, relying instead on handouts from headquarters. Change would not be simple, Browne feared, and if he didn't play his cards right, it could become downright messy. A major collapse of morale at the company's flagship paper was exactly what he didn't need right now.

The company's stocks were in decline, not alarmingly so but a well-placed analyst on the Street had warned him about rumblings the previous week. *'Word has it you're going gray at the temples,'* he had said, eyeing him over a lunch of red snapper with lemon and capers at Cipriani's. His conciliatory comment later as he tucked into a generous portion of triple-layered chocolate cake - *'There's no need to worry, all print media are in the same boat'* - did little to alleviate Browne's worries. It was hardly the fillip he had hoped for but the analogy made him realize even more that the key lay with the Kansas City paper. It was the cornerstone of the company, at least in terms of years, and if it crumpled, the rest could follow. The fact that the newspaper's development mirrored – indeed was responsible - for his own, only served to complicate matters. Sentiment in business spelled danger. It must be kept outside, a ghost at the door forbidden entry. All these factors contributed to a sleepless weekend. Not only did he not know if he was making the right decision but if he was making it for the right reasons.

But insomnia has its own peculiar advantages, offering an abundance of uninterrupted time for thought, and out of thought comes ideas. His came just after 4 am. It was a long shot, but he had a gut feeling it might work. Much would depend on what happened over the next few hours.

The elevator whisked him to the top floor and stepping out, his feet sank softly into the rosette motif of thick Persian carpet. He glanced at his watch: 7.46. He had time to relax and review his strategy, analyze the numbers again, prepare his opening words.

"Good morning, sir," a chirpy voice said. A sparrow of a woman - her petite stature not too dissimilar to that of the feathered species with a small, beaked nose to match - greeted him. Darting forward on tiny, thin legs – she stood before him, gazing dutifully and unflinchingly up at him. "I trust the traffic wasn't too bad."

"Not at all," he replied, the question making him realize how he barely noticed traffic anymore, his attention being devoured by a pile of newspapers meticulously laid out on the back seat for him every morning. New York's traffic had many disadvantages but for Browne it meant arriving at work well-versed on the latest business and political developments from Toronto to Tokyo. Slipping off his coat, he moved to a soft elongated sofa beside the floor-to-ceiling window. His espresso came duly served and he sat undisturbed for several moments looking over the cityscape, watching groups of morning joggers in Central Park – tiny moving clusters of dots far below him sweeping around the ten kilometers of Park Drive.

Beyond, the slow, rhythmic progress of tugboats, barges and sailboats along the Hudson near Battery Park past tall gantries and lean cranes out to the Atlantic soothed his senses. For a few minutes, he eyes and ears closed to the noise and grime of the city and its million space-sucking concrete cubbyholes. He reflected on the one chance he might have had to be different and wondered what life might have been like for him if he had chosen that road instead.

Chapter ten

Ernie's gaze moved slowly along the entire length of the island from the craggy outcrop of bare quartz rock to the dense dark slice of bog and back again. Nature's wrath was plain to see. Shapeless heaps of rubble lay where sturdy, solid stonewalls had stood. Boulders that had once embraced each other closely like old comrades-in-arms had been cracked by age-old glaciers, torn from their centuries-old clasps, rolled along the ground and banished among the reckless, unruly grass and weeds.

The short rows of remnant houses that remained resembled a mouthful of broken teeth, bits and pieces missing or askew. Collapsed half-chimneys, broken doorways. Partial roofs displaying the sharp edges of gray-blue slates, their middle mere gaping holes open to the wind and rain. A few skeletal timber beams lay haphazardly in the air, flinging shadows here and there like gossamer.

Walls of some houses were cracked by the elements and sagged like tired, mutilated bodies after a battle. Others had vacant eyes for windows, the glass having splintered long ago, their tiny slivers spread on the grass verges below. For others, the struggle had been altogether too much and they had retreated, giving up another part of themselves with every assault until they had finally capitulated, leaving little behind but a few jagged shards of stone foundation.

The debris of centuries, Ernie thought. Boneless fragments of past lives. Where weeds abounded, he remembered verdant pasture for sheep and cattle. Where emptiness lay, he recalled the carefree, endless-summer calls of children. Where a front door hung lopsided on its rusty hinges, he pictured his mother gazing out to sea on a warm summer's day, waving at a neighbor, unruly hens kicking up dust balls at her feet. Along these stony paths, in a time long ago, men walked sturdily, their boats high on their broad shoulders, herring and crab and lobster jerking spasmodically in woven baskets. Here tears were shed as the mighty ocean claimed its rights, a small graveyard a grim remainder of its supremacy. Here laughter and the buzz of conversation once rang out, echoing along the shoreline, as births led to marriages and marriages to births and the cycle of life rolled on like the surf-flecked waves beating upon the distant shore.

Ernie pulled his cap further down over his forehead as the first splash of rain struck his cheek, large heavy droplets that made the swaying grass twitch as if a surge of electricity had passed right through them. Above him hovered a squally scribble of purple clouds, a bunch of bruised fruit, pallid at the edges. *It'll be a wet one today, alright,* he murmured to himself.

"If da place was made of sugar, sure we'd all melt inta tha sea." The voice came out of the silence, as if carried on the rising wind itself. Ernie jerked round quickly, taken by surprise. A small, bearded man stood close to him, a faded corduroy coat hanging loosely off his shoulders like a blanket drying on a washing line. Its pockets bulged with this and that.

"It's yourself, Seamus. Ya saw me comin' I suppose."

"No need for eyes, a chara. Sure, haven't I the best ears in the county. I can hear grass grow."

"Indeed, ye can. When ye want ta, that is."

"Aye so. And yourself, are ye grand?"

"Middling so, can't complain."

"Sure who'd listen anyways."

"Right so. Ye're here with the supplies then?"

"I am, right enough. Second time this week. Was told just to leave them up outside at MacSuibhne's old house. Bit strange if ye ask me. The goings on here."

Ernie listened, feigning not to. He didn't mean to reply.

"Not that I'm worryin'," the man went on. "Pays grand so for a return crossin'. I'm after hauling four wooden boxes over on the boat. And another the day before last. Marked '*Fragile*' and '*Feed*.' What does that mean, ah ask ye?"

The man hesitated, his intent clear. Gathering information was like panning for gold. Each nugget worth a pretty penny in the poorhouse, as they used to say. Now worth a pint in the pub. No response coming as to the contents of the mysterious boxes, he tried harder.

"Feed for what? The seagulls? Sure, there's not much else to be feeding aroun' 'ere."

Ernie kicked a stone, idly scratching some stubble on his chin as he looked down, keeping his tongue tied to its moorings.

"Ah well, sure there's no harm in it," he said finally. "So long as ye get the price of a pint or two out of it."

"Right so. And yon fella. Have ye seen him? A blow-in right enough. Bit touched if ye ask me by the looks of him. His hair looks like it just came outa washing machine. The Insect Man, they're sayin', down at Hiudai's. Doesn't say much. Be easier gettin' water fro' a stone."

Ernie raised his head, tempted to speak, but resisted the urge.

"What brings ye over then? Its outa yere way a bit," Seamus continued.

"Oh, just checkin' on a few things, tha's all."

Silence ensued as the two men looked beyond each other, searching for the meaning behind the words between them, like grains of sand between toes.

"Well, ah better be off," Seamus said finally. "A northwesterly headed this way. Bad time to be passin' the Three Sisters. Ahv a stutter in ma engine'll need fixin'. Catch ye later so."

Ernie watched as the man made his way swiftly down along a grassy pathway past large flat yellow rocks into which the sea had carved deep incisions leaving it looking like giant pads of butter. He stopped at the edge of a narrow stone pier and waited until Seamus had reached a small boat bobbing gently on the rising tide there and loosened the rope tied to the iron ring in the concrete wall. The outboard engine sputtered, coughing up a plume of black smoke, then started on the second attempt. Man and boat faded into the gray waters offshore.

Ernie turned, moving upwind towards the abandoned houses, the bog moss soft underfoot, brown water oozing out from under his heavy boots with every step. He felt strange, as if he was trespassing on sacred ground, walking a place he didn't belong to anymore. In the distance, he could see fog approaching, a fluffy gray pillow rolling gently along the sky. He watched it creep silently landward. It was as if the floating mists carried wisps of memory curled in their spidery nets. As if ghosts were coming ashore. Out at sea, in the caesura between waves, an eerie lull lurked. He remembered the wailing winds and the loneliness. He shrugged off the thought. He wouldn't stay long. A quick check things were fine. He'd promised. Then he'd be gone. He took a folded sheet of paper from his coat and opened it. Two lists were typed neatly on it, one on each side. He scanned the first – '*Arthropoda - cockroaches, millipedes, termites, earwigs, crab-spiders, grasshoppers, dragonflies.*' He flipped the paper over. '*Lower Invertebrates - ribbon worms, mussels, anemones, hydra, jellyfish, slugs, limpets, cockles, moss animals, abalone.*'

Above him lay a menacing sky. He had to be up at the house before dark. He'd promised Patricia. He fingered the keys in his pocket. He felt trusted but an inexplicable sense of apprehension rushed over him, of events out of his control. Secrets were hard to keep around here.

Chapter eleven

Browne glanced at his watch. It was still an hour before the board meeting. Muffled noises behind closed doors ahead of him mirrored Martha's military-style maneuvers. She had been in action all morning, ordering her team around.

"Over here, over here, what did I tell you, not that way, this way," her terse words, her no-nonsense tone was reassuring. He could hear the results of her efforts - the constant ping-ping of the photocopying machine, the rustle of documents, the squeaking of furniture as it was polished and moved around the room.

Yes, preparations were well in hand. Martha knew what was needed and how to get it. He hoped in a couple of hours he could say the same of himself.

Her assuredness was obvious. He had taught her well. Strange then that he himself was not so sure any more. The numbers looked poor and the prognosis even worse. The golden days were well and truly over. Leland was cash-strapped, worse, deep in debt, and today, ten people led by him, would sit around a table and struggle to find a formula for a wide-ranging financial restructuring acceptable to the company's shareholders and lenders. With a deadline looming next month for payment of a tranche of bank borrowing, time was not on their side.

Going over the numbers was a most dispiriting exercise. He had not faced such an acute financial imbalance in years. And there wasn't any end in sight. But he had faced crises before and the experience gained would help him deal with this one. He had set up the agenda for the meeting very carefully to suit his purposes. He had considered every possible board resolution and its implications, rerunning possible scenarios in his mind. He expected much discussion – after all, it was one of the gravest crises the company had to face – and while he hoped there'd be full agreement on the overall plan, he had sat in on enough board meetings to know that one could never be sure. Sometimes, he recalled, the darnedest, most frivolous decisions, took way too much time, leaving the key ones to be agreed in an instant without barely a word of debate - not that he himself hadn't used this simple strategy once or twice in the past when the situation demanded it.

Remembering past meetings, he could almost swear sometimes that a change of weather or poor constitutions, a bit of indigestion, hell, even the color of the rings on Venus, had more to do with conclusions on major matters than details on the issues themselves. As some board members were getting on in years, he prayed they'd all eaten well this morning, had enjoyed regular bowel movements and that no bouts of heartburn would flare up before the meeting. Or, even worse, during it.

Having made up his mind on Kansas City, he wasn't much in the mood for prolonged discussion. Other reasons aside, saving it would give more time to restructure the company, bring it firmly into the digital world of the 21st century. He clicked on a file marked '*Media Plan*' on the computer screen in front of him. '*Hunt for online news income heats up as ad sales plummet.*' He focused his attention on the article for the third time. Its content made board agreement even more important.

'*As newspapers struggle with declining readership and advertising revenues, executives at Rupert Murdoch's News Corporation are planning meetings with publishers about forming a consortium that would charge for news distributed online and on portable devices – and potentially stem the rising tide of losses in the newspaper business. Chief digital officer Jonathan Miller has positioned News Corp. as a logical leader in the effort to start collecting fees from online readers because of its success with The Wall Street Journal, which boasts more than one million paying subscribers. He is believed to have planned meetings with such major newspaper publishers as The New York Times, The Washington Post, Hearst and The Tribune, publisher of the Los Angeles Times.*'

Browne was a graduate of the old school, starting his career when slugs were made of lead and a Mac was a hamburger, but this idea excited him. Dead tree media, as he termed old thinking, treated new technology with disdain but this idea could be the difference between print dimes and digital dollars. Tech tapeworms in the intestines of the Internet, they may well be, recalling colleagues' invective against news aggregators such as Google, but they can't be ignored. Every newspaper editor worth his salt knew that.

Erect pay walls and collect fees for digital news distribution by combining resources through a single on-line registration for readers to use across key news sites and track the stories each person reads. Together with demographic and geographic data, this anonymous reader information would be valuable to advertisers seeking to reach a particular consumer. It could be the solution to the broken business model most newspapers now worked under. Offset the double-digit drop in print ad revenue over the last year. Keep the stock market hyenas at bay. Would enable him to invest in new technology, give Leland's titles a stronger presence on the web. As a member of Murdoch's exclusive club, he'd gain benefit from strength in numbers. It might be the only way to turn things around. Firing people wouldn't save much. Staffing had been cut to the bone anyway. Editorial content was already suffering because of it.

There was just one problem. How to get in on the act? The Australian billionaire and any other top international publisher would probably look askance at him if he called about wanting to join the consortium. Try as he had, Leland Publications simply wasn't in the premier circulation league. Never had been, probably never would be, not unless there was a swift takeover, an unlikely scenario in the present print media climate, and even that didn't automatically mean higher circulation. So that road into the consortium seemed closed. He needed added leverage.

Browne bowed his head, drawing his fingers together in a steeple and resting his head on them, the leather of the ox-blood armchair adjusting to accommodate his body movement. His mind raced.

His options were limited, he understood that, but he refused to believe they were non-existent. One just had to be on the lookout for them. He wished, however, they'd come sooner rather than later. There wasn't much time. Cardiac massage on a corpse, after all, was an exercise in futility.

Circulation figures were not good enough to put Leland Newspapers in the premiere league but brand and prestige could. That's where his hopes rested and that was the crux of his embryonic idea.

Chapter twelve

Senator Edward Clarke knew by the number of empty seats that he had much work still to do.

Some members of the Committee on Energy and Commerce, he knew, were there simply for constituency-building purposes, to be seen on C-SPAN as committed watchdogs on consumer health issues. But a sweeping gaze around the cavernous, wood-paneled room, with its green marble and bronze lamps, also showed he'd attracted more faces than before. And they weren't all party colleagues either. Health had the power to divide party ranks.

Seeing his nemesis, Senator Joe Barden, arrive early made his political heart leap, with equal measure of triumph and trepidation. It meant – to use medical parlance – he'd touched a nerve. The question was: which one, and how? From what he'd heard earlier, his presence shouldn't have come as a big surprise. Keeping secrets in Washington was an impossible task and, my oh my, what he'd not give to have been a fly on the wall in the back room of Art and Soul on New Jersey Avenue the previous night.

'*Seating for six,*' his aide de camp had told him that morning, his face beaming with pride at the juicy morsel of gossip he offered. '*Well-dressed, middle-aged. All men. All arriving separately, some chauffeur-driven. Hungry.*'

'*For information, I dare say.*'

'*Food also by all accounts. And lots of it. Seared black bass, maple glazed veal chops, Pan-fried Chesapeake Bay oysters.*'

Unfortunately, while the waiter had delivered the goods on food –– he hadn't delivered much else. Indeed if it hadn't been for the poor tipping etiquette of Senator Barden and his entourage, Clarke might not even have known of the meeting.

"The waiter said it was all hush-hush," his aide added, explaining the dearth of detail. "They made sure the door was closed tight after food was served. No chance to eavesdrop. But he was sure he heard the word '*cosmetic*' mentioned."

That they'd met was itself a tasty tidbit, one that made Clarke's political antennae vibrate faster than the wings of a humming bird. Lobbyists for the cosmetics industry meeting with their key supporter on the evening before his address? The thought had rankled him all morning. He juggled three Cs in his head. Celebrations? Perhaps, but a bit premature. Hearings were still ongoing. Though he desperately needed a silver bullet and they well knew it. Concerns? Hardly. Bottomless pockets gave them the best lobbyists money could buy and an inside running track through Barden. Coincidence? There was no such thing in Washington. Those thinking so ended up as dogs' dinners.

Something was in the air. Something his office had overlooked. Something out there they simply didn't know about. Whatever it was, he needed it, and fast.

'*Man the phones, make calls to friendlies, arrange meetings,*' he'd ordered senior staff that morning. '*We're on high alert. I want every lead followed-up, no matter how remote. Tie our researchers to their desks. Go through every report produced on the issue. Double check stats, re-read witness statements, look out for anything or anyone that seems out of place. Something's afoot and we need to find out what it is. Quicker than quick. They're worried about something. We need to find out what.*'

Clarke shook the myriad possibilities from his mind. Regardless who was or wasn't here today, he was determined to push ahead for greater regulation of the cosmetic industry. For decades, he'd forged a national reputation in healthcare second to none but time was no longer a friend, especially since... he jerked the thought away. The situation was dark enough as it was.

He cleared his throat. "Ladies and Gentlemen, fellow committee members, many of you have heard me speak about this subject before, some of you more than once. To come to hear me again is highly commendable. Firstly, I thank you for your patience. Secondly, I thank you for your interest. And thirdly, I hope I'll soon be thanking you for your support for my proposed Safe Cosmetics Act.

***

Clarke's words caused the last vestiges of conversation in the room to fade, absorbed into the carved ceiling high above. Everyone had turned their eyes to him except one. In the middle row a pot-bellied man with a florid face bent down and lifted a briefcase that lay at his feet and unclasped its ornate buckle, a distinctive red and blue swallow-tail flag with the single word '*Buckeyes*' on it. Senator Barden didn't need to look at the speaker. He knew full well to whom his remarks were aimed. Their predictability jarred his patience. Truth be known, this game of sniping had begun to bore him a long time ago. It would be better for everyone if his esteemed colleague would acknowledge the writing clearly on the wall and simply roll over. To arise again another day, on another issue. That was the essence of politics. Surely if he had learned anything he had learned that much.

Glancing down as he pulled out a document, seeing the inscription on his briefcase, '*With God, all things are possible,*' he remembered. Clarke slipping discreetly into the Senate chapel earlier that morning. Surprising. Catholic, yes, but his colleague's religious convictions hardly extended beyond the cathedral on Saint Patricks' Day in his south Boston constituency. A secret strategy meeting in the most private of places? Such nefarious scheming was not unheard of in the annals of the nation's highest chamber. Or maybe - smiling at the thought – a penitent seeking a miracle to get his bill to the floor. Fat chance, it'd be DOA at best. But the rumor he'd heard over dinner last night bothered him. He couldn't take anything for granted. The sardonic grin that lay effortlessly upon his face in the past listening to Clarke's ramblings on the FDA did not come so easily now.

He shifted his backside on the padded seat and made his sizeable bulk more comfortable. He'd be here for a while. The rumor meant he'd no alternative.

Chapter thirteen

Barden waited half-expectantly for his nemesis to indicate he knew. But as the minutes ticked by, he detected no change in his demeanor. His words had fallen into a predictable pattern. Either Clarke was blatantly unaware or he was an accomplished actor, which, after thirty years here on the Hill, he certainly should be. But it takes one to know one and he could detect no sign of play-acting. Nuances rarely escaped Barden's notice. Recognizing them, after all, was a sign of political adroitness.

"The FDA wields immense influence on our lives," Clarke was saying, leaning closer to the microphone. "It regulates roughly a quarter of America's economy, including food, drugs, medical devices and cosmetics. Yet despite a long-standing reputation for operating above politics, the agency has been roiled with problems of a political nature: self-serving political interests; a partisan approach to the Plan B contraceptive drug; the recent finding that marijuana has no medical benefit, despite evidence that it does; and the mysterious resignation of a commissioner who served for only two months."

Though Barden had heard similar sentiments a hundred times before, he was relieved hearing them again now. Focusing on the nation's leading food and drug agency surely meant Clarke was in the dark about the other thing. Otherwise, wouldn't he'd have pulled the rabbit out of the hat here and now, halted the hearings in their tracks? He felt the muscles in the small of his back begin to relax, the threat of a headache ease away. He decided to enjoy himself. After all, while unintended, Clarke's talk of the FDA was an indirect compliment to him. It had taken years and some rather astute planning, with a little help from financial backers of course, but the goal had been achieved. The cosmetic industry was the music maker and the FDA danced to its tune. What else could it do? Operate above politics? The naivety of it made Barden smile, recalling how its advisory committees hummed with conflicts of interest. He should know, he'd sat on most of them and like any right-minded politician had taken full advantage, learning a few lessons from tobacco along the way. He leaned back.

"Agency officials face frustration, not just on the funding front, but also in terms of authority," Clarke was saying. "Their scope of investigation is limited. Little wonder, some of the very people we put in place to protect the nation's health cross over to work for the very groups that oppose such protections."

Barden jotted down a name, mouthing a silent 'Thank you' to the unknowing speaker as he did so. Favors given, favors returned – the way of Washington. Jim Milton was just the man to give him the inside scoop he might need. Moving him from the agency to the cosmetic association for double the salary and generous benefits had been a masterful stroke. Now was the time to reap the informational reward.

"Difficulties faced by the FDA are no more obvious than in the field of cosmetics," Clarke continued, taking a long pause.

At last, thought Barden, the nitty-gritty.

"It has only two people working on labeling and packaging of cosmetics. Most of the thirty people in the FDA Office of Cosmetics, work on the regulation of color additives, not on content."

Keep the eyes of the enemy off the ball. That had been his policy and it had worked a treat! Color additives? What colors? Primary colors, secondary colors? Multi-colored rainbows? He'd have painted them red, white and blue if they'd asked him. Instead - Barden reveled in the thought - they were green, glowing green, dollar-bill green.

"The reason for this underwhelming presence is simple: the FDA has put limited resources into the cosmetic program because they don't have adequate legal authority to address cosmetic safety. If you can't enforce the law because there's no enforcement authority and because the standards are basically nonexistent, you aren't going to squander valuable personnel when there are drugs and medical devices to approve and foods to keep safe. If the FDA suspects a cosmetics safety problem exists - as they do today with the use of alpha-hydroxy acid face creams – it faces high hurdles bringing any kind of regulatory action."

Barden was ready to burst. How much of this could he take without sniggering? But with C-Span there and maybe one or two network feeds, he certainly wouldn't do that. It was one thing to outmaneuver an opponent, quite another to revel in the eye of the beast. The first showed confidence, the second arrogance. And the camera rarely forgives. With effort, he shaped a thoughtful expression and continued listening.

"With limited personnel, the FDA also bears the burden of demonstrating by its own testing that a cosmetic product is injurious to health. It cannot make the company demonstrate it's selling a safe product. It cannot even require companies to register their product formulations."

Barden jotted down a few phrases. *Free enterprise. Cornerstone of capitalism. Fear of foreign competition. Need for corporate discretion.* They'd make solid foundations for a rebuttal later.

"So today, the FDA knows how many milligrams of aspirin are in a tablet, how much sodium in human and animal food and can require disclosure of this information to consumers, but it knows very little about the toxic elements in thousands of cosmetic products linked to side-effects ranging from cancer to neurological disease, birth defects to development problems. The industry uses roughly twelve thousand unique chemical ingredients in personal care products—the vast majority of which have never been assessed for safety by any publicly accountable body. Americans use an average of 10 personal care products each day, resulting in exposure to more than 126 unique chemicals yet the agency can't even require companies to disclose what's in each product."

Barden sensed what was coming. The Achilles' heel of his carefully laid strategy, which, if what he heard last night was true, had the potential to jeopardize things.

"A mother of a six-year-old girl in Oakland, California found out about the dangers from everyday cosmetics when she applied a hair product to her child that resulted in second degree burns on her ears and neck," Clarke said. "A 59-year old Oklahoma woman almost died from an allergic reaction to hair dye. The hair of another caught fire as the result of an inflammable treatment gel, leaving her severely scarred. For every one million cosmetic products purchased, there are more than 200 visits to the doctor to treat cosmetic-caused illnesses. These are only the tip of the iceberg. The General Accounting Office says estimates of cosmetic-related injuries do not accurately reflect the situation as symptoms may not occur until months or years after exposure to the toxins."

Barden wrote down the examples. Worth having his public affairs officer follow up. Clarke hadn't named names. Either to protect privacy, or he lacked solid scientific evidence. Or his staff hadn't managed to get on-the-record testimony. Such generic cases would never sway the vote.

Unless people themselves walked into the chamber and spoke to the committee.

He tried to imagine how desperate Clarke must feel up there right now. Clutching at straws. And with just a few days to go, he'd remain that way. Paying the price for overstepping the mark, not playing by the rules. He'd tossed his dice recklessly into the dust, the political sin-bin of failed causes. Washington was full of such carcasses. End-to-end, they'd stretch along the Mall from the Lincoln Memorial to the front steps of the Capitol itself.

"You may wonder why the FDA has not expanded its resources in light of the problems with cosmetic safety. I suggest we look to ourselves for the answer: we hold the purse-strings, we pass the laws."

If heads had turned, Barden wouldn't have been surprised. For as he uttered the words, Clarke gazed directly at him, barely disguised disdain on his face. But Barden was not known as '*the Bulldog*' for nothing. He met his opponent's gaze head on and held it, secure in victory. There had only been two previous attempts at reform in the seventy years since the Food, Drug and Cosmetics Safety Act had passed. The first in '73 by Senator Eagleton of Missouri, the second in '88 by Senator Wyden of Oregon. Barden still cradled fond memories of the political battle that had ensued - more of a massacre really - after he and his high-flying friends flexed their muscles.

"A classic example," Clarke continued. "A few years ago, the agency proposed a cosmetics hotline for consumer complaints because cosmetic companies' own voluntary adverse event reporting systems had dismal compliance rates of well below 40 percent. But mix a twenty billion dollar industry, politics and some heavy lobbying together and you get a Congressional prohibition forbidding FDA from establishing a hotline."

Barden pursed his lips to conceal the smile that threatened to slip out. It was like listening to excerpts from the political memoirs of someone very close to his heart. He was surprised Clarke chose the figure of twenty billion rather than fifty, the universal figure. Maybe he didn't want to over-emphasize the size and slaying ability of the giant in their midst.

"Outside the United States, regulation of cosmetic companies is superior to our own. The European Union requires full ingredient listing on packaging, documentary proof of good manufacturing practice and similar proof that extensive testing has been carried out on all products."

Didn't Clarke realize how tedious he sounded? There probably wasn't a single Senator in the room, Republican or Democrat, who didn't have a sneaking admiration for anyone who could keep regulations in abeyance in one of the most consumer active nations in the world in the midst of a maze of regulations elsewhere. Barden felt like standing up and taking a bow.

"In the Federal Food, Drug and Cosmetic Act, there are one hundred and twenty-six pages devoted to the regulation of drugs and devices. Yet, less than two pages devoted to cosmetic regulation - two pages for a twenty billion dollar industry."

Had almost got it down to one, recalled Barden, but the font was too big. They'd all laughed afterwards over raw oysters washed down with a veritable barrel of choice Chablis, '96 JM Brocard Montmains followed by several glasses of smooth Lagavulin 16-year-old Islay malt and a couple of Monte Cristos someone had managed to slip past customs.

"We need a bill that closes a gaping hole in regulation and prevents production of cosmetics with harmful chemicals in them that we use every day. The industry seems to believe that for purchasers of their products, ignorance should be bliss. Right-to-know has become right to no information. No warning labels. No information that a product contains carcinogens or causes severe allergic reactions. No 'Keep out of reach of children' labels. No notification that a product has been recalled because it is dangerous or adulterated. We've known for years that as much as a third of cosmetic chemicals are toxic but we've done nothing to strengthen consumer protections. Instead, we'd rather weaken state consumer protections. It is plain wrong and shows the extent to which the cosmetic industry will go to ensure profits."

Barden smirked. A team of like-minded people was already putting together a bill to prevent individual states from establishing requirements relating to public information on safety of products. It would give almost carte blanche power to the industry. He glanced at his watch, silently urging the speaker to hurry up. He'd needed to find out more about this annoying development he'd got wind of. Find out how much danger it posed, if any, and what was being done to stop it.

Clarke's tone lowered. Barden recognized the sign. He was coming to an end. Talking loudly for an hour took its toll, especially if you're a septuagenarian. With a well-honed instinct for sound bites, Clarke's habitual tactic was to ease off the volume peddle a few sentences before the end, save his vocal resources, then finish with a powerful flurry of upwardly sweeping words that could be easily canned and fed to the networks.

"It's up to each one of us as democratically elected representatives to make sure profit does not take precedence over public safety and a first step in doing that is to give greater power to the Secretary of Health and Human Services to achieve the following." Clarke raised his right hand with a flourish. A dramatic ploy, Barden thought, granting reluctant credit to his foe's cunning eye for TV visuals. Counting off one finger at a time, Clarke intoned slowly, pronouncing each word fully in measured rhythm. "Set proper standards. Authorize a recall or cease distribution of an adulterated or misbranded cosmetic. Review and evaluate cosmetics that are marketed in interstate commerce. Require manufacturers to submit safety data for ingredients listed on labels that will then be published in a database. And finally, establish an Interagency Council on Cosmetic Safety."

He paused for effect, then added, "I look forward to your support in passing this key act which will amend the Federal Food, Drug and Cosmetic Act thus providing stronger protection for all our consumers."

A respectful - but Barden felt - raggedy round of hand-clapping broke out as Clarke stood back from the microphone. He joined in. Gently. No need to be spiteful. Wouldn't hurt his image to be seen politely acknowledging the views of an opponent. It showed strength and a firm belief in the mores of the finest democratic system in the free world. He glanced again at his watch and almost felt a collegiate sense of gratitude towards his Massachusetts colleague. He still had time to catch up on the latest gossip in the 'The Hill' before lunch.

Slipping out of the chamber, he had to admit. For someone on the back foot, Clarke had put on a credible performance. He wasn't going to go down without a fight. If truth be known, his address had unnerved him a bit. Set off that questioning voice in his ear again. What if he knows about the other thing? What if he's just waiting? But for what?

Chapter fourteen

All eyes fixed on him as he spoke.

"A new world is upon us. Old media is in decline. We must make tough decisions or we'll go down." Pleased with the effect his words had, a boxer softening up his opponent, Browne started peppering his listeners with a volley of verbal bullet-points, letting each land full and hard unmercifully upon the faces of those seated around him.

"After a century of publishing, The Christian Science Monitor will no longer print a weekday paper. Time Inc. Olympian home of Time, Fortune, People and Sports Illustrated, will cut hundreds of jobs. Gannett, the largest newspaper company in the country – owner of eighty-four dailies and more than eight hundred small, non-dailies - is cutting ten per cent of its workforce, three thousand people gone, and probably more to come. The Tribune has reduced the newsroom of The Los Angeles Times, leaving it half the size it was just seven years ago. For a newspaper in the home of Hollywood, it doesn't even have a solitary full-time movie reviewer on staff. TV Guide, one of the most famous brands in the magazine sector, was sold for one dollar. Less than the price of a single copy."

Browne felt his audience recoil from the unsavory details, his staccato of words making his listeners crouch uncomfortably in their seats, chastened children fearing worse punishment still to come. While he knew all of them were aware of the malaise affecting the industry, he also knew citing bald specifics would help hit home his message: the need for immediate action. Hopefully, in the manner he wanted.

"Fitch last week predicted the outlook for newspapers across America is so dire that many will begin to default on their debts and go bust. Many of our cities could be left with no daily newspaper within the next few years."

Browne paused, allowing his litany of bad news to sink in. "One doesn't need to be a financial insider to know what is happening. But to analyze some specific figures and help us understand better, I've asked Dave, who heads up operational finance, to give us a quick run-down."

Browne nodded his head in the direction of a plump, bespectacled man seated at the far end of the room, documents spread out before him on the smooth ebony table. Taking his cue, the man stood up uneasily.

"Thank you, Richard. Yes, mmm." He hesitated, as if unsure where to begin, then plunged on as if considering it best to have bad news out fast.

"The picture is not rosy. Prolonged declines – both in circulation and in advertising – have placed us in a challenging position. We have several key financial issues to deal with and the sooner we act, the better both for future credit purposes and stock price stability. In short, we have an unpaid bond of $200 million and a bank debt of $50 million that requires repayment next month. Unfortunately, that's not all…"

"Dave, sorry for interrupting…" A middle-aged woman, in a light-colored linen suit, her blonde hair gathered in a tight bun, had raised her hand, a sheaf of papers clutched there. "…but due to the excellent work you and your team have done, we have the figures right here in front of us and can interpret them for ourselves. We're well aware of the urgency required in dealing with this unfortunate situation. The question uppermost in our minds is: What is the best way forward?"

Dave fidgeted with the documents before him, patting them as if he was preparing pie dough. "It's quite a complicated scenario and being a financial analyst, not an industry strategist, I don't know what the long-term future holds for the print media market. In terms of finance, however, I'd urge the bondholders and the banks to sign up to a standstill pact over the unpaid money, maybe extend the maturity of the debt…"

"What's black, white and red all over?"

The question, loud and curt, leaped like a cat on to the table. The sardonic voice uttering it made heads turn. Having captured the room's attention, it soared, ever more confidently.

"Newspapers in today's economic environment."

The answer to the riddle hovered in the air. Nobody laughed. Everyone remained stone-faced. Like the others, Browne knew full well who the voice belonged to, the clipped tone of Brian Kemp was unmistakable. He'd expected such an interjection but was surprised it had come so early in the meeting.

"So let's just jettison some of our titles and save lots of money."

The idea was gift-wrapped and tied neatly at the edges but there were no takers. The middle-aged man, greying at the temples, who offered it, stood up slowly from the table, releasing a button on his navy, pinstriped jacket as he did so.

"We all know we cannot continue like proverbial ostriches with our heads stuck in the sand. We're hemorrhaging money, staff and paying readers and unless the government decides to offer direct sponsorship or tax credits to the entire print media industry, both highly unlikely scenarios, the situation will remain that way for the foreseeable future. In fact, probably worsen. Between what Richard and Dave have said and what we've seen in the financial report before us, there seems but one way forward."

The others remained quiet, expecting him to go on. Without missing a beat, Kemp obliged.

"A discounted rights issue would, of course, bring in necessary cash to help deal with the debt situation. But that's just a Band-Aid when what we need right now is radical surgery. Amputations. For company shares to be of any lasting value, we must trim our sails to suit the prevailing wind. And do it right now, not when forced to do so out of desperation, not when the storm rages, when creditors start telling us what we can and cannot do. That makes a mockery of the term independent media. We have little breathing space. Off-load our more burdensome titles. Lighten the ship and keep it afloat."

"And in your opinion, what titles would those be?" a jowly man in a heavy dark jacket piped up.

"Well, looking at the numbers, the *Kansas City Guardian* is the first obvious choice. An old-style paper way past its prime that's been run into the ground. A stumbling zombie."

Browne stiffened at this glib remark, sending his mind racing back to a time when such a description would have been utterly laughable. A more pleasant place thirty years before, when he, a bright, young executive brim-full of zeal and ambition, had been given the task of overseeing the Kansas City operation. A time when enthusiasm bore rich harvests. Ad revenue doubling within five years. Success there had opened the golden gates, sending him scurrying up the corporate ladder faster than anyone ever expected, not least himself. He recalled being regaled in style on his frequent visits to the Midwestern city on the banks of the Missouri. Chauffeur-driven from airport to grand suite at the Raphael on the ornate Spanish Plaza. Sumptuous dinners with the city's County Club set – the Halls of Hallmark; big-time developer, Miller

Nichols; pharmaceutical giant, Ewing Kauffman. Tributes flowed aplenty. Unveiling Oscar Neman's memorial to Winston Churchill at Brush Creek. Doling out prizes at the annual American Royal down at the old stockyards in Kemper Arena. Throwing the switch on the Thanksgiving lights. Announcing the newspaper's latest donation to the Nelson-Atkins Museum of Art. Invited as an honored guest to the Royals changing room after Bret Saberhagen's 11-0 shut-out of the Cardinals during the famous 'I-70' World Series. Sitting with the Chiefs' owner Lamar Hunt, in Tulane Stadium in New Orleans when they overturned the odds and whipped the Minnesota Vikings in the team's only Super Bowl triumph.

The moments, the memories, the magic, they rushed at him like images off an old photographic reel. He'd carried the torch for the city, facing down high-flying East and West coasters who dismissed it as a backwoods frontier town that time had forgot, a place one flew over on the way to somewhere else. Fuel from the blazing success that was *The Kansas City Guardian* had given him self-belief, propelling him to the top of Leland.

And now here he was – torn between pulling down the shutters or making a last-ditch effort to resurrect it. Kemp was right, of course. Hefty savings would accrue but damage to the Leland brand through closure of its flagship paper could be irreparable with a corresponding slump in its stock price. But if he was to be honest, it wasn't just practical considerations that colored his view. The idea of overseeing the paper's demise was anathema to him and sentiment played a prominent role in his thinking. And not just out of nostalgia. An historic occasion was fast approaching - the venerable newspaper's centennial next year, for which he had grand plans.

A glittering 'who's who' of social and political titans, coast-to-coast financiers, publishers he'd rubbed shoulders with at national newspaper conventions for years. It was to be his professional rite de passage into the media hall of fame. Like the Chiefs that fateful day, he wanted *The Guardian* to overcome the odds and defy doom merchants like Kemp. The question was how. Much needed to be done and quickly, starting with a clear-cut board decision today.

His attention returned to the room full of people to whom Kemp was providing a rationale for his slash-and-burn strategy. It was as if he was reading his mind.

"Let's face facts," he was saying. "The San Francisco Chronicle was founded 145-years ago in the wake of the gold rush. Its illustrious writers included Mark Twain himself. Yet Hearst - a company, I would remind you, much richer than we - is on the verge of closing it. So what if *The Guardian* is our oldest paper, or if we had Ernest Hemingway on staff – it was but a few short months anyway. We can't rely on past glories. We can't let sentiment get in the way of healthy finance and mature decision-making."

Mumbles greeted his words. Kemp resumed, cutting a wide berth through them.

"How can we sit here as experienced board members of a prominent national media company and say with straight faces that our reputation is tied to a single newspaper that is losing more money than any of the others?" He turned and looked directly at Browne.

"We must wake up to reality. It had its day, that day is now gone."

Browne felt an uncomfortable tightness in his chest. '*Out with the old, in with the new,*' this had been his colleague's favorite mantra since coming on the board, and a handy stick to beat Browne with. Handsome, charismatic, confident Brian Kemp gazed calmly round the room, snug self-confidence in a silk Armani suit. An ad man through and through and a successful one at that he had to admit. Someone who considered Leland did not sleep enough with the companies filling the paid-for spaces, who considered editorial quality of minor importance.

"Aren't they the rails upon which carriages carrying ad revenue run?" he had once asked mockingly.

For twenty years Browne had fought a sharp, at times testy, battle with him for the most prestigious sales and marketing managerial awards in the media industry. Before his retirement, Kemp had signed one of the most lucrative below-the-line telecom contracts with Sprint for McCann Erickson, thus sealing his '*can-do*' reputation, thus bringing into sharp focus - in the narrow space of a single room - a rivalry spanning many states, many years.

Financial success meant Kemp lacked for little in life. While indulging his love of golf and sailing, these twin hobbies weren't enough to take the edge off his hunger for professional recognition. A place on the board was fine but it wasn't enough. The seat at the head of the table was what he most craved and demise of the Kansas City paper, especially if it led to re-invigoration of company finances, would be quite the feather in Kemp's cap, a promising election platform ahead of the next AGM.

That's why Kemp's outburst, said with more bravura than ever before, unsettled Browne. Aware of the fickleness of board members facing raw, depressing financial figures and shareholder value to protect, he knew he had to step in smartly before the board meeting got out of hand and he was left outvoted. But he needed to walk a thin line, to appear to agree with Kemp's analysis, but disagree with his strategy. Browne's recurring nightmare was of a forest of weeklies and dailies, many of them freebies, popping up like mushrooms, stealing not only his middle-class suburban readers but also the rural, one-street towns in Kansas and Missouri. But he didn't tell the board this.

He intervened swiftly, swinging heads back his way.

"As Brian points out, the situation in Kansas City is deteriorating," he began in a slow, even tone. "If we don't do something about it now, we never will, because it'll be too late. With circulation and ad rates falling and while the newspaper is approaching its hundredth year of operations, celebrations at this point seem merely misplaced sentimentality. It is showing its age, and so, I'm afraid, are some of the people leading it."

Browne saw surprise at this unanticipated support, then triumph, sweep across Kemp's face.

"The 'must-read' symbol on *The Guardian*'s masthead is becoming tarnished," Browne continued. "And not just because of seven separate metropolitan radio stations and three TV stations running a diet of news and views throughout the day. Our demographic data shows people still want to read about local news in the region - if they have something worth reading."

He paused for effect.

"That's the nub. While the newspaper stumbles, circulations of suburban weeklies in Missouri and Kansas, are rising. Or at least maintaining their numbers. They're sneaking exclusive news stories from under our noses while holding on to ad revenues. To add insult to injury, they've even poached some of our more promising journalists and sales reps. Seeing the gap in our business coverage, a business and financial weekly has started and has launched a metropolitan distribution system that places their newspapers in pay boxes close to our own. Impertinence, yes. Confidence, yes. Both virtues we sadly lack there. But that doesn't mean we should be alarmist and close the store."

He watched eyes watching him, noting Kemp's face darken with suspicion.

"While some of you may think we don't need the Kansas City paper, that we have fifteen other publications across the country to maintain our position, just keep in mind – if one plum falls, our detractors will say the whole tree is rotten." He let his words sink in.

"Also, let's not forget, once upon a time in Kansas City, nothing moved without the paper's say-so. Politicians and financiers were in and out of the building as if on a merry-go-round. Unfortunately, that's not happening anymore, so something dramatic must be done to shine up our badge again."

He paused, then changed tack. "Gone are the days when surfing meant getting your hair wet and browsing was done in bookstores." Puzzled faces greeted his words. "We, and newspaper groups like us, are fading in the light of a new dawn. We live in a brave new connected world of limitless information called the Web. Is it a blessing or a curse? Does it lend itself to oligarchy, a new elite? These are philosophical questions for another time. But be under no illusion. Pernicious and merciless in its brilliance, it is destroying established traditional newspaper business models like our own, and it will continue to do so. Will we be eliminated? Maybe, but that maybe becomes a certainty if we don't get on board fast. We'll be dumped in the dustbin of history."

Browne thumped his fist on the table causing his coffee cup to rattle, "If we don't get in on the Internet power block soon at the highest level, we'll be left outside clutching a begging bowl, emaciated, living on scraps from the table of the new, mighty media. And sadly, we'll be eliminated from the greatest, most challenging game on earth since time immemorial – the creation of knowledge – for it will be colonized and controlled without us. There are new gatekeepers, new hierarchies, and we're not among them."

His eyes, blazing, swept around the room, from one taut, worried face to another, with a look that said he'd vanquish defiance wherever he found it.

"So this is what we must do," he said confidently into the silence.

Chapter fifteen

Colm had hoped he might have been able to catch up with the Mondeo but by the time he'd maneuvered out of the crowded parking lot she'd had too much of a head start.

But the name on the photograph in the doctor's files was imprinted in his memory, 'PATRICIA ROBERTS, WESTON, MISSOURI.' Not a big town, finding the address was easy.

That's why he was exiting I-29 and swinging on to a secondary road that snaked past groves of fruit trees and scattered patches of cottonwoods and Chinese elms. His mind was a buzz. Who was this mysterious woman? Why would she, living in a quiet out of the way place like this, be chased by national media? Even stranger, how come he had never heard of her? Or had he? Could she have had another name? A married one? A maiden one?

So many questions, so few answers. But maybe things would be clearer soon enough, for a big sign up ahead was announcing his arrival into Weston. He braked, glancing at the name on every street he passed. Within a few minutes, bingo, he had it. He turned slowly into it, parked and got out, finding himself standing car-side in the middle of a quiet, deserted cul-de-sac under a hot unforgiving midday sun. All he needed was a Stetson, a holster and six-gun. This was Jesse James territory after all and he half-expected tumbleweed to roll by and a swarthy man in tight leather chaps to step out of the shadows, a cheroot hanging from the corner of his mouth. Colm shrugged off the image. Guns harbored bad memories. He'd had more than enough of them. It was part of a past he wanted to forget.

There were four houses on the street but none had numbers on them. Not knowing which was the one he wanted, he took out his cell phone and called the number he'd got. Seconds later, he heard a faint ringing sound. He spun on his heels. It was coming from the house immediately behind him. A two-story detached, with white stucco walls, the blinds on the windows completely drawn. Seemed nobody was at home. He let it ring for a few minutes. No answer. Disappointed, he was about to hang up when a low mumbling came down the line.

"Mmm."

His pulse began racing.

"Hello, hello," he said quick-fire.

The response was the same but more drawn out. "Mmmmmmmmm."

"Is this the Roberts residence?" he asked urgently.

"Ysssscannehelpyou?" The words came out all strung together, like the slurring of someone with too much drink taken.

"I'd like to speak with Patricia Roberts, please."

Nothing. No response. Sensing the person might just hang up, he added quickly, "I've come from the University of Kansas Medical Center."

It pricked his conscience to say it but necessity prevailed, erasing guilt. Under a strict definition, what he'd said was true. He had come from the medical center. It didn't seem to matter anyway for all he got was more silence. Fearing he might have said the wrong thing, he tried desperately to think of a fresh approach, then suddenly she was back on, "Did you say you're calling from the medical center? Or you've come from the medical center?"

"From…" Colm answered quickly. "Just arrived. I'm here now. Just outside your house. I didn't think anyone was home. I hope I haven't disturbed you."

"No. Well, a bit. A touch of migraine. Kills me dead sometimes. Blocking out the light helps. That's why I drew the curtains."

"I see."

"You probably called earlier," the voice continued. "Sorry about that. Took the phone off the hook for a few hours to have a nap. I still get calls, you know. Journalists. New York, Los Angeles. Wake me up at all hours. I mean, 'do they ever sleep there?' "

Colm felt his heart skip a beat at her words. His imagination leaping into overdrive, questions rushing at him this way and that. And the person was more talkative than he'd expected. That boded well.

"These headaches weren't so bad until all this trouble started," the voice continued. Colm heard a quick intake of breath. Fearing the woman had seen right through his ruse, he half-expected the line to go dead.

70

Then she was back.

"I just realized. You said you were outside and here I am babbling on and you standing in that awful heat, melting away to nothing. I'm so silly sometimes. I'll come right out and unlock the gate."

Colm breathed a sigh of relief, but mixed with uneasiness. Would she recognize him from the gift store? If so, how would she react? Panic? Run back into the house? Lock the door? He couldn't just rush after her. She might call the police, say he was a stalker. If caught, they'd ask who he was, what he was doing here. They'd talk to the newspaper, even his editor didn't know he was here. He had been too excited to call. What would he have told him anyway, '*I'm rushing up I-29, chasing after a mysterious woman.*' If this got out, Stubbs would have a field day. Being revengeful, he'd demote him to obits. Not long ago it had seemed such a good idea to come here. Now it seemed the worst idea in the world. A voice in Colm's head told him to make a beeline for his car, crank up the engine and hightail it out of there as fast as possible. Nobody'd be the wiser. He hadn't given his name so couldn't be traced. Chalk it down to experience. Keep it for his memoirs. He was half inclined to do so but before he could act, he heard a noise. The front door of the house was slowly opening, a few inches at first, then wider. A head popped out, then part of the body. He squinted in the glare of the sun, unable to make out details of the figure behind it. Then he saw her, or at least part of her, the top half. Head, face, shoulders. He raised his arm in greeting but stopped halfway, rooted to the spot, staring wide-eyed in shock.

***

She smiled self-consciously as she walked slowly down the narrow pathway to the iron-gate. Colm watched, astonished. This couldn't be true. How could his eyes have deceived him? Where had he gone wrong? There was only one Patricia Roberts in the telephone book for Weston. This had to be her, but…?

It simply wasn't the woman he'd expected. He felt deflated, empty.

"What did you say your name was?" She was looking straight at him. His mind in such a whir he couldn't think fast enough to give a fictitious name.

"Colm. Colm Heaney." He hoped she wasn't one to remember reporters' bylines. Then added to reassure her. "I was with Doctor Gray earlier today." His conscience radar barely registered the ambiguity.

"Ah, Doctor Gray. A wonderful man. So helpful, so kind."

As the woman fidgeted with the gate latch, Colm took the opportunity to examine her even closer. Unless this was a case of a skin procedure gone badly wrong, this was not the person he had hoped to see. The pretty oval-shaped face of the woman in the photograph, her smooth, flawless alabaster skin, was still etched indelibly in his mind. This woman's face was plump, with a thick layer of make-up partially covering blotched and puffy skin. The woman in the photographs, in the gift store, was mid-20s, beautiful. This woman was middle-aged, overweight.

His expectations, so high, collapsed in a heap, a high-flying kite having lost wind.

"Is everything okay?" she said. "You look a bit... lost."

She had opened the gate and was waiting for him to approach.

Colm untangled his thoughts.

"Yes, yes, I'm fine," he mumbled. "It must be the heat."

"Let's go inside. You'll feel better there. I've put the air conditioning on full blast."

She shot a furtive glance up and down the street. Seeing surprise on his face at her gesture, she added, "Can't be too sure."

As he walked alongside her up the path, his eye ran over the fence with sharp metal edges that ringed the garden.

"Ugly, I know, thought it would help keep photographers away," she explained, noting his gaze. He nodded, still none the wiser.

"Sorry you couldn't get through on the phone," the woman continued, guiding him through the doorway and along a dimly-lit hallway into a dining room. "I hope you didn't need to speak to Patricia urgently. She drove straight to the airport from the hospital. She's probably already on board now."

At mention of the name, Colm shot her a quick glance.

"She should arrive in Belfast this evening."

Colm's eyes snapped open. Belfast? What the hell? Was this a joke? A set-up? Images from the past rushed headlong at him, ones he'd fought long and hard to forget. Before he could recover from the onslaught, the woman spoke again.

"What part of Ireland are you from?"

The abruptness of her question caught him off-guard. He didn't know what to say. He'd already given her his name. Now this. A voice in his head – the same one that had urged him to hightail it out of there - told him this was too weird. That there were too many coincidences. That the past he had tried to hide had come roaring back to haunt him.

He wrestled with the idea of saying nothing at all. Isn't that what he'd done back in Belfast? But there it was different, that was almost expected when you're dragged into an interrogation room and accused of being a terrorist. If he did it here, it'd seem really strange and this woman, whoever she was, might indeed call the police. Then there really would be hell to pay.

"Belfast," he blurted out finally. What else could he say? He'd already told enough half-truths to get him into trouble.

"Really, well of course, you're working on the project, right?" she replied.

Colm's mind was a muddle of convoluted thoughts. Did the doctor know more about his background than he'd let on? Was this a set-up? But for what? What had happened then was so long ago. Surely nobody here would know about it.

"I've not been but Patricia says she'll take me one day when this is all over," the woman was saying. "A lot of trouble there, I heard. Terrible."

"Not any more," he replied automatically, his mind hurtling back in time, to the barricades, the bombs, the shootings. He thrust the images away. "They've put away the guns. Or at least most of them."

"Well, its lucky anyway she doesn't have to stay in Belfast. But I still worry. She's used to all this travel. Cannes. Paris, London, Berlin, Milan. But they're big places and everywhere she goes there's always lots of people around, plenty of bright lights. She's fussed over, protected. But up there, in Donegal, it's just too quiet for my liking. Hardly anyone lives there? It's tough for her especially after all she's been through."

Colm listened intently.

"Bloody Foreland," the woman continued. "For goodness sake, even the name sounds awful. Makes me shiver just thinking about it. And my little girl there, all alone." Her face began to crumple with emotion. "I mean, why would anyone set up a laboratory in a remote place like that. It's bizarre. Like something out of one of those science fiction movies."

Colm stood stunned. A special research lab established in one of the most remote parts of Ireland and now this mysterious woman hiding out there. What was going on?

She looked at him, expecting an explanation. Getting none, she waved off his silence with a shake of her hand.

"I know, I know, she's told me, you guys can't say much. Top secret. But it seems too high a price for her to pay. When she first mentioned this idea, I just couldn't believe it, then I realized it could be the answer to all my prayers. She'd at least be away from all those nasty media people and get some treatment."

She shook her head. "But now I'm not so sure. You're here, I'm here. Doctor Gray's here. We're all here. But nobody's over there with her. Nobody. It must be so lonely."

She stared at him, a look of defiance in her eyes.

"If Patricia's guilty of anything, it's being born beautiful and that's no fault of hers. If anything, that's God's fault. And mine. But my daughter's not guilty of what they accuse her of. She wasn't responsible for that crash. It wasn't her fault."

She swallowed hard, clamping her eyes tight. Colm dearly wanted to ask. "What crash? What project?" but he was supposed to be from the medical center, supposed to be a colleague of Doctor Gray's. He was supposed to know all this already. He couldn't take the risk and make her suspicious. He stood bewildered, not knowing how to react.

"It's more a curse, than a blessing," the woman continued. "I can see that clearly now though I wish I'd seen it all those years ago. I thought she could have the chance I didn't. What I did, I did for the right reasons. Nobody can accuse me otherwise. We have to forgive ourselves, move on. That's what I'm trying to do. I don't know if Patricia is. Or can."

Her chest started heaving. Then the dam broke and tears flowed freely.

In a blinding flash, it seemed to Colm he'd inadvertently walked on to a movie set. Stranger still, the script seemed to have been written just for him. But why? And by whom?

Chapter sixteen

"When will you go see her?"

"I'm not sure. When I find time I suppose."

"She's pretty miffed, you know that."

"What can I do? I'm working my ass off dealing with a mess and barely have time to go to my own home."

"Mess? I hope it's not related to the committee."

Larry didn't answer.

"Look, the last thing we need is a problem right now. Not when the hearings are almost over. What is it anyway?"

"They have documents."

"They? Who's they? And what documents?"

"Consumer types. They've got something, some materials that could hurt us."

"Can you get them, have a look-see?"

"That's what we're trying to do."

"We? Who's we?"

Larry stared at his fingernails as if evaluating the manicure he'd had just an hour before. But that was far from his mind. Instead, he was deciding whether to answer, and if so, what answer to give. From out of nowhere, conflicting emotions surfaced and swept around him, sheets billowing in the wind. He hated being questioned like this, as if he was a kid. He'd never liked it, even when he was one, now even more so. He'd earned the right to be his own man though the help he'd had still hung over his head like a noose. But debts shouldn't be forever. That's why he disliked these meetings. They made him angry, so angry he felt like taking the belt to the man who'd taken it to him so often.

"It's not important who."

"Really? Says who?"

Though his attempt at avoidance hadn't worked, he didn't want a head-on clash. That wouldn't help matters any. He tried a different tact.

"I made a call."

"To whom?"

"You don't want to know. And in your position, it's probably best you don't."

The older man glanced surreptitiously around the half-empty restaurant. With a grunt, he swept up the double whisky and soda in front of him in his pudgy hand.

"I've bad feelings about this," he said, swallowing hard.

"Keep 'em to yourself. I really don't need 'em right now."

"I mean there's a lot more to all of this than you know. We've been movin' campaign funds around. If the net widens, we could find ourselves entangled in it. That'd hurt the party big time. PACs would get offside quick. State as well as national. Our financial supporters don't want no truck with that kind of stuff."

"Don't worry."

"Remember, that man in the White House is using more executive orders than any previous president. He and his host of goody two-shoe regulators won't be slow to use one against us, especially if it's about consumer health and we are stupid enough to present them with a golden opportunity."

"Take it easy. Everything's under control. I'll know more tonight."

"Call me," the older man said curtly, standing up to go. "No matter the hour." He started to walk off. Then, remembering something, turned back to his younger companion, now seated bent over, head in hands at the table.

"And for Chrissakes son, call your mother. I promised her I'd have you at the ranch this weekend. I don't need the hassle. I've had enough of that on the Hill after Clarke's performance yesterday."

Larry glanced up, nodded curtly, then watched his father turn away again and lumber off. He didn't fail to notice - and not for the first time either - how the sculpted muscular shape the man who had come to be known as Senator 'Atlas' Barden had turned to undulating layers of fat that seemed to cling to his middle, making him seem like he was swaying from side to side not walking. Slithering, more like it, an inner voice hissed at him, an image his mind wasn't quick to quell. Not much belting left in those arms any more, he thought.

Feeling dispirited by these thoughts and the fact they still troubled him after all these years, Larry yanked the cell phone from his coat pocket. Still no message. That made him feel worse. It was getting late. The job should have been done and dusted by now. What was the hold up?

Chapter seventeen

Seated on the wooden bench, Patricia watched Nature at play. Breezes swept around the cottage this way and that as if gift-wrapping it in threads of invisible silk. The salty taste of sea air nipped at her tongue. Fluffy clouds floated on the far horizon like giant clumps of candy floss.

The long trans-Atlantic flight with stopovers and the tiring drive up here meant she'd slept late. Would have been later had it not been for the cheerful chirruping of chaffinch, dunnocks and song-thrush around the garden feeder. Sleeping so long, breaking the habit of a lifetime felt invigorating. A small victory. Wasn't that what they'd said recovery would be? A series of small victories. She chalked this one up, remembering routine snatches of sleep on LAX-LHR red-eyes, early morning fittings, make-up sessions, photo shoots. Like old photographs they now faded into sepia. How had she managed so long? No wonder what happened had happened, a snake in the grass pouncing when she was most vulnerable. No snakes around here though, she thought, gazing across at the potatoes, cabbages and carrots all in neat rows. Not quite a Garden of Eden, but close enough. Not that she was in a hurry to play Eve. Once was enough, the memory of it leaving her with a lingering sense of ignominy. A promo for exotic lingerie. Wearing nothing but a slice of rabbit skin across her pelvis and nipples. Hardly an auspicious occasion. Hardly the basis for a lifetime achievement award.

Harnessing her newfound control skills, she banished the memory, diverting the torrent of stress that threatened to cascade down upon her and scatter her into tiny fragments. *'Simple things. That's what you need. The simpler the better,'* Doctor Gray had advised. *'You've been in the fast lane too long. Peg yourself down there. Enjoy the tranquility.'*

'Peg yourself down,' the perfect description, especially during those first lonely weeks. She'd felt tied hand and foot. *A fetus-like creature*

undercover unable to move a muscle, she'd penned during her worse moments. *Mere flotsam in the river of life.* That had described her brooding frame of mind then. Well, hadn't they advised her to keep a diary? That she should be perfectly frank and honest in it. At times, writing it, she felt like a hormone–ridden teenager.

From the madcap rush of cosmopolitan living in the city that never sleeps to the quietest of backwaters that does nothing but sleep, she'd written one rainy day. From flashing neon lights to an almost complete lack of lights. Where before she had no time, now she had plenty. Time she didn't know what to do with. Dealing with the hard work of doing nothing left her exhausted.

'*It'll feel strange at first, like you're shedding your skin*,' Doctor Gray had said, trying to boost her morale, adding, with a mischievous wink, '*But you'll wriggle through.*' That made her smile. He had the knack of doing that.

And thus it had come to be. So much so she sometimes felt itchy all over as if she was indeed undergoing a physical transformation. Like backstage costume changes. Only this had taken more time, and alone.

Her fast-moving, transcontinental world had shrunk. Now this little wooden bench was the fulcrum around which her slow-moving one revolved. From here, if the weather was kind, she'd gaze over her *île flottante*, a phrase she'd coined for the trio of islands, Inishsirrer, Inishmeane and Inis Fraoigh, nestled snugly in the swaying curtain of the Atlantic below. The phrase reminded her of what she'd left behind. The all-night Parisian parties. The glittering shows. Haute couture with skinny jeans, soft silks, floral prints. Punks, portraits and precious jewels. Thai traditional, American Indian. Minis, micros, megas. pharaohs, high priestesses, Goths, gladiators.

Hard to believe sitting here they weren't the wild imaginings of a lonely mind. Ironically, she recalled, in the very city of its making, île flottante was exactly what she could never have there. Not if she'd wanted a size zero and slip into Vivienne Westwood denims or tight black secretary skirts. How things were different now. In fact, to flaunt her newfound freedom, she'd treat herself to that very dessert this afternoon. The idea pleased her no end, deliciously decadent. At least it was better than being as thin as a toothpick with bones jutting out at all angles. Remembering, a wave of shame rolled over her. Covert trips to the bathroom. Not that anyone cared. They all did it, taking turns, laughing about it in the dressing rooms later. Musical chairs they called it, an affable name for an ugly act. She'd told Doctor Gray when they'd talked about diet and nutrition. She'd never seen him so angry, he usually so calm and cool. *I'll absolutely not tolerate it,* he'd said, *do that and you can find another doctor.* Seeing her eyes fill with tears, he'd melted. His voice quivering with emotion, he'd told her. His story had left her shocked. Even now, she still found it hard to believe. The trouble they'd both been through had helped create the strong bond between them. It was the reason they'd hatched their strange plan together which, if it went wrong, could bring both their worlds crashing down around them.

Anyway, here she was, from the City of Light to Donegal, where there was hardly any at all. No gleaming limousines. In fact, hardly any cars at all. No well-heeled crowds. In fact, hardly anyone at all. Man and nature, it seemed, had called a truce, gone their separate ways, leaving her to contemplate, the ancient, rolling landscape. The purple-heathered hills behind and the brown-black turf bogs beyond Cnoc Fola bedecked with pipewort, knitting needles as Ernie liked to call them. The murderous sundews, the tireless, ever-flitting dragonflies and the inseparable pair of plump, pied-plumed magpies sweeping overhead on the lookout for shiny things.

Not that she had the discipline to abandon all the trappings of urban life. That'd be asking too much, specially the one sitting snug in her hand. The Clooney special. Thanking the cuddly actor under her breath, she sipped slowly on the pungent-smelling espresso, then thought back over the last few days.

The news in Kansas City had been encouraging. '*You're making great progress,*' Doctor Gray had told her. Not mere bedside words of comfort either. He'd meant it, and she could feel the change inside, something palpable, renewing. A part of her awakening that had lain dormant for so long. She could almost touch it, feel its rising rhythm. No more so than right now as the sun's rays warmed her face, caressing away cares, ushering in quiet waves of contentment on a gentle tide. The worst of the worst was over, the baggage of bitterness was floating out to sea, its sourness curdling as flecks of foam around the craggy, Three Sisters, the last rocky outposts before the broad sweep of nothingness.

A comforting feeling settled around her like a shawl. It was as if Nature was lavishing its bounties on her for her sole and exclusive benefit. The slowness of time here had been a friend, providing a balm for her bruised emotions. Though the physical pain had receded, she still found herself fingering her neck gingerly, feeling the scaly hardness of the scar tissue. With the treatment she was receiving that would fade. It was the internal ones, however, the ones deep inside, the ones that corroded her heart, they would take longer to heal. She understood. That's why she was here.

She stretched out her legs, her bare-feet caressing the soft strands of horsetail – faery flowers, folks here called them – that poked out between stones. Closing her eyes, she let the silence seep into her senses. Moments later, a familiar sound made her open them again. The mellow warbling of a blackbird hopping around, its tail straight up. Hearing its sharp notes rise and fall, a practicing chorister in full voice, she watched it flutter its ruffled, unruly feathers then tame them with a meticulous rub-down with its rich orange beak. It's primping and pampering reminded her of pre-show preparations. The hum of hairdryers. Rouge on cheeks, dark and glossy on lips. Light foundation with a slight shimmer. Brushing, stretching, tweaking. Smell and sweat, sweet and sour. The illusion of glamor.

She looked up, the sky a rich aqua shade of blue with smudges of eggshell white speckling its edge. Like the finger-size porcelain teacups her mother kept behind glass at home, lined up neatly along the shelf. Admired but never touched. Fragile. For display only. Just as she had been. A fragile four-year-old. For display only. Admired but never touched.

She struggled but wayward thoughts scurried forth like spiders out of corners. Her mother's face. Shapely, oval, younger. Clear, flawless skin. Tresses of thick auburn hair. Hazel eyes, arched forehead, high-cheekbones. Sensuous lips. The same features a daughter would later inherit. The curse of overabundance. Beauty that had brought so much success, so much hurt. They'd cried together when she'd left, the doctors said that was progress, but it was hard to forget. Even harder to forgive.

She remembered when the notion first hit, when candy became illicit. Shopping Saturdays, M&M mornings. A little girl rushing down the aisle, tracing the clown's face on the wrapper, slipping it into the shopping cart. Her mother smiling. But not that day. Examining her mouth where a tooth had fallen out. Her frown. "*A small imperfection in an otherwise perfect face,*" she'd said, frowning. "*They'll make you fat like a big rubber ball, you'll come out in horrible yellow spots we'll have to pop every day.*" The candy went back on the shelf.

New rules brought in overnight. Rigid, unwavering, even on birthdays. No parties with fancy-hats, pop-sickles, balloons and cake. Instead a regime of exercise, sleep and sugar-free foods.

"*Stay away from the park. You might fall and bruise your skin.*"

Pageant days were worse. No school. '*I promise not to play during break*,' she'd cry. She never kept that promise. Was never given a chance to. She was kept away.

Crying sprees ensued. Hunger strikes came and went. Protests were attempted, her prostrate at the front door. All failed to melt her mother's determination. Alas, she learned, escape routes for an only child are distinctive by their absence. Shuffled into a green pink sequin dress in Spring, a butterfly flower halter variation in Summer, she'd perform *'I'm A Little Teapot'*…over and over and over.

Grooming was endless. *'Stop shifting, you don't want to look like Widow Twanky or the Cinderella sisters, do you?'* her mother would shout. *'I'm doing this for your own good. So you won't have to starve, or worry about money ever again. Look at Christie Brinkley and Elle Macpherson. You'll be adored, you'll be rich. What more could a woman want?'*

But she wasn't a woman. She was a little girl. And she was never convinced. Not the money. What did a child know, or care about that? No, what she wasn't convinced about was that this was about her. She'd look at her mother and see with a child's discerning eye this craving for winning, this yearning for success, was not hers. Only much later did Patricia realize just how vital a role *'tiaras for toddlers'* had been in filling a gaping chasm in her mother's life, how it elevated her above the dreary existence into which she had fallen. A job at the supermarket check-out hardly provided breath-taking excitement. Evenings at home meant quiet, except for the drone of the television. Her father had left long before. Since then nothing seemed to interest her mother much. Except the pageants. The little girl had no choice. Deep down she knew. If she didn't go, a hole would open up and swallow her mother. Then it would swallow her too.

She remembered standing in polished black patent shoes with silver buckles, a blue ribbon placed over her head for third place. Filled with pride, she'd gazed deep into the audience, seeing tears in her mother's eyes. Her skin tingled with excitement. She longed to be in her arms, be hugged for what she'd achieved. The curtains closed, she stood backstage, waiting. Parents arrived excitedly, laughing and chatting, leading their children out, some being carried high on shoulders. They'd congratulated her. But still her mother didn't appear. She'd begun to worry. Took off her ribbon, folded it carefully, stored it neatly in a special little suitcase that she kept her clothes in. Still no sign. Soon there was nobody left except workmen clearing away chairs and tables.

Later, alone, even stage hands gone, she'd pushed nervously through the heavy curtain. The hall was empty. Some seats had been moved out, leaving large gaps. She imagined she was a dentist looking into a mouthful of broken teeth. Then, as she turned to go back, she noticed a movement in the shadows. Someone stood alone there. She recognized her mother's coat. Maybe she had been on her way back-stage and fell. Maybe she was hurt. She clamored down. It was high, she had to go down on all fours, drop her legs over the edge. She walked along the narrow aisle, holding her dress up at the waist to stop it trailing dust, shouting out, 'Mommy, mommy' excitedly. No response. Her mother didn't even look up, her shoulders shaking. The little girl slowed down, unsure, sensing something was wrong, but not knowing what. Then she stopped altogether, watched closely. Her mother dabbed at her wet eyes with a tissue, covered her face with her hands. Was this a game of peekaboo, the little girl thought, and when she touched her would she have a big, bright smile as a reward and laugh and take her in her outstretched hands and tickle her and smother her with kisses and hugs for her success in her very first try. But nothing like that happened. Instead, her mother lifted her handbag from the floor and buttoned her coat tightly around her. And walked away.

Sipping the last of her espresso, Patricia shivered, recalling the little girl's fears, the nervous trembling of her body.

'Mommy?' The word was more a plea than a question.

No answer.

'Mommy? Are you okay?'

Without speaking, her mother turned, grasped her hand roughly and led her out of the theater. The little girl's heart sank like a stone, the truth slowly dawning. She hadn't won the tiara. Ever since, Patricia recalled, her main aim in childhood was to win. To make her mother smile again.

Getting through high school wasn't easy. Crunch study between pageants. Long, lonely rides on the Greyhound. Not even allowed to lean against the window. "You're cheeks will swell, you'll blotch your dimples." Wheat-fields and water-towers. Kansas City. Omaha. Des Moines. Denver. Rodeo Queen. Miss Stars and Stripes. Heart of America. Darling Dolls. Quick overnights in cheap roadside motels. Tiresome, boring, nothing much to do. Then the little girl grew up and New York beckoned. She escaped. They grew apart. Months without speaking. Then the accident. Out of the ashes of separate lives rose hope. Feelings woke from the deepest of slumbers. Two pitiful people facing prying eyes. They lurched towards each other, tentatively at first, then with all-consuming urgency born of desperation, finding there a refuge from the accusations and innuendos being flung their way.

'*It could be a new start for us,*' her mother had said one day, more in hope than confidence, pouring coffee into her prize porcelain cups.

They cried. Then smiled. Awkwardly at first, as if exercising unfamiliar facial muscles. But they were smiling. That's what mattered.

'*The hounds still smell blood,*' Patricia explained later about leaving for such a strange place as Donegal. '*There are only fish where I'm going. And they really don't care.*'

Her mother accepted her words without question. It was the price to pay for peace. Explanations would come later.

Chapter eighteen

Karen glanced at the closed door for the fourth time. She was only a secretary, what could she do? Fingers of light seeped out from under it and she could see a shadow flit past now and then and hear the soft sound of footfall on the carpet inside.

It was a quarter after the hour. If she waited any longer she'd be late. And David would be less than pleased being caught in rush-hour traffic.

Doctor Gray had been working a lot of late hours recently. Too many. Something important though she didn't know what it was.

Reluctantly she put on her coat and headed out along the narrow corridor leading to the back parking lot. On each side of her, a line of white doors remained firmly closed, everyone having left. Emptiness and silence greeted her. She didn't feel comfortable walking here. With the constant movement of people up and down during the day, she was fine. But at night, deserted as it was, she felt a ghostly atmosphere pervade the place. Hearing it had once housed the morgue, that cadavers had been stored here many years before, hadn't eased her concerns any. Overhead lights were dimmed automatically in the evenings to save on energy, making its spookiness even spookier.

Suddenly, an unfamiliar sound snapped her out of her reverie. She stopped to listen. That's what was strange. There was nothing to listen to. Before she could react, before she realized the power generator had gone off, she found herself standing in complete darkness. She stood stock still, every muscle stiff. She felt faint. Holding out her hands, she searched for the wall, slowly, tentatively, as if fearing she'd touch something she didn't want to touch. Then she heard it, not the soft purring sound of the transformer starting up, but footsteps and the whishing sound of a door not far behind her. She spun round fast, almost falling over, but could see nothing. That's when she dropped it. She fumbled around, her heart fluttering wildly as if it had sprouted wings. It began pounding, sending prickles of pain through her chest. Sweat clung to her forehead.

Then out of the silence, the piercing squeal of a car horn. It made her almost jump out of her skin. Her senses overloaded, she became disoriented, on the verge of sobbing. Then, with a great surge of relief, she realized what it was. She rushed forward in the darkness, expecting any second to smash into something solid, a wall, a door, a dead body even. Instead, after twenty bounds, she found herself twisting madly on a handle and rushing out into the starry night headed for a parked car, its headlights blazing. She yanked at the door with both hands, banging her knees with it as it flew open.

"Someone's there," she gasped breathless as David, her boyfriend, looked up bewildered.

***

While his fingers drummed an urgent rhythm on the cover of the thick file on his desk, Dr. Gray's mind raced elsewhere. He didn't like what he had done or the way he had gone about it but as he saw it, he really didn't have much choice – either for Patricia or for the mission. It was only a matter of time before the paparazzi found out where she was and grilled her and he didn't know if she was strong enough to take that, so better a serious, sympathetic reporter like Colm than one hell-bent on sensationalism. As for the mission, committee hearings were coming to an end. Time was against them. This might be their only chance.

Colm had called as expected, his tone a mix of excitement and anger. He may have missed Patricia but he hadn't missed the chance to meet her mother. They'd had a long talk. He'd learned most everything. He'd calmed down after a while, seeming to understand his refusal to break patient confidentiality. He'd warned him if he went, though there was no certainty he would, he'd have to be really sensitive. Patricia was fragile. She deserved a break. She'd had her fill of snooping journalists.

He opened the file, the first page an introductory letter. All too familiar to him now, but one that marked the beginning of this entire saga. He skipped quickly through it –

Dear Doctor Gray,
...honor to write ... admirer of your consumer advocacy work ...patient in question ... car accident...other woman ...head injuries...

coma.

... prominent models ...fashion and cosmetics.... Miss Roberts, driver ...dizziness, severe irritation... pain in eye... momentary black-out, lost control ... initial suspicion ... human error ... tiredness or/and excess alcohol or/and drug consumption... late-night party.

Blood and urine analyses ...alcohol levels ...below legal limit... no traces of benzoylecgonine for cocaine or THC for cannabis.

Mild corneal disruption ...pupillary dilation...ongoing eye problems ... ...resisted repeated antibacterial treatments... thoroughly investigated... astigmatism, blepharitis, conjunctivitis, corneal ulcers, uveitis, acute glaucoma, diabetic retinopathy.

... infection remained mystery... reviewed notes ... interesting possibility ...particular field patient in... products used daily...significant factor... thought of you.

...enclosed documents...list of elements ...complete list impossible....

... discretion...sensitive information ...confidential...

...coincidence...Roberts... Missouri... Weston...near Kansas City.

Sincerely Yours,

Dr. George Watkins,
Chief of Ophthalmology

He remembered the palpable sense of excitement he'd felt first reading it, even more so after examining the test results attached.

How quickly things had changed. An urgent call to Dr. Watkins, a review of Patricia's condition. The flight to Boston.

Now, bathed in a penumbra of light from the floor lamp, his mind shot back to that trip. He was to meet Patricia in a private room at the end of a long corridor with a glass observation deck above. He went to the deck first. He wanted to study her as she approached. Watching her unnoticed would help him gain invaluable insights into her state of mind after the trauma she'd been through. When she appeared with a nurse, she looked gaunt, almost skeletal, her walking bereft of the confidence to be expected from someone who literally walked for a living. The nurse was trying to engage her in conversation, but Patricia paid scant attention, her eyes darting nervously in every direction as if ghosts flew around her head. A wraith-like vision of uncertainty - frightened, vulnerable - she resembled an alcoholic, a drug addict in recovery. A far cry from the picture-perfect image of vitality, elegance and beauty plastered across glossy magazines. With an intake of breath, he realized who she reminded him of and tears filled his eyes. He took a deep breath to calm himself. One of them needed to be strong. Healing skin damaged by burns, he sensed, would be the least of the challenges he was about to face.

Then as he walked down the stairs to meet her, it happened.

"I'm Doctor Gray. I'm from Kansas."

He held out his hand and smiled. She stared at him, her gaze unwavering, full of suspicion, her eyes those of a cornered animal. Suddenly, she let out a gasp and tears began to fall. She slumped against him as if she no longer had the power to stand. All he could do was wrap his arms around her, hold her. Her shoulders shuddered against his with the sheer power of the heavy anguished sobs that wracked her frame. It was as if mention of Kansas had swept her back in time, to a time of innocence, a world away from the ugliness she'd had to endure.

And so it was. A bond forged in seconds. One that enabled him to overcome two of the three most difficult obstacles he'd envisioned – persuading her to return to the Midwest for a battery of tests and then to travel outside America '*away from the maddening crowd*' as he'd termed the chasing paparazzi. The third obstacle, however, remained unresolved. That's why he sitting here at his desk, pondering.

Turning back to the opened file, his desk light flickered and went out. A blanket of blackness consumed him. Taken aback, he sat motionless, staring directly ahead, trying to see through the inky void. There was no sound, no movement. Remembering he had a flashlight, he rummaged in his top drawer, found it and switched it on. It gave off a wan, buttery stick of light. Should have checked the batteries, he thought, annoyed at himself. He stood up and maneuvered slowly around office furniture. Making his way to the door, he opened it, closing it gently after him. Seeing the reception area also in darkness, he recalled Karen had just left. Thinking she might be stuck in the long corridor - a scenario he knew she wouldn't relish - he began moving in that direction.

"Karen? Karen? Can you hear me?" he said as he went.

Halfway along, without warning, he stumbled on something. Pointing his torch downward, he caught it in a pale arc of light. Recognizing it immediately, the first stabs of anxiety gripped him. Then he heard the ssssh of soft footfalls. Not far away but fading quickly.

"Karen, is that you?"

He swept the torch in a wide arc along the blank walls of the corridor but its beam fell only upon a row of identical white doors, all tightly closed.

Before he could investigate further, music started playing. He wondered what it was, then realized and fumbled in his pocket.

"Doctor Gray?" said a breathless voice when he'd put the phone to his ear.

"Yes, yes, that's me. Who's this?"

"It's me Karen, your assistant."

"Oh, hello my dear, I didn't recognize the number or your voice."

"I'm calling from another phone."

"But your voice, it sounds strange. Is something wrong? And where are you?"

"Outside, in the parking lot. The lights all went out. I thought I heard footsteps behind me. I ran. Are you okay?"

"Yes, yes, no need to worry. Actually, I'll let you in on a secret but don't tell anyone. I'm enjoying a second childhood in here, reliving old 'Secret Seven' adventures in the dark." Hearing no chuckle, Doctor Gray continued, more soberly.

"Actually, I came looking for you, young lady, but it seems you left in quite the hurry. You left something immensely valuable behind."

"Yes, my handbag. Oh, thank you."

"Knowing how much you love this corridor at night, this power outage must have given you quite a fright. I must say, it does seem a bit eerie in here."

"You're in the corridor?" Her tone conveyed disbelief.

"Yes, I thought you'd be frightened and might require an ally against the dark forces of evil. With the doors all closed and no windows here in this corridor, you probably can't see my Star Wars sturdy lance of shimmering light."

Doctor Gray heard the urgent exchange of voices on the other end of the line.

"Hello?" he murmured, confused. Silence.

"Hello? Karen? Are you there? Is someone with you...?"

"Yes, yes, doctor, I'm here, with David, in his car. But..."

There was concern in her voice.

"Yes?"

"I can see a beam of light. "It's coming from...," anxiety rose in her voice, "...your office."

"Oh, but that's not possible. I've just come from there."

Doctor Gray felt the muscles in his shoulders tighten.

"It's moving now."

Silence.

"To where?"

"Towards the corridor."

"You must be mistaken, I'm standing in the middle of…"

Karen heard a muffled sound, then a dull thud, like something falling. Then nothing.

"Hello? Hello? Hello?"

Her urgent cries went unheeded, sucked up in the void of silence.

***

In the darkness, Doctor Gray could see very little. From his prone position on the floor, he could see even less. What he did see for an instant above him was a delectable slice of Cheddar - a particular item of food for which he had a lifelong fondness. It had a small irregular bite taken out of one side as if nibbled at by a small animal and it hovered in the air above his head tantalizingly. It was a brief image, lasting no more than a few seconds, then, just quickly, it had vanished.

He was delusional, his right lobe in the ascendency. He needed to put on his thinking cap, switch lobes. His snap diagnosis was mild concussion. His cerebrospinal fluid had probably gone for a spin and his brain cells, depolarized, were firing all their neurotransmitters at once in an abrupt cascade, flooding his brain with chemicals and ions. As such, the hanging cheese tit-bit was probably not an entirely accurate depiction of what he had seen. More likely it indicated deadening of receptors associated with learning and memory. Thus, probably more likely something more relevant to his present situation. Classical textbook learning told him his brain, suffering from constricted arteries and lack of oxygen, craved a shot or two of sugar glucose to provide healing energy, but he also knew this would spell disaster. A metabolic crisis would ensue. Thus, he decided, best to remain exactly where he was on the floor until the world stopped spinning, then gently exit the surreal world the sudden thump had sent him sprawling into. What he didn't know was just what quantity of brain cells had been damaged and how long it would take for blood flow to return to normal. However, staying horizontal would help this most important of organs remain in a quiescent condition.

Having decided on this rather well-considered plan of inaction, he was therefore confounded when the juicy yellow morsel appeared once again to taunt him. In fact, it grew bigger, relentless in its provocation.

Then he heard a door closing and the cheese disappeared yet again. A voice whispered in his ear.

"Doctor Gray, are you okay?" The tone was familiar, reassuring.

"Yes, well at least I think so. I had a bit of a tumble."

"Well, you're safe now. Can you stand up?"

"I think so."

"Are you sure?" Now, he knew who it was.

"Yes, my dear Karen. I thought I was concussed. I saw a lovely slice of cheese dangling there. I was ready to pluck it and devour it. Now I realize what a foolish thing that would have been. Trying to eat a chunk of the moon. Lucky the Chancellor didn't see me."

"Sorry about that, doctor, but at least you're safe. I promise I'll bring you a whole box of cheeses first thing Monday morning, how's that. But now, let's get you on your feet."

Doctor Gray felt several pairs of hands help him to a standing position. Just then the lights flickered and came on again, blinding him momentarily.

"Did I trip? Fall over another discarded woman's accessory?"

"No, sir, we think you were pushed." It was David, Karen's boyfriend. "We saw someone rush out of here and disappear into the trees beyond. We've notified security. They're searching the grounds."

"Well, well. How strange. Why would anyone…?"

He stopped, his mind clearing in an instant.

"I need to get to my office," he said turning quickly and heading back along the corridor.

"Doctor Gray, you can't possibly think of going back?" said Karen, her eyes wide with concern. "You may be concussed. We need to get you to a doctor."

"My dear, how easily you forget." His tone benevolent. "May I remind you? I am a doctor."

Karen's face went red. "I mean…," she mumbled. "What I meant was, what I mean is, well, you doctors may be experts at treating others, but sometimes you don't treat yourselves very well."

Seeing her resolute, sensing this could reach the ears of his wife, Doctor Gray sensed a compromise was in order. "Okay, my dear, okay. I'll agree to come peacefully but first let me take a short walk to my office. Just to check everything is fine."

Karen sighed, there was little she could do to stop him. Side by side, the three of them headed back.

He didn't need to enter his office to know. He remembered closing the door behind him, now it stood wide open. His empty desk confirmed his worse fears – the file was gone. There was no turning back now.

Chapter nineteen

Finding a computer in a quiet corner of the newsroom, Colm quickly typed *'roberts patricia'* in the Google search bar. The first link selected was to a knitwear company based in London, then several biographies, none of which was what he was looking for. Beneath them, a headline caught his eye.

'Late night road tragedy, emergency services called to crash scene.'

Clicking on the file he was confounded to find it wasn't a local story but a one-paragraph brief in *The Cape Cod Times*. He read on.

'Two young women, thought to be in their mid-20s, were injured late last night in a single vehicle accident two miles north of Hyannis. Police named the two women as Patricia Roberts and Christine Scott. Paramedics at the scene said the first woman they saw was stumbling around outside the car holding her eyes, which were found to be swollen and bloodshot. The other woman had suffered head injuries. Citing patient confidentiality, hospital officials declined to release any information on their condition saying they had both undergone emergency medical treatment. Police said they will issue a full report once their investigation is complete.'

Could this be her? Impatient, he hurried on to the next entry. A much longer article, from *Fashion News*, with head and shoulder close-ups of the two women as illustration. Broad, beaming smiles, perfect complexions, bright seductive eyes staring confidently into the camera lens. Colm recognized her instantly. The face a little fuller than the one he had seen in Doctor Gray's medical file but unmistakable. While both looked beautiful, they were different in many ways, none more than in their hairstyle. Patricia's hair was thick, auburn. The other a close-cropped 'Joan of Arc' style, and blonde.

Colm read slowly.

Leading models still recovering in hospital

Former Miss America, Patricia Roberts ... Colm's eyes snapped wide reading this - *who stole the catwalk at the recent Paris Spring Fashion, and Christine Scott, who scooped the Miss California title last year, are still recovering in a Boston hospital following a car accident.*

Citing patient confidentiality, hospital officials said they could not release detailed information but described the condition of the two women as 'stable.' Family members, who rushed to the hospital after being notified, also declined to comment.

According to 'Fashion News' sources, Roberts and Scott had left a private party in Hyannis following the official launch of the perfume 'Stay Awhile' when the accident occurred in the early hours of Thursday morning. Police said the car, a dark-blue Lamborghini Murciélago (see inset photo), had gone off the road and hit a tree, adding that a full report will be issued when the investigation is complete.

'The car's a real write-off,' Jimmy Sweeney, a mechanic with Limbaugh's Garage Services told a local radio station. 'I wouldn't like to have been the person inside.'

Industry leaders voiced their concern about the condition of the two women, who were believed to be in the line-up by Gucci and Louis Vuitton for the Milan autumn fashion show.

Catherine James, who garnered the title 'Queen of Couture' after her Dolce and Gabbana collection last Spring that featured the two women, told 'Fashion News,' 'We were shocked to hear the news. My thoughts are with Patricia and Christine and their families at this very difficult time. They are both divas of the catwalk, sheer magnificence no matter what ensemble they wear - exquisitely tomboy, hippy sheik, maximal, minimal. It doesn't matter. There was no limit to what they could achieve.'

Colm greedily scrolled down the pages, eyeing headlines, clicking on entries, devouring details of the celebrity drama that unfolded on the screen before him.

At first, the sheer number of articles made a mockery of his proud newspaper reading abilities. How could he not have heard of her? Then he realized. The stories were in the celebrity glossies, hardly his daily diet. While it was an accident, the key ingredient of death was missing, thus insufficient gravitas for bigger play in broadsheets. Also, none of the reports mentioned Patricia being from the Midwest, instead indicating she was a New Yorker.

As he read on, he became increasingly enthralled, drawn in by the fickleness of fame in the world of fashion. His eyes narrowed, then snapped wide open with each new surprising twist to the tale. He leaned closer to the screen, one elbow resting on the desk, his hand supporting his chin. Most articles carried the same details on the crash but it was the abundance of non-sourced industry gossip that fixed his attention. Christine Scott being seriously injured and unable to speak, the unanswered question became the extent of Roberts' responsibility for the crash, especially as reports said road conditions were normal and that no other vehicle was involved. With Roberts declining to make a statement, the rumor mill went into overdrive, culminating in a dramatic photo from the front page of *Celebrity Watch* with a bold single-word caption, '*Innocent?*' splashed across it.

Though intrigued, Colm was left puzzled. He simply couldn't understand the link between the photo and the caption. Patricia, easily recognizable, was seated at a table, her hair cascading down the back of the oyster colored chiffon dress she wore. Around her were other women, equally well dressed, equally beautiful, all looking chic, sassy and sexy in sumptuous silks and satins. They were all laughing, obviously enjoying a humorous remark someone had just made. But Colm couldn't see anything unusual, simply people in high spirits. Having a good time was hardly a sin so why the inference in the caption? Heightened curiosity was obviously the desired effect the magazine editor aimed for, enticing people to buy the magazine by promising drama inside.

Colm did as thousands of readers had done before him, he jumped to the next page. There a second photo appeared, a close-up of the table around which the beautiful women all sat. It was cluttered with an assortment of beer, wine and champagne glasses and bottles. The page designer had made a few enhancements to the photo. Circled in black was a set of car keys attached to a silver-colored ring ornately shaped into the letters 'PG'. Colm's eyes widened. They widened even more upon seeing a second object circled in black. Hard to recognize at first, partially hidden as it was behind a half-filled wine glass. Colm leaned closer to the computer screen wondering what it was. Then he realized. A narrow three-inch long glass cylinder. And beside it, a thin line of white powder. A hand and bare forearm rested across the table, nudging against them. Without having to look again at the large front-page photo, Colm guessed who's arm it was.

He clicked quickly on the story.

Roberts-Scott crash investigation reviewed
Sources say police are reviewing media reports linked to their

investigations into the car crash that caused two of America's most well-known models to undergo emergency medical treatment. Captain George Carmichael, spokesman for the Hyannis Police Department, said officers from the traffic division were re-examining the accident file following the release of a photograph indicating what looked like quantities of cocaine present at a party attended by the two women on the night of the accident. Police have requested the original negative be handed over for inspection.

Sources say police have detected no mechanical problems with the sports car and are investigating what they term 'other factors' that may have contributed to the accident.

'The accident could have been caused by any number of things, so we would prefer not to speculate until we have analyzed all the information at our disposal,' Captain Carmichael said. 'The area was a rural one so there is even a possibility that wild animals or low-flying birds were a contributing factor.' Asked if blood from animals or birds was detected on the vehicle, he said 'not as yet, but tests are still ongoing.' Weather reports indicate conditions in the area on the night of the accident were 'dry and clear.' Captain Carmichael said, 'any ramifications arising from publication of the photograph should be tempered with reason and common sense. The photographic image may or may not be of an illegal substance and, even if so, it is certainly not proof that such a substance was used by person or persons attending the party. It must be emphasized that no blame for the car crash is being apportioned to any individual at this time. We are simply re-examining certain information as a matter of course. It is normal police procedure in such situations.'

Celebrity Watch then quoted anonymous sources, a fashion designer, saying, *'It is common knowledge in the trade that so-called 'after hours' parties often feature a range of, how should we put it, 'interesting substances.' I say 'common knowledge' but nobody actually talks about it, for good reasons. Like most stars of the entertainment world, models work hard and party hard. There is a lot of social pressure and such get-togethers are considered a fun way for them and their entourage to relieve stress.'* And also paramedics at the scene saying Patricia was *'stumbling around the car, her eyes swollen and bloodshot.'* Colm re-read the photo caption: *'Patricia Roberts (left) enjoying a product post-launch party. Police say they are re-examining the circumstances of a car accident in which she was involved.'*

He noted the way the magazine stepped nimbly around a potential legal minefield by not commenting directly on the photo, leaving it tantalizingly ambiguous.

"C'mon, give me a break." The short, sharp voice broke the silence, a whiplash snapping Colm out of his cyber world. A bearded, bespectacled man in a crumpled sports jacket was leaning over him, smiling. "Give it up there, my friend. You've been on it for over an hour. A case of cold Coors and a double-header at Kauffman's Stadium against the Padres is on the menu tonight. A perfect time for you Europeans to learn about our nation's favorite sport. "

It was Tony Miles, the federal court reporter.

"Tony, hi," Colm mumbled.

"A hot potato, eh?"

"Maybe, who knows. Now just a hunch," said Colm, logging off. But he knew it was more than that. And it was all his.

"So, are you ready for the ballpark?"

"Will give it a miss I'm afraid." Colm was too excited to spend the evening watching boys batting balls back and forth. Anyway, soccer was his game.

His colleague's face registered disappointment.

"Next time. I promise."

As Colm stood up, someone passed close to him.

"You're too excited for your own good," Pratt said coldly. "After what happened before, don't go thinking I'm open to one of your so-called enterprise stories. Stick to the basics and stay out of trouble."

Colm attempted to speak but Pratt turned on his heels and was gone.

Chapter twenty

Evening was falling gently, the bright blue of the sky turning slowly to steely grey. He opened the refrigerator and grabbed a cold Grolsch. Pushing open the screen door and stepping on to the wooden porch, he was met by a warm breeze and a noisy chorus of cicadas.

He sunk down on the rickety rocking chair.

Darkening clouds meandered overhead, forming and re-forming patterns, producing an ever-changing jigsaw puzzle. The sun set directly in front of him into a crimson ball, then a vague rim of the moon appeared, faded, almost transparent at first, then a rich buttery yellow. He'd been given a front row seat and a bowl of fruit for the evening, he mused, a giant grapefruit and a slice of banana to marvel at.

He drank deeply and lay back, setting the rocking chair into lazy motion. Talk of Ireland earlier with Mrs. Roberts had sent a wave of nostalgia washing over him, unwanted reminders of the place he'd left and what he'd left there. In spite of his efforts, barriers erected to the past faded away. His mind wandered through half-forgotten alleyways of thought he had hoped not to visit again. He closed his eyes. A familiar face appeared to him, haunting him, filling him with deep sadness.

One of the most beautiful girls he had ever seen. Before bombs and bullets and burning buses. When the days were long and hours seemed timeless, suspended in a summery soup of youthful innocence. Jet-black hair, gleaming even in fading sunlight. And the brownest of eyes, hazel nuts, he'd called them. Said she should be careful going through the park from school, squirrels might attack. Her face so perfect, he wanted to caress it forever. As if he had a beautiful, small bird in his hand but was afraid of letting it go, of letting it fly away – because it might never come back and he'd be left forever far below on the ground among all the other ordinary people gazing up at the beauty he could never touch again, his hands together, but with nothing inside, nothing at all.

Colm didn't hear the sound of footfall.

"Good evening, Master Colm." The shock of the disembodied voice biting into the silence made him jump in his chair.

"Look as if you've seen a ghost," the voice said calmly, unfazed by his reaction. Looking up, he saw Lu, his old neighbor and landlady, smiling benignly. She seemed to have materialized out of thin air. With a bonnet tied tightly under her chin and a pair of worn dungarees billowing at the waist, she looked dressed for stealing corn from the farmer next door under cover of darkness.

Colm stared at her unable to speak, his mind in another world entirely.

"What's wrong? Cat got your tongue?"

Slowly the power of speech returned.

"You scared the living daylights out of me," he said catching his breath and settling himself back again on the rocking chair. "You shouldn't go sneaking up on people like that."

"Sneaking up?" she said, a grin spreading across her face. "I was making as much noise as that darn raccoon around the garbage can every night. Are you going deaf?"

"No, you caught me thinking, that's all."

"Hurt did it?" she asked cheekily.

"Just a bit," he replied, warming to the duel.

"No harm done then."

She waited expectantly. "Well?"

"Well?"

"Well, what were you thinking?"

"I was thinking what a bloody nuisance you are."

"Oh, tough talk, and for such a little person," Lu shot back. "Anything else?"

"Oh, things. The usual, you know."

"If I knew I wouldn't be asking now, would I?"

"I suppose not."

"Anyways, the only things boys like you think about are sport and women. And as you haven't a clue 'bout baseball, I guess it's gotta be women."

He didn't say anything but silence was an answer.

"Telepathy, eh. Not just a pretty face, kid." She stopped as if reveling in her insight. He could almost hear her purring with satisfaction. "Who was she then?" she asked finally.

"Oh, no-one special."

"Really now." She bent close. "By the look on that face, I'd say she's more than that. In fact, I'd say she might have been the one."

"Mmmm."

She cocked her head to one side. "That bad, eh?" She clucked her tongue. "Hard to believe. I mean a man like you's got to have more women stacked away than you'd find in the maternity wing of Trinity Lutheran Hospital." His smile encouraged her, "And most of the children there are probably yours too."

He stuck his tongue out at her, which she took as an invitation to stay awhile.

"Here, take my chair," he said starting to get up.

"No, been sitting all evening, need to crack ma joints a bit," she replied, resting a hand on his shoulder. In the silence, they watched a pair of shooting stars break through black velvet.

"So, you're telling me one of them there ladies I've seen hanging around here done gone robbed your heart?" she continued.

" 'fraid so. But not from around here. A long time ago."

"By the looks of you, all forlorn and all, it couldn't have been that long."

"Years, many years."

She gazed at him quizzically.

"Are you being straight with me, honey, or just plain ornery as usual, having fun pulling an old witch's leg?"

"Back in Ireland," he continued, sitting upright. "And don't you go being jealous. Was long before I met you." He winked at her playfully.

"Tch, tch." Lu made a pretense of shooing him away with her hand. "I tell you, you're so full of it, it's coming out your ears." She looked at him again, closer this time, a blend of kindness and concern in her eyes. "G'wan, get it off your chest, kid. Make my day. I'm bored watching 'ER,' too many wet eyes and canoodling for my liking. And NYPD, all re-runs, and I've seen most of 'em. Know who's the murderer before someone's been murdered. Anyway, I'd rather have a real live situation like this to get ma teeth into." She hesitated, "But let me settle myself proper before you begin. Wanna be real comfortable for this one."

She shuffled slowly round in front of him, careful on her feet, her age showing in the sharp bony angle of her back. She took his outstretched hand and eased herself down on to a cane chair that stood against the wall.

"Ok," she said, patting down the front of her dungarees and leaning

100

back, hands in her lap. "I'm all set now. You can begin anytime you like."

"I'm not telling you anything, my dear. If I do, the whole town will know before breakfast."

"Cross my heart and hope to die."

"You wouldn't be interested."

"What woman wouldn't be interested in a bit of romance. Long as it's not too gushy."

"You really want to hear about it?"

"Of course. Am all ears. I won't interrupt. But don't go disappointing me. I want the whole kit and caboodle. No half measures. I didn't come over all this way stumbling in the dark for nothing. Coulda been eaten by a ground hog on the way and you'd never have known."

Colm gazed at her with tenderness. She could be so beguiling. A soft fruit with a hard skin.

"She was a girl I'd known since we were kids playing in the street."

Lu nodded her head as if she too cherished such memories.

"Then the war in Belfast began and we all changed, fast. We all grew up and went off and did what we did."

Lu glanced over, puzzled, her mouth a pout. "Call that a story," she scolded. "That's the beginning and end all in one sentence. What do you mean, 'did what we did'? What a peculiar thing to say?"

"Not really. Not if you know Belfast, and certainly not if you knew it then. A rough place with no escape. Street riots, bombings, shootings. You name it, we had it."

"And you kept in touch with each other through all that?"

"Became close friends. Went to university, not many did in those days in our area. Lots of chat on the bus coming and going. Philosophical stuff. How we were going to be big and change the world. Even went on a few holidays together." He looked up, hearing a tut-tut sound. "Not alone," he added, "you didn't do that in those days in Catholic Ireland. A crowd of us all together, students."

"Go on, hurry up, get to the juicy part," she said, urging him on. "I'm just about old enough to hear it."

"Well, I guess, the inevitable happened."

"Inevitable? When you've lived as long as I, kid, you learn nothing and everything's inevitable. But go awn anyway, whatdya mean?"

"Well, we started dating."

"Ah, now we're getting to the good stuff." Lu rubbed her hands together and shuffled in her seat to get more comfortable. "Do you remember your first kiss?"

The question came at him fast, leaving no hiding place, a dart in the dark. He hesitated, "You promised you wouldn't interrupt."

"I know I did, but I was lying." She waited expectantly. "Well, do you?"

She was a stubborn old mule, he knew. He'd never get away without answering, so might as well come clean. "It was a typical dull day in Ireland, drenching wet," he began, images flooding back to him as he spoke. "Raining hard and heavy, no end in sight, we were sitting on the bus, our faces buried in our overcoats and scarves, the steam rising off us, peering out, she through one window, and me beside her, just staring at the strange patterns it made slapping and sliding down the glass, deep in our own thoughts. Then we turned, at the very same time, turned to say something, and caught each other's eyes, embarrassed, both our mouths open ready to speak, and then I just leaned in, and she too, and well, that was that."

"Oh, honey, that's beautiful, I can see it as clear as daylight." The catch in her throat made him turn. In the wan light of the moon, old Lu seemed angelic, translucent, her skin as thin as parchment paper. This wrinkled dwarf of a woman, with her bent back and her bony hands, staring into the darkness, her eyes shining. She coughed softly, clearing her throat.

"Did you stay together long?" she asked.

He took a deep breath. "Long enough," he said.

"What happened? Did she go away somewhere?"

Colm had hoped she wouldn't ask. Emotions, long dormant, rushed up inside him clamoring for attention, pushing him this way and that. He tried hard, breathed deep, held them down, kept them out of harm's way, but they just kept coming, wave after wave, clambering, a marauding army laying siege at the castle gates, climbing up from his heart, invading every fiber of him. He felt a tremble but wasn't aware until he felt a skinny hand gently touch his own. He glanced down. A handkerchief in an open palm. He took it. Then looked away. Everything around him became a hazy blur.

Chapter twenty-one

The chubby man seated at the head of the table was waving two sheets of paper in the air as Larry and Jackson entered the room. He motioned impatiently for them to take a seat.

"This is what we're up against," he said sternly. "We must be vigilant. We cannot underestimate the power of their message. If we do, we lose momentum and before you know it, we've lost the battle. We have fought this before and won, and we have the money to do so again but we are not invincible."

As Larry sat down, still mulling over his father's warning the previous day, the gathered department managers smiled over at him, except one, the woman opposite, who pointedly ignored him. No big deal. He'd not have to put up with it for long anyway. Unfazed, he folded his hands on the table. When the CEO of Bellus, Dick Covington, spoke, everyone listened.

"Have you seen this, Larry? Whadaya think?"

Covington slid the sheets of paper across the table. Larry lifted one. It was a color photograph of a pretty child examining her face in a mirror. She held a tube of lipstick in her hand. The caption ran, *'Putting on Make-up Shouldn't Be Like Playing with Matches.'* Beneath were health warnings and a list headed *'Culprits.'* Larry didn't bother reading them. He knew the toxins alphabetically off by heart. He picked up the second sheet, blank aside from a single paragraph.

'Propylene glycol is a key ingredient in car antifreeze, so dangerous the EPA requires workers to wear protective gloves, goggles and clothing working with it. It was removed from cat food because cats were dying of liver failure. Beware! You spray it under your arms as an antiperspirant. You spread in on your body for a better suntan. Stay away from this product.'

"They're trying. So what, that's their job," he said dismissively. "What we're doing is even better. Taking the lead as consumer educator."

"But is it enough?" Covington queried. "Using their own tactics to beat them may whip right back in our faces."

"It couldn't be worse than it was," the woman's voice broke in. Larry bristled. Slim, her thick, jet-black hair caught up in a bun, the ebony-skinned woman seemed not to notice his reaction, or didn't care. "Attack mode didn't work. Saying they were interested only in publicity and donations backfired on us. Calling them *chemical terrorists* and trying to muddy the debate waters with *junk science* as some sort of a magic catchphrase won us few believers. Probably lost us converts."

Larry swallowed the bile that rose in his stomach. He didn't need any reminding of his misdirected campaign. And certainly not by this bitch. Surprised their dueling had re-started so soon, he hit back. "I've lined up some persuasive independents, strengthening our message on product safety."

"Do we have hard data to show that?" the woman's voice was unyielding.

"Of course, results from focus groups conducted by Luntz Research show it's working." Larry countered, turning from her and addressed himself directly to Covington. "You'll remember Frank Luntz from his polling on the Republican *Contract with America.* We used his *dial technology.* People turn dials to show their responses to phrases and images in videos. One video featuring an epidemiologist that we paid received especially high ratings."

"We're all familiar with the technique, we don't need a lecture on it," the woman snapped back. "There's a danger we'll be tied to tobacco in the public mind, with people thinking, *'Didn't the tobacco industry's scientists lie to us for years?'*"

"Our consumer website will deal with that," Larry said, barely able to contain his anger. He didn't care if Cathy had been communications manager for the last ten years, it didn't give her the right to piss him off. "On test promos we say we're using the latest technology to provide consumers with safety information about our products and ingredients, as well as educational information on how the industry conducts its safety reviews and testing. It'll leave the Environmental Working Group's *'Skin Deep'* site in the shadow."

"That's exactly what I mean," Covington cut in. "We're doing what they've already done. Seems we're playing catch-up. That *Campaign for Safe Cosmetics* crowd has gone and created an annoyingly popular interactive site that provides toxicity information and regulatory status on thousands of ingredients in more than fifteen thousand cosmetics. For Chrissakes, they even estimate a 'safety score' to guide consumers on what they should and shouldn't buy."

"Don't worry, we'll beat them," replied Larry, trying to make himself sound more confident than he felt. "Just like *Skin Deep* we're drawing on government, academic, non-profit and professional reports and databases. But we'll have more information. We're recruiting academics to provide exactly what we need. We'll update it daily. Theirs will look static, dull and out of touch."

"Imitation is the highest form of flattery." The sarcasm in the voice was more than obvious. He felt like boxing her ears. Ignoring the interruption, he added, "We'll also have what we're calling, 'a consumer commitment code' with a tagline reading, 'to reaffirm the industry's commitment to safe products.' We're telling consumers to report what we're terming 'serious' or 'unexpected' adverse reactions saying we'll make ingredient and product safety data available to the FDA."

Seeing concern flash across Covington's face, he added quickly, "Of course, as we define what is 'serious' and 'unexpected,' we're giving nothing away."

"There's also that report they produced last week," Covington said. "They said fifty-two of the seventy-two cosmetics, deodorants and perfumes they tested contained phthalates. It's giving momentum to their National Compact Campaign. More than three hundred companies have signed up."

Instinctively, Larry knew how that information had reached Covington's desk. Out of the corner of his eye, he could see a smirk of self-satisfaction spread across his nemesis's face, a deep-seated pride in the success of a drip-feed information campaign of her 'anti-consultant' strategy. Like everyone in the industry, he was well aware of the compact. Based on European standards, some companies had agreed to inventory the chemicals they used in products and replace those banned by the European Union with safer alternatives and publicly report on progress.

"That's going nowhere," Larry replied. "There may be three hundred but they're tiny, Mom and Pop corner-shop operations. The blue chips refuse to sign up."

"Yes, but first it was that Healthcare Without Harm crowd and now this," Covington said. "It's worrying. They're gaining momentum. Pushing Congress hard to do something. PR Watch says other groups are signing up – the Breast Cancer Fund, even something called the

National Black Environmental Justice Network."

"As I said, tiny groups," replied Larry. "Whoever heard of the National Black Environmental Justice Network? It's probably a single room, a chair and a computer. In a basement somewhere in the back of beyond."

There was a cough from across the table. They both turned.

"For your information, the National Black Environmental Justice Network isn't a chair and a computer in any basement," Cathy's anger was barely disguised. "It's a major health and environmental network with affiliates in thirty-three states and the District of Columbia. Its members include some of the nation's leading African American grassroots environmental justice activists, researchers, lawyers, public health specialists, technical experts and authors."

"Whatever, it's still not a threat," Larry replied.

"Listen, all of you, and listen good," Covington said, stepping into the fray. "Self-regulation is our Holy Grail, and we want to keep it that way. We don't want our ingredients evaluated by overeducated idiots from outside agencies. Millions would have to be spent on re-labeling every product and jerking around with content to meet convoluted standards that'll certainly be brought in if we lose our status. Sales could suffer, our stock could slide under the table, competitors would see our formulae. The resulting mess doesn't bear thinking about."

Larry didn't need to be reminded. EU officials had banned more than a thousand substances from cosmetic products, including chemicals still allowed in U.S. and had passed legislation requiring manufacturers to provide data on potential health and environmental hazards before products were sold.

"We're on top of things," he said, sensing an opportunity to score points by emphasizing his high-placed political connections. "My Republican friends tell me they'll derail any attempts to copy our European cousins. We've got people on key standing committees. They'll not let us down. We pay a lot into the PACs. They'll characterize the move as too costly, burdensome, complex, anti-free enterprise. Also, I'm confident of Grahams crossing over. Over dinner last week, his eyes brightened like a rabbit finding a pile of lettuce when I described our welcome package. Without him, the FDA goes blind in one eye."

"And what about that other thing?" Covington interjected. "We don't need that hitting the media specially with Friends of the Earth and the International Center for Technology Assessment already pushing the feds to monitor nanoparticles more closely."

"I'm having it checked as we speak," said Larry. "We should get the information we need later today. Then we can decide what action to take."

"Remember, I want the association kept out of it."

"What's this about?" Cathy interjected, a quizzical look on her face. "What information? What media? Is this something I should know about?"

Larry said nothing. It was Covington's call.

"No, nothing that concerns you. It's on a simple need-to-know basis."

Cathy's face dropped, her displeasure obvious. She opened her mouth to protest but Covington moved the conversation on quickly, "Today's event. Give us an update."

She hesitated, uncomfortable about not knowing but seeing her boss's fixed expression, she reluctantly moved on. "*The Hill* give us a mention in this morning's edition."

Larry fought back a smirk. If this was her way of saying she was well connected, Covington should stop delaying and hand the reins over to him.

"Fragrance Day remains the title. We considered other options but this is the best. Neutral, ambient, positive. No mention of cosmetics. We've got gift-wraps for everyone. Creams, perfumes, sprays, lotions. And a testing table."

Covington nodded for her to go on.

"The event will open with a VIP reception, by invitation only, for Congressional Members, then an open house for staffers."

"How many do you expect?" he asked.

"Hard to know. I've a team tying down numbers today. They're working on secretaries, offering free samples in exchange for a bit of boss lobbying. I'd guess well over a hundred."

"Sounds promising," Covington said. "The committee's almost finished its hearings. We need to come up smelling roses. What about Senator Clarke?"

"He'll be there. One of the first to confirm. With a few senior staffers."

"Strange," Covington's eyes narrowed. "If I didn't know any better, I'd think he was up to something. Keep a close eye on him. The gloves may be about to come off."

Chapter twenty-two

Whitsmith stood alone as if in a trance outside the swing doors of the newsroom when Colm reached the top of the stairs.

Seeing him, the pint-sized photo editor's brown eyes brightened like that of a squirrel finding a ripe nut among a pile of dead leaves.

"Unbelievable, just unbelievable," he said excitedly, shaking his head from side to side. "How did he manage to keep it so hush-hush? That's what I'd like to know. How did he manage it?"

"What are you talkin…" Colm's attempt to speak was cut off by a flurry of words.

"I mean, Je'es. I thought I was plugged into the circuit but this just blows me away, just blows me way over the top. What da'ya think, my friend? What da'ya think?"

"Think? About what?" The vacant expression on Colm face went unnoticed as Whitsmith rattled on.

"You would think we'd all know about it, wouldn't you? I mean people like you and me. We work in the news business after all. We're communicators. We're supposed to know things, right? I mean, we know what's happening in Tel Aviv and Washington and Dar El Salaam but no, not here, not fifty meters away at the other end of the room."

Colm blinked. There was little else he could do. The man's arms were flapping so wildly now he half-expected him to take off and crash land three floors below.

"At least, the waiting's over. That's a blessing. Small mercies, eh. It's a long time coming though… " Seeing utter non-comprehension writ large on Colm's face, his flapping slowed to a flutter. "You don't know what the hell I'm talking about, do you, my little pea?"

Colm shook his head in bewilderment. "Haven't a clue."

"Oh my! You poor lost soul. You look so, so… lost. I feel like cradling you in my arms and telling you everything's going to be alright."

Knowing Whitsmith's personal preferences, Colm took a step back, just in case.

"We've got a new editor."

Colm swallowed hard. "A new editor?" he mumbled, still confused.

"Yes, isn't it great? Out with the old, in with the new, that's what I say."

"But…" Colm couldn't find his words.

"Yes, I know, hard to believe, isn't it? They finally did it."

"But…who, who is it?"

"Try guessing. He's one of us, one of the best. Journalism in the blood. Father a printer…" Whitsmith didn't get a chance to say more for Colm had him round the waist, whipped him into the air and was dancing with him in mad circles around the floor.

Seconds later, they heard footfalls from the stairs below. They stopped, gazing intently downward. McCarthy's face appeared. He shot a quick glance at both men. At Whitsmith's beaming face. At the excitement in Colm's eyes. He lowered his shoulders and covered his face with his hands in mock defense.

"Honest, guys, I couldn't say a thing. They told me to keep it quiet until…," but his words were drowned out in a whirl of movement and voices as they rushed upon him smothering him noisily with embraces and pats on the back.

Hearing the hullabaloo, two secretaries popped their heads out of their offices. "Men," one muttered to the other, "they never grow up."

Chapter twenty-three

To say Pratt was not happy was a complete understatement. He was pissed as hell.

He was being sidelined in the newsroom and he didn't like it one bit. He wasn't used to it and he had tried to deal with it as best he could. Stirring discontent in the ranks was one way that eased his frustration but it wasn't enough. And as time went on, he sensed what he once thought was unshakeable loyalty by certain editors, some hired under his watch, that he had personally interviewed for their jobs, then promoted, was fading fast. Ungrateful bastards.

With McCarthy officially in charge now, his own options were limited. His attempts at rousing mutiny had caused some damage, but not enough. A deliberate slow-down meant a few deadlines had been missed but the paper had still gone to bed, late sometimes though it might have been. Some stories were lost but readers didn't seem to notice and circulation remained steady. He needed it to nosedive, then he'd be called in to out the fire.

Something else needed to be done, and fast if he was to reclaim his throne. The problem was he couldn't think of anything. Even his closest lieutenants couldn't come up with any ideas during brainstorming sessions thinly disguised as card-games at his home. And if truth be known, they were more concerned about their own jobs and their place in the pecking order at the newspaper than a full-scale revolution.

He was in a foul mood when the call came in. A voice he had never heard before and a first name that meant even less, did little to cheer him up.

"Mister Pratt, my name is Larry, we've never met, but I believe we can be of mutual benefit." It was an east coast accent but he couldn't place exactly where. If he had to hazard a guess, he'd have said upstate New

York. "I wondered if we could meet. Soon. To talk."

Not used to such blunt directness, Pratt was momentarily taken aback.

"Who is this? What's this all about?"

"I will explain everything, but I'd rather do it in person so there's no misunderstanding. I'm willing to fly to Kansas City and sit down with you somewhere quiet," the voice said, business-like but non-threatening.

But Pratt was a Midwesterner and Midwesterners are, if anything, conservative by nature. "But I'll need to know who I'm talking to and what I'll be talking about," he said, his curiosity rising.

"Let's just say I am well aware of your difficulties at the paper and believe I have a way to correct that. Rather quickly."

Pratt glanced up from his desk, nervous. Was this a trick? Was someone playing him for a fool? His gaze swept around the newsroom seeking out suspicious ears and eyes. No one was taking any notice of him. They were all engaged in their daily routine chores. He looked towards his old office, saw McCarthy. It was something he'd probably pay someone to do, just for the satisfaction of seeing him squirm. But he was sitting at his desk reading sheets of paper spread out on his desk.

"Are you still there?" the voice said, a hint of urgency obvious.

"Yes, I am, but I need to know…" He was cut off mid-sentence.

"Mister Pratt, with all due respect, I don't think you have time to waste, and I certainly don't. Name the place, and I'll be there tonight. I'm sorry to say this, and please don't take offence, but as I see it you have nothing to lose. And everything to gain."

This rankled Pratt and he was about to snap a sharp response down the line, but…

He waited a few seconds. "Okay, no harm in listening," he said, adding with false bravado, "I'm a journalist after all and we're supposed to be good at that."

Larry smiled. The first part of the plan complete. The rest should be easy.

Chapter twenty-four

"Are you sure our prime piece of evidence is safe?"

"Positive. I bagged it myself."

"And the tests are all verified?"

"Yes, done and dusted. Signed off by three different department heads."

Doctor Gray sighed with relief. He'd been trying Jack on his phone all evening, growing frantic by the minute. Ever since the theft, his concerns had magnified. He had two emergency calls to make but couldn't get through to either person. At least now, one matter was being dealt with.

"You seem upset. Is something wrong?" Jack asked, worry in his voice.

"There's been an incident."

"An incident? What kind of incident?"

"Someone broke into my office. Stole the report."

There was a momentary silence. "Are you okay?"

"Yes, a few minor bruises that's all."

"Bruises? You were attacked?" The voice was etched with shock.

"Not quite, but I won't go into that right now."

"But you're safe?"

"Yes."

"Look Gray, this is becoming dangerous. You never know what could happen. A lot's at stake. We need to tell someone."

"Who?"

"Someone in authority. What about the Centers for Disease Control?"

"Why? It's not a disease we're dealing with."

"What about the FDA? Those guys'd be interested."

112

"They don't seem to be. If so, they'd have done something by now to regulate the cosmetics industry."

"But you have a smoking gun. They can't ignore that."

"I'm afraid that's what they might well do. Or, more likely, bureaucracy being what it is, take so long to investigate, it'll be too late."

"Too late?"

"To influence the Senate committee in Washington."

"What else can you do?"

"Well, I met with that reporter I mentioned."

"And?"

"He's interested. In fact, he's already seen Patricia. Here at the hospital when she came for a check-up."

"He knows everything then?"

"No, he didn't actually speak to her but he visited her mother and learned where she is in Ireland. He asked me a lot of questions afterwards but I can't cross that line. It'd be unfair on Patricia. Best he finds out himself when he gets there. I told him about Ivan."

"So he's going over?"

"Seems so."

"So what do we do now?"

"Wait and see, I guess. Not much else we can do."

"Have you spoken to Patricia? It's important she knows."

"I've been trying, believe me, but no luck. Phone keeps ringing but no pick-up."

"Speaking of trying, do you think they'll try anything?"

"They?"

"Bellus."

"Like what?"

"Well..." there was hesitation in Jack's voice. "Knowing from the report where she is right now, they might... well... I don't know.... do something. Drastic. To keep it under wraps."

Gray shut his eyes tight, sensing a severe headache coming on. Jack was right. There was enough at stake, nothing could be ruled out. Not just millions of dollars in product investment by Bellus. But high-powered careers on the line as well. What might they do? How far would they go?

Chapter twenty-five

"I didn't see anything," Chris said, his voice an exasperated whisper as he glanced furtively around making sure nobody was within hearing distance. It was lunchtime and First and Second Avenues were chock-a-block with pedestrian traffic.

"Well, it was there for you to see," Clarke replied.

The two men were walking briskly along Constitution Avenue towards a broad building up ahead. Reaching it, they turned through a main door and into a large atrium. Sweeping legislative reorganization during the 1970s expanded Senate staff and stimulated construction of a third office building, named after Michigan Senator Philip A. Hart. But rather than adopt the neo-classical style of the first two office buildings, the architect gave the Hart Building a more distinctly contemporary appearance, with a marble façade in keeping with its surroundings. The nine-story structure is the largest of the three Senate buildings, so large it houses not only fifty senators but also three committees and several sub-committees. Clarke liked it because a two-story duplex suite meant most of his staff could work in connecting rooms, allowing a free-flow of information and enabling him to keep a tight rein on communications. He also liked the fact that it was designed for modern telecommunications. Removable floor panels permitted the laying of telephone lines and computer cables, which greatly aided him in rearranging his office over the years as computers rapidly altered staff functions.

Recognizing the two men, the uniformed guard inside smiled as they approached but thoroughly checked their IDs nonetheless before waving them through. Homeland Security had issued stiff regulations and it wanted them carried through to the letter. Lax follow-through was a firing offence.

In contrast to the other two Senate buildings, Russell and Dirksen, where offices ringed open courtyards, Hart featured a ninety-foot high central atrium with walkways bridging it on each floor. It also had sky-lit semi-circular staircases but the two men ignored these, crossing the atrium directly towards the elevator banks at the far end. They walked in silence, moving apart to circle around a small knot of visitors gazing up open-mouthed at the monumental Mountains and Clouds sculpture towering above them. Completed in 1986, Alexander Calder's superb work, combining painted black aluminum clouds suspended above similarly painted steel mountains, the tallest peak suspended fifty-one feet above, never failed to impress. Acknowledging how its sheer size and intricacy contributed greatly to enhancing the status of office-holders above in the eyes of both constituents and potential campaign donors, Senator Clarke - as had all Senators - designated it a must-stop on every introductory tour for selected constituents and fund-raisers.

"See what?" resumed Chris, stepping into the empty elevator behind the Senator, his exasperation increasing by the second. "I saw nothing."

"Exactly."

"I don't get it."

"It was a nothing event. Yet, they were all there."

"Who were?" Chris asked confused, pressing the elevator button for the seventh floor.

"His senior staff," replied Clarke as the doors closed with a swish. "They were all there. For what? Scent on the Hill? Please. A routine publicity stunt. A perfume-smelling freebie? There's a zillion things for them to be doing here in the inner sanctum of our nation's most important political institution other than that. Even during the quietest of times."

"But we were there too."

"We were there for a reason."

"Maybe they were there for that reason also."

"Exactly my point."

Chris looked at Clarke, his face a blank sheet.

"I don't get it," he said finally.

"They were there to see us."

"Why?"

"To find out if we know anything."

"About what?

"About what they know."

"But we don't know."

"Exactly, that's why it was good for us to be there."

"But we still don't know anything."

"But they don't know that."

Chris fell back against the wall of elevator trying to make sense of the riddle. "Let me get this right, boss. We don't know what they know but they don't know that we don't know?"

"Almost."

"Almost?" Chris almost yelped with frustration. "Ya gotta help me out here. You're driving me nuts."

Senator Clarke liked Chris. He was loyal and hardworking, his biggest strength being an insatiable hunger for detail, a gift that had helped him master the intricate labyrinths of Capitol Hill. Dealing with Washington's endless rules and regulations, the overwhelming minutiae of legislative reform, had caused many a politician before him to falter on the verge of greatness, especially those lacking an able public affairs assistant. It wasn't the first time walking these hallowed halls that Clarke had felt himself caught in a time-lock, not a member of the world's leading ultra-modern democracy but in some anachronistic institution, a throwback to the regal courts of an early seventeenth century France. But there was a downside to his assistant's gift for detail. He sometimes ended up missing the big picture. And while this could drive Clarke mad, he had learned that anger was a last resort, not a first-choice solution, and usually led to even greater confusion in the mind of his young protégé. He smiled paternally.

"They think we might know," he said gently. "That's why they think we were there."

"Know what?"

"I don't know."

"But if you don't know and I don't know, how does that help us." Chris looked bewildered.

"Because we can pretend we do."

"Huh."

"Then they'll get nervous." The Senator smiled confidently. "Then they'll make a mistake."

Chris looked even more bewildered.

"Then we'll know."

The two men stood side-by-side in silence for a moment as the elevator engine continued to hum. A tinny sound began as the button above the floor numbers blinked and the doors slid open. They stepped out on to a long corridor covered with thick carpet and as they turned to walk down it, Clarke stopped.

"We know as much as could possibly be known about the cosmetic lobby, about the chemicals in the products, about the FDA's lack of control, about those who are for us here and those who are against us, right? I mean we've been fighting this behemoth for an eternity."

"Tell me about it," exclaimed Chris. "I could write a book on it. In fact, maybe I will one day."

"That's why we need to shift our attention," said Clarke , ignoring his assistant's literary aspirations.

"Shift our attention?" Chris exclaimed." To what? Transport? War on terror? Balancing the budget?"

"Of course not, let others do that. Healthcare is our bailiwick. The single biggest issue on the domestic agenda right now and we helped put it there. It's manna from Heaven."

"I'm lost."

"Don't you see? We're looking in the wrong place."

"Wrong place?"

"Yes, why would they be so keen to come to see what we know if they already know what we know."

"Boss," Chris's voice had an edge of apprehension to it. "You're sending me in circles again. I'm gonna get dizzy and fall down this elevator shaft….. or I might just jump and be done with it."

Clarke ignored the idle threat. His mind was elsewhere.

"There must be something they're very worried about, something so big they sent out a posse of people to a silly event to check up on us." Chris knew Clarke long enough not to interrupt. His boss was thinking out loud, not talking to him, a thing he did often. Usually it had tangible results. He waited silently to find out what they'd be.

"We all know chemicals in the products are bad for us. We all know regulations are lax and need to be tightened. But what else could be so important that they want to keep it hidden? Something relatively new relating to chemicals in cosmetics. And big money."

"Taxes?" Chris piped up. "That idea making the rounds to adjust the corporate rate, to reduce fiscal relief for R&D activities?"

"Too general. Anyway, I'm not involved in that. It's got to be something to do with the products themselves. Content? But we already have a comprehensive hit list of rogue chemicals in most of them. Delivery avenues? Creams, lotions, sprays?"

Chris jerked upright, his eyes ablaze with excitement.

"I know, I know, I think I know," he blurted out exuberantly.

"You do?"

"Yes."

"What?"

"Nano," he said triumphantly.

"Nano?"

"Yes, nanoparticles. They've been used in other industries, textiles, steel, medicine – but now cosmetic companies are in on the act. They're small enough to go anywhere inside the body, even across the blood-brain barrier."

Clarke's brows knit, his expression encouraging him to go on.

"Cosmetic companies are putting a helluva lot of money into specialized research on them. They say they transport material inside the cells of the skin, helping keep it young and fresh. But some scientists and medical types are apprehensive. They say their efficacy is uncertain. That not enough tests have been done. Products are already on the market, much more to come."

Clarke's beaming smile was the kind of reaction Chris liked to see. Sensing what was coming next, he braced himself for the heavy arm flung over his shoulder.

"You know what to do, my boy. Now go do it."

There was nothing Chris liked better than a mission, a search for details. Before Clarke could say another word, he was bounding along the corridor, a racing greyhound out of a trap.

Left alone, the Senator stood wrapped in thought. He plucked out his cell phone, pressed a number and waited. "Doctor Tompkins please…"

Chapter twenty-six

"You asked me to call you if I had any information that might be of help."

The voice was strained, almost a whisper, muffled as if the owner's hand was cupped tightly over the speaker, so low Larry thought he could hear the rumble of conversation in the background. He recognized the voice immediately - the flat Midwestern tone unmistakable – so he slipped into his best collegiate tone. He didn't want this man backing out now, not at this critical moment, not with plans on several fronts well underway, didn't want him having second thoughts, believing it a Faustian agreement and telling his publisher everything just to recoup lost kudos. Larry had taken a risk, mainly on instinct, but he was under no delusions as to who'd be the fall guy if things came tumbling down around him.

"Good afternoon," he said, infusing his voice with cheeriness. "You must be feeling good today. I saw the Royals whipped the Cardinals in a double header at Kauffman last night. That'll teach 'em who's king of the I-70."

"Yes, I was there, a great night. We whipped their asses."

His simple ruse was working. He could almost feel the body of the man on the other end loosen up, his voice relax, safe on familiar territory, on a subject he remembered only too well from his visit that Pratt loved to wax lyrical about. He felt a surge of pity, seeing him for what he was - a petty man of selfish interests and limited vision. But he needed him right where he was.

"If the beer was Budweiser, the taste of victory must have been even sweeter, I'm sure," he said rhetorically, recalling that Anheuser-Busch was headquartered in St. Louis.

"You betcha," came the boisterous reply.

"Anyhow, my friend." Informalities over and time being money,

Larry's mind had turned to business. "Do you have anything for me?"

"Sure do. First of all, someone's been assigned to chase after your model. A reporter called Colm Heaney."

Larry sat up straight. "Really. When?"

"Few days ago."

"Who is he? What's he doing?"

"As I said, chasing the girl. He's the paper's medical corr. Got the green light to go to Ireland and search for her. Should be arriving soon."

Larry's hand clamped tighter on the phone. This piece of news complicated matters. A lot. But not wanting to come across as too worried in case it spooked his informant, he changed tact.

"Anything more on the doctor?"

"Yeah, did a bit of digging around here and found out something pretty interesting."

"What's that?"

"His only daughter died last year."

Larry was confounded. "Okay, so what?"

"From cancer, malignant melanoma."

None the wiser, Larry's patience began to fade fast. He disliked roundabout answers, except when it was he giving them. But for relationship sake he decided to wait a few minutes before ending the call.

"Related to sunscreen lotion."

Something in Larry stirred. An instinct, nothing more.

"Go on," he said, his tone changing.

"Gray believed she was killed by chemicals in the lotion. He sued the company."

"And?"

"Well, naturally, there was no way to prove such a crazy allegation so it was tossed out of court."

Pratt kept on rambling, but Larry barely registered what he was saying. He'd heard enough. He got off the phone quickly. He didn't want Pratt thinking the tidbit of news was more than ordinary. But he knew, without doubt, it was. If placed in the wrong hands, it was dynamite. Even more so if placed in the right ones.

He stared blankly ahead then hurried out of the special office he'd been given to work full-time on what he now called 'Project Patricia.' He sped along the corridor and up a flight of stairs, taking them two steps at a time. Striding confidently towards Covington's broad-windowed office directly in front of him, he ignored the protest from the pretty secretary sitting nearby. Such recklessness was something he'd normally not risk, but the bounce in his step mirrored his confidence, indeed his certainty, that the announcement he was about to make would thrill his boss no end.

This nugget of news with a smidgen of poetic license could undermine the doctor's credibility. The phrases came tripping off his tongue, luscious and tangy, like his favorite walnut ice-cream. *'Despondent father desperately seeking revenge,' 'twisted medical mind,' 'reckless with truth,' 'manic manipulation to achieve madcap ends.'* A bit over the top perhaps, but something he and a certain CEO he knew could work with and shape for their own ends. Yes, he thought, pushing open the thick glass door, this development is just too juicy to be told over the phone.

"We just hit pay-dirt," he said stepping boldly into the room, surprising Covington at his desk.

Chapter twenty-seven

"Please make sure your seat backs and tray tables are in their full upright position and your seat belt is correctly fastened. Also, we advise you that all electronic equipment must be turned off. Thank you."

It was still hard for Colm to believe he was sitting on the tarmac at JFK about to cross the Atlantic. Once officially installed as editor, McCarthy had lost no time in making his views felt, instilling a renewed sense of purpose in editorial staff to chase enterprising, potentially award-winning stories. And Colm's, he believed, was a classic. Even more, he'd told him yesterday in confidence, it could be a blueprint for what others could achieve. Already filled with trepidation about his journey back to Ireland after so many years, this made Colm even more anxious. Failure was not an option.

Making himself comfortable in his seat, he glanced at the three words scribbled on the cover of a thick file across his knee – 'The Forgotten County.' His Internet searches had revealed many quaint names for the strange place to which he was headed, both in Irish and English... *Tir Conaill,* 'Land of Conal,' one of the twelve sons of Niall of the Nine Hostage; *'Dún na nGall,'* Fort of the Foreigner….. but this one had captured his imagination more than the rest. He flipped open to the first page.

Tucked away among the mountains and the sea, northwest Donegal is a remote region cut off from the rest of the country by narrow ribbons of dizzying roads zigzagging across soggy marshes and lake-lined bogs. A place not easy to get to. Or to leave. And forgotten by most except those who live there.

Through a narrow gap between two leaning towers of jagged rock and you're bound for another world, leaving behind traffic lights, McDonald's, apartments, office high-rises, doorbells and elevators. And, to a great extent, people. It's bloody wonderful. And it's easy to tell when the real world ends and the surreal begins. As houses disappear, so does the road. Into a layer of mist, thicker than an Irish stew. Instead of everyday noise, there's an eerie silence. And a long, twisty, empty, bumpy, pebble-filled excuse of a path ahead daring you to continue into the unknown. Before you, a landscape stretches to the far horizon that resembles nothing less than the face of a distant planet as you might imagine it to be. Stunted clumps of purple and yellow heather flourish everywhere, the only vegetation capable of withstanding this alien climate and the smooth, bald silver slopes of the majestic Errigal Mountain in the distance, a reminder of scenes from 'Close Encounters of the Third Kind.' And the wind, everywhere yet rising from nowhere, howling banshee-like, bending marshy brown reeds backwards over huge, splintered granite rocks, millions of years old, dumped here since the dawn of time. That's the beauty of the place. It's ancient in every way.

Then you approach Glenveagh National Park, a gorgeous landscape that almost sings with the music of nature. Vibrant with deer, badger, thrush and lark, a refreshing waterfall that plummets down sheer cliffs and a romantic 19th century castle at the head of a lough bathed in colorful flower gardens. The only catch to arriving in 'The Forgotten County' is timing your arrival to the lifting of fog so you can see through the curtain to catch a glimpse of the darned thing. But it's well worth the wait.

Upon first reading it, Colm was left wondering. Was this from a travel book or a sci-fi novel? *The Forgotten County* – the phrase rolled around tantalizingly in his head, hinting at intrigue and dark secrets. Some of the very hallmarks he hoped might soon characterize his own story-to-be.

He skimmed through his notes, wondering why he had never visited this esoteric corner of his native country before. Maybe he too had forgotten it existed. He remembered going west, he obviously hadn't gone far enough. Celtic ancestry… Pagan rites… Rich mythology… pre-historic burial chambers… Dolmens… Superstitions… Fairy trees… home of the Gaeltacht… staunch Irish-speakers …dizzying, drop-dead scenery... labyrinth roads.

He smiled. His education in Belfast might just save him from wandering around in never-ending circles. His grasp of Gaeilge was precarious, but key phrases he could cobble together might help him over the worst - '*Tá mé caillte. Cá bhfuil an baile?* (I am lost. Where is home?) and '*An bhfuil uisce beatha agat?* (Do you have any whisky?).

He turned to another page. '*Thanks Be To God We're Not Made of Sugar.*' It was a headline he'd found too comical to ignore. Colm needed no reminder of Ireland's limitless capacity for rainfall – barbecues under cloudless skies in the Sunflower and Show-Me States were regular reminders of how little he missed the rarely-changing national weather forecasts of *'overcast skies and scattered showers'* aka *'pissing rain.'*

I had heard of Donegal's proclivity for wetness, the travel writer had penned. *But wasn't prepared for what I experienced. It only rained twice last week. First for three days, then for four. 'Thanks be to God we're not made of sugar,' one farmer said, telling me it had been so windy the week before, one of his chickens had laid the same egg twice.*

Colm was even more intrigued by his final destination, literally a dot on the map. *Bun na Leaca, or Brinaleck for Anglophiles, a clump of homes in the shadow of Bloody Foreland, a stark, heather-laden escarpment overlooking the broad Atlantic and a spray of rocky western islands dotting the coastline. It's old, and I mean old. Not old like ravens. Or old like Jesus Christ or Helen of Troy or Tutankhamen or Tyrannosaurus rex. Much older. Imagine 420 million years, and a great body of rock melting deep underground during a massive collision of continents, then Ice Age glaciers scouring out the whole area, cutting deep into the granite. A place with as many legends as there are twists in the road. But let me not spoil the surprise. Go there, see the place. Then try telling me if there's any place closer to Heaven you might want your withered bones to lie.*

A shiver ran down his spine. Either the writer was on something not normally prescribed, or winter gloom had overwhelmed his senses. He hoped summer would provide a warmer welcome for him, but then realized - summers in Ireland were just winters by a different name. He leaned back considering what challenges might lie up ahead. The weather would be the least of them.

***

Soft noises, then sudden movement. He opened his eyes. He was staring into a huge inkwell. He felt disoriented. His hands splayed out automatically seeking a hold on something, anything. He touched soft fabric either side. He gripped the material. Panic rose. What happened? His chest tightened. Beads of sweat prickled his skin. A feeling of helplessness fell over him, a heavy weight that seemed to squeeze energy out of him. He felt an overwhelming sense of weariness. More than anything, he wanted back to the place he had just been, a quiet, warm, cocooned place.

"Quick," a voice urged. "Wake up."

He tried desperately to find his bearings, but failed, the pit of blackness defeating him. A body beside him was moving with surprising agility. He felt it clamber across him, then scamper over other inert objects lying nearby.

"Christ, watch out," Harsh cursing, a string of expletives. The objects were moving, they were people.

"Let's go, let's go," someone ordered in hushed tones.

Bleary-eyed, he obeyed, not thinking. Struggling on to his elbows, he sensed others moving around him, rising wraith-like in the dark, drowning in their own muddled thoughts. A pair of piercing brown eyes fixed on his, mere inches from his face, anxiety writ large there. Fear gripped him. What was happening?

"Don't worry, I'm not the Devil, just a wee bit devilish." It was a woman's voice. And a pretty face with a warm smile center stage. It warmed him to see it. He opened his mouth to say something but wasn't given a chance. Lips were pressed gently against his.

"Don't talk. No time. Later." A whisper. Intimate. Encouraging. A light went on. He cupped his eyes to hide the blinding glare. "For Crissakes, turn that bloody thing out. They'll be on us before we've even started." The same woman's voice, but husky now, bold, inviting no protest. He felt breath warm on his cheek.

"C'mon Colm, you'll have to move. We don't have much time."

Just then, another banging sound. Silhouettes shifted around him in the gloom. One, two, three, four… they seemed to grow in number the more he watched. Rising from a maze of makeshift beds shoved randomly together, like one amorphous being. They started to get ready, their movements stiff, awkward, as if unfamiliar with the operation of their limbs. Men, women. Single, in pairs. Yawning, stretching, murmuring.

"Guys, you're like zombies," the woman's voice again. "What are we waiting for? Let's get out there, show 'em who we are, what we stand for." A pep talk. For what? Then, he knew, in an instant. His brain, hitherto a shrunken shadow, became a blazing bulb. Urgent knocking on his door at midnight. She standing in the drizzle, a hood covering much of her face, head bent, not wanting to be seen. Their hurried conversation. His glancing up, seeing the huddle of people across the street. Pilgrims for the cause. "Just until morning. Your folks'll never know. We won't leave a trace. Promise. There's nowhere else to go. It's safe. We're told the Brits have been ordered back to barracks. There'll be no house searches tonight. No street patrols." Him agreeing. Of course. How could he not?

He'd have agreed to anything. All she had to do was ask. Brave, outspoken, beautiful. Cat and coy. Those eyes, brown, mesmerizing. Like autumn leaves. Dark flowing ringlets, gypsy-like, break any man's heart, they would. She signaling. The huddle trooping across the street, weary, wet, wiped out, as if they'd just finished a long march, which maybe they had. Self-conscious, embarrassed by the late hour, they nodded their thanks awkwardly, each passing through the doorway in turn. Him pretending not to notice. Hard not to, solid shapes stretching the fabric of their coats, snub metallic noses sticking out below. He'd lived long enough in Belfast to have seen a few.

She knew her way around the house. He put the kettle on. Tea, Irish salve for every wound. Coats and weapons hidden carefully under the stairs. Within easy reach, just in case. Tension filled the air, a keg ready to blow. Had been that way for years. Newspaper headlines, radio commentators, television pundits, all predicting more violence to come. A bundle of Semtex and walls would come tumbling down, lives disappear, names carved in stone. Death at the door and they all rushing to embrace it, eyes half-closed. Not even dawn now and they were all downstairs. Someone had opened a side-door. Rifles, guns, coats passed from one hand to another. Colm went for his anorak. He felt a hand on his arm. "You're not involved." The tone wasn't stern. More a request than an order. He turned to look. Dark hair cascading over her shoulders, sharp eyes gazing into his. "Involved?" he shot back. "If we're not involved what are we then?"

She tweaked his cheek and smiled. "You know what I mean."

"I don't. You'll just have to stop and explain – in great detail as we go."

"Good try mo chuisle mo chroí, but alas no time, no time." Seeing a mix of disappointment and concern in his face, she added reassuringly, "When I get back. Promise. Cross my ..." She stopped abruptly, the phrase spilling out in silence.

"No way," he replied. "I'm not letting you go out there. Not alone."

Her eyes shone, a hint of cheeky humor there. "Remember?" She nodded around the room. "I've got plenty of company. We're Belfast C company." As if in support, a communal shuffling began around them, a last snap and pull of buttons and belts, a tying of shoelaces.

"Anyway, you're not authorized. No reporters allowed. OC's orders. Don't want publicity. Not yet anyway." She spoke gently, but it still irked him. He felt like a scolded child. Before he could respond, she added. "Anyhow, you're way better with a pen than a gun, and I'll need a nice cuppa when I get back. And an even nicer hug to go with it." She put her arms around him, kissed him warmly on the lips, lingering there, then buried her face in the pocket of space between his neck and shoulder, letting out a sigh of contentment as if finding something there she had long searched for.

Just then a door opened. In a flash they were gone, rabbits out of a hole. Or into one? He wasn't quite sure. Left there alone, they disappearing round a corner, close together, one behind the other, he wondered. Involved? Should he be? What did it mean anyway? He gazed up, watching the day wake from its slumber. A tantalizing smear of crimson, as if from an artist's palette, enlightened the bluish-grey sky. A nice morning lay in store though a chill still lingered. It clung to his bones, making him shiver. He turned to go inside. Suddenly, an almighty explosion ripped through the air. His body shuddered.

***

The shuddering continued, shaking him ever more strongly. He felt himself falling sideways. Then, oddly, into his senses wafted a smell, a bittersweet smell. His eyes were closed, lids heavy. He prized them open. A pretty stewardess, her dark hair caught up in a bun, stood over him, coffee jug in hand. Then he realized. He'd dreamed the dream again. He ran his tongue over his lips. Could almost feel the moist of her parting kiss but knew it could never be. The knowing burnt a hole in his heart.

Chapter twenty-eight

"Any problems getting those documents?"

"No, the operation was as smooth as cream pie."

"So? Tell me."

For the first time in all the conversations he'd had with Covington, Larry didn't feel intimidated, even seated as he was in his boss's teak-paneled office. In fact, he wore an air of confidence. Not about the final outcome. Not at all. There were too many variables, but certainly in this little tête-à-tête he was king. The way the man opposite leaned that bit closer across the table towards him - not enough as to seem conspiratorial – but ample proof of heightened interest, even a sense of reliance. Basking in this newfound power for a tad longer was too rich to deny himself. Larry lingered a few seconds before answering.

"It's not pretty…" he said finally, watching Covington's eyes snap open with concern.

"…in fact, may be worse than expected," he added for good measure.

"How?" Covington began massaging his temple.

Larry pulled the string tighter.

"The test results on Patricia. The doctor completed them. They don't look good…"

For emphasis, he rested his gaze on the chocolate brown file lying on the table between them.

"…verified by several labs, ones with gold-plated reputations."

Silence. That was good. Might be easier to sell him on his ideas. But first he needed to know more. Covington was eyeing him warily, stretching out his hand to draw the file towards him. Then seemed to have second thoughts and stopped. Larry took his chance.

"I hope you don't mind me asking," he began. "But as I'm involved in trying to fix this, I suppose I should know as much as possible about it."

No response. He interpreted this as an invitation to continue. "If this product is dangerous, why not just discontinue it?"

"Dangerous?"

"Well, you know. These tests. They seem to show big problems."

"Big problems?"

Larry felt a wave of uneasiness. Had he gone too far? He wasn't a manager in the company – not yet anyhow. Rather than risk, he stayed silent.

"Eating oranges makes some people come out in rashes, peanuts can shut down a person's entire immune system, kill them in a matter of minutes," Covington said. "Does that mean we should ban them?"

Larry didn't answer.

"They can't be absolutely sure what caused her black-outs," Covington continued. "Could have been a thousand other things, including what she had for breakfast that day."

Larry felt emboldened. "Hardly, I mean, the evidence..." he pointed to the file. "It's all there, at least it seems to be."

"Seems is not quite the same as is, is it?" Covington growled, glaring at him. "And it's not a bloody vaccine that requires FDA permission for human clinical trials either, eh?"

With his tone turning accusatory, Larry sensed a swift dose of diplomacy was in order. "I understand, but would it not be better to withdraw the product? Do more tests just to be safe. After all she's the only person who's been using the product regularly, right?"

"And risk losing a fortune as our stock hit the floor?"

Larry pushed on. "Right, but if the FDA guys see this stuff..."

Covington cut him off with a sharp wave of his hand.

"Enough." His voice rose with impatience. "Is the whole report here?"

Larry nodded, feeling a tang of bitterness at being so chastised. "Everything we managed to snatch from his office."

"I'll read it later."

Much as he loathed being the bearer of bad news, especially in a situation as sensitive as this, Larry had no option. What he knew was important. Maybe the most crucial piece of information he had to give. "They've got the product..."

Tiny muscles around Covington's mouth grew taut.

"...but I don't know where they're hiding it. We..."

Covington didn't speak but color drained from his face. Larry had never seen his boss so bereft of words. The change in him was startling.

Then, as if aware of the impression he was giving, Covington cut in.

"What about this editor?" he said, quickly changing the subject. "Did he say much?"

Larry responded just as quickly, eager to move on to better news, safer ground. "Plenty. Not much persuasion needed. A small advance payment. For services rendered, was how he put it. And a coupla Jack Daniels and a T-bone, rare. With a mountain of peppercorn sauce. Hereford House. A Kansas City eating house, the kind ya might read about in a Wild West novel. I half expected a stage-coach to pull up outside."

His attempt at humor failed. Covington's impatience with trivialities was writ large on his face.

"Not reluctant then I take it?"

"Not at all. A loss of status thing with him. Being demoted doesn't suit him. He badly wants his broad butt back in the plush seats at Arrowhead stadium."

"Big sports fan, eh?"

"Not just, big ego to match."

"So? What'd you learn?"

"A lot. Here's what we're dealing with. A reporter is tracking our girl. Colm Heaney. Young, ambitious, emigrant Irish. The new editor sent him, fella by the name of McCarthy. Ink in his veins, father a printer. Browne is the group publisher, based in New York. He moved Pratt out of the top seat. Like everyone in the newspaper industry, he's counting dwindling pennies, watching helpless as digital grows ever larger."

"Mmmm. Anything else worthwhile?"

"Worthwhile? More like invaluable," Larry said with gusto, knowing full well the importance of what he'd just found out.

"We've hit the bulls-eye. Got the name of the place where our lady friend's hiding out. In the backwoods of Ireland of all places. No family link to the reporter, we don't think, though a helluva coincidence."

Larry saw Covington's face relax, pleased they'd found her.

"And in return?"

"His old job back."

"That's it?"

"Yep, plain and simple. He wants us to do a hatchet job - on McCarthy and the reporter."

"I hope you didn't promise something you can't deliver."

"No, though I did hint it might be possible."

Covington's eyes narrowed with suspicion.

"I had to offer him some kind of incentive," Larry said, part apology, part defiance. "Money won't be enough."

"You're making me nervous. If he expects that and we don't deliver, we could be in even worse trouble, regardless of whether it was a promise or a hint of a promise. In his eyes, there's no difference. And if he's pissed off enough to speak out…"

"I've thought about that…"

"Have you any idea what's at stake here?" Covington said, pushing forward, scraping his chair on the floor noisily as he did so. "This is not just about a single product going to market. We've invested big in this, years in the making. If things go smoothly, we're talking major league, a big score in the last quarter that puts us in the play-offs. A public stock offering would bring in hundreds of millions. With investment funds lush and looking, they'll rush to us, arms outstretched. In no time we could be building new manufacturing plants, expanding product line, strengthening exports. If we win this race, we'd send shockwaves through the nanoworld."

He paused, fixing Larry with an unwavering gaze.

"But if things go pear-shaped because of this whacky doctor and his personal crusade, we could lose so big we could be out of business altogether. Bullish or not, investment funds'll be quick to distance themselves from any kind of adverse publicity. We can't allow anything - and I mean anything - to go wrong. Da'ya hear me?"

"Of course I do," Larry replied, feigning insult. "Why do you think I've put so much effort into this? Everything else in my life's on hold." He stopped then, a smile ripe with self-satisfaction escaping from his lips. "I've a couple of ideas I think'll work. Call them Plan A and Plan B. But with so much at stake, I think we should put both into action at the same time."

"I'm listening."

"Plan A involves you."

A dark cloud fell over Covington's face. "They should all involve me. I don't want anything that doesn't. Is that clear?"

"Of course," Larry's said defensively. "Rather than involvement, let's just call it your direct participation."

"Go on."

"Brown, as I mentioned, is counting pennies."

"So?"

Larry opened his mouth to explain but seeing a gleam of understanding in Covington's eyes, knew there was no need.

"Okay, okay, what's plan B then."

Larry bent over and lifted his briefcase off the ground. Opening it, he pulled out several glossy magazines, fanning them across the table.

"What's this?" Covington said, reading out the titles with barely concealed derision. "*Celebrity Watch. Inside Scoop. Revelations.*"

"Tabloids, supermarket trash yes, but read by millions," Larry replied, watching his boss flick through pages randomly.

"With news and entertainment inseparable these days, they're the only side of print media that's not dropping like a rock in a pond," he added.

"Stop beating about the bush. You've two minutes to make your point."

"There are highly-prized news tidbits in there," Larry said, waving his hand at the magazines. "Enough to start a coast-to-coast media circus. If the right thing is dropped in the right place, that is."

"So what?"

"So, if you can't deal with the truth, deal with the witnesses."

"You've got one minute."

Chapter twenty-nine

"Seemingly she was vivacious."

"Hard to believe, looking at her. Lying there, lost to the world. Poor soul. The spark's gone clean out of her."

"And so beautiful. Staff nurse Gilmore showed me the photos in a magazine. Most women'd die to have half the looks she had."

"So much ahead of her. Fashion shows. TV. Maybe even Hollywood."

"Yeah, a terrible shame. I mean, I know it's a shocking thing to say, but I wonder what she'd think if she could see herself now. I mean would she say, 'Let me go, please, just let me go.'

"Too young even to think of a living will."

"Worse on the father. Lost his wife a few years back, and now this. Here almost every day, just sits there at the edge of the bed. Staring at her. But mostly just into space. Sometimes I wonder who's more lost, he or she? It'd break your heart, it would. I pop in regular like and ask if he wants a cup of coffee and a cookie, but really…"

The nurse broke off and leaned over to move a loose strand of hair that had fallen across the inert woman's closed eyes.

"I know what you mean," the other said. "Not one life ruined but two. I hear he has to travel about a hundred miles here and back. Must be so lonely in that car."

"I've never seen him cry, though I thought I heard him sobbing once," the older nurse said, wiping the patient's hands gently with a damp hand-cloth.

"Probably all cried out," the younger one replied, gazing at the pallid face on the pillow.

"She was an only child. Spitting image of the mother I'm told. Must be doubly bad for him when he sees her looking so peaceful. Morbid thought but must make him think of his dead wife in her coffin."

"Has she shown any signs at all?"

"Not since I took over duty four weeks ago. Very low on the Glasgow Scale. Though Nurse Crossan told me one time after she'd gone out of the room to check on sanitary supplies she'd heard a moan. Rushed back and could have sworn her head had moved. Said it had been facing the wall but when she came back it was turned to the window, where the sun rises. Thought there was the beginnings of smile on her face. Spooked her big time. Ran out of the room right quick. Dragged the duty doc down here right away."

"And?"

"Nothing, no change, same old. Doc said she must have imagined it."

"They'll have to make a decision sometime."

"They say it's not likely she'll improve. But it takes ages to get through the courts. Terrible burden on the father."

"Starving someone to death. Shocking."

"They'll have to disconnect the ventilator first. Then maybe the IVs."

"Same thing, isn't it, whatever button you press."

"Suppose so. But who wants to play God?"

"Better settled one way or the other. Minimally conscious? Vegetative state? Is there a difference, really?"

"Was a woman back in Missouri, read about the case in nursing school. Car accident. Head trauma. Just like this. Was in a coma for years. Family had to go all the way to the Supreme Court to disconnect the tubes. Father committed suicide later, emotional exhaustion."

"I heard there's something else going on here, all the same."

"Really? What?"

"I'm told there were a lot of white coats in here at the beginning. Took a lot of samples. Hair, facial skin swabs, tear ducts."

"What was that all about?"

"Haven't a clue, but the girls say it was more than just head injury treatment."

"That's real peculiar."

"Yeah. Did the whole lot. EEG, CT, MRI. And a lumbar for cerebrospinal fluid, looking for water on the brain. Seems they couldn't make up their minds what it was. Encephalitis, meningitis, hydrocephalus. Even checked for West Nile and St. Louis."

"All sounds a bit bizarre."

"Anyhow, my dear, none of that's our concern right now. Let's you and I give this nice lady's hair a good brush and put some make-up on her. Her father'll be here in an hour. She may not be as beautiful as before but at least we can make her look presentable for him."

The younger nurse nodded in agreement. She took a last long look at the inert woman on the bed, crisp white sheets pulled up around her neck. They were both about the same age. The thought saddened her. In a couple of hours, she'd be at The Merry Go-Round, downing tequila shots and dancing to Madonna and Britney Spears.

And Christine here wouldn't have moved a single solitary inch.

Chapter thirty

All hands on deck. He'd been preaching the mantra a lot recently.

That's why Browne agreed to the meeting. Under normal circumstances, he'd have told his group sales manager to deal with it, a new client wanting a network ad deal. But in the current financial situation he couldn't ask others to do what he wasn't prepared to do so himself. It was national, after all, and the numbers relayed to him were big. The message was that the man would only speak to him.

With declining financials and multi-million dollar bonds due for maturity soon, investors holding them were beginning to howl at the door like hungry wolves. If he couldn't boast new revenue, they'd take even greater control and extract new terms. And that would be the very window through which Kemp might clamber to claim the throne and kick-start the break-up of the media kingdom Browne had created so diligently over the years.

Instinct told Browne there was more to this mysterious caller than simply a national contract. After all, it was the company's CEO who wanted to meet him.

'...*to discuss a major advertising arrangement*,' was exactly how his own secretary had put it after taking the call from her counterpart earlier.

Browne found the word '*arrangement*' intriguing. And disconcerting. If there was the possibility of muddied waters, and he sensed there might be, he'd best deal with it than learn about it second-hand from a subordinate. That's how mess happened and mess was the last thing he needed right now. Image was a key ingredient as stock merchants on the Street were well aware. Like sniffer-dogs, they were trained to smell problems, so avoiding unsavory odors, no matter how slight, was paramount. One falter would add more fuel to the fire of Kemp's rising ambitions. In fact, his nemesis might be the shadow behind this mystery.

He needed to be on his guard.

With meeting time at hand, Browne's curiosity had risen exponentially. He'd talked with every industry insider he knew. What he'd found out about the company created an emotion in him he was not particularly proud of – envy - that particular brand one struggling CEO feels towards another, more successful one, a feeling exacerbated by the belief that the other's success wasn't related to experience, quality of leadership or strategic management ability, not even to that quirky element business textbooks refer to as 'emotional intelligence.' Bellus - and by extension, Dick Covington, the man he was about to meet - was doing particularly well because the whole sector was doing particularly well.

And therein lay the reason for Browne's rising curiosity. Riding a market wave, Covington nor Bellus needed favors from the struggling print media. It just didn't make sense.

Time for Browne to think more about it had run out and if truth be known, he was glad. He was getting tired lately of thinking so much about the 'what-ifs' of life.

Hearing his secretary in the outer room taking the call from reception that his guest had arrived, he tidied up the sales account sheets on his desk. Crunching numbers mid-afternoon could give the wrong impression. Anyway, an untidy desk made for an unorganized mind, and he sensed he'd need his to be crystal clear.

***

It was his guest's blunt statement, '*I believe we can be of mutual benefit,*' midway through their meeting, that indicated the real reason they were seated opposite each other.

Until then, Covington, suave and silk-suited, his shoulders broad and muscular indicating he might have been a running back in earlier years, had meandered this way and that amiably enough but with no fixed purpose. Sitting over leisurely afternoon coffee, they'd remained on safe ground – macro-stuff: inflation, the federal budget, the yawning deficit, international exchange rates, the nation's declining competitive advantages. The sort of chit-chat high-level executives meeting for the first time often feel obliged to mull over in an ambling sort of way to proclaim their worldliness before getting down and dirty and talk about what they really want to talk about – defining their business relations to achieve that at all-important symbol of mutual benefit – profit.

Of course, as expected, their conversation was sensibly devoid of politics, nothing being more likely to scupper ambitions and create acrimony than a slip of the tongue on this most sacrosanct of subjects, the one topic, next to religion, most likely to bring the whole house toppling down.

While neither of these sacred grounds was violated, another was. One even more sensitive; one that presented him with perhaps the toughest decision of his entire career. Media ethics.

Thirty minutes into the conversation, with healthy almost dizzying, ad buy figures mentioned, Browne was poised to have his national sales manager march right in, blank contract in hand and for the three of them to down a glass, nay a bottle, of vintage Dom Perignon kept in his cabinet for just such auspicious occasions. Forty-five minutes in, his mind was in such a swirl, this was the last thing he wanted to do.

The strategy adopted by his guest was a deft one that shifted the conversation from the macro to the micro – to the world of cosmetics.

"We're a fast-growing sector," he began. "There's barely been a downturn in the market in decades. New products constantly coming on-line keeping things fresh. Consumer demand never seems to waver."

As he listened to the flow of impressive statistics, Browne couldn't help but think of his own sector, about how his guest's air of confidence matched his own in the heyday of print media. With that thought, professional envy poked out its beaked nose and a mood of mild despondency settled about him, a mood exacerbated by his guest proceeding to wax lyrical about why his industry was so important.

"We're one of the biggest contributors to national GDP, not to mention an extremely important source of tax revenues. We also account for one of the highest percentages of overall exports."

At this point, Browne was struck by a revelation that eased him out of the fog of despondency enveloping him. His guest was sounding like a salesman ready to pitch, but he had no idea what bag of goods he was being sold. The thought - emerging more from instinct than reason - made him feel stronger. It was as if the tables had turned and he was the leader of a thriving, profitable company whose expansion plans knew no limits and his guest was the one who had fallen on hard times and had come seeking succor. As he bathed in this rather incongruous thought, his guest began talking about the multifaceted benefits his company bestowed upon society.

"We support a wide range of civic programs, especially in the area of mother and child healthcare but also in the environmental and education fields."

At this juncture, it crossed Browne's mind that his guest, believing, with some justification, the media to be liberal in its outlook and that he'd also somehow found out he himself had entered the profession through the editorial portal before migrating to the dollars and cents side of the business, was appealing to that particular sentiment as part of his build-up. A build-up to what Browne sensed was a more demanding request than simply supporting a civic venture. But what?

"With all this in mind," his guest continued. "It would be most discouraging for such a fine record to be stymied in any way... for expansion plans at Bellus in particular and the cosmetic sector in general to be hindered in any unfair manner..."

"...just when the industry is about to embark on one of the most exciting periods in its entire history, utilizing the latest in nano technology...and just when Leland Newspapers could be... a key place for promotion of our company's rapidly developing products - if things go unhindered by unnecessary, and unjustified, media interference."

Browne's initial reaction was to raise his hands in the air and admit ignorance. While he was kept well-informed of controversial stories in the group's publications, expensive lawsuits being something he was keen to avoid, Bellus's name had never come up. But then again he couldn't know every single one of them and maybe this one was pending.

"I'm not sure what you mean but believe me..." he began, his tone neutral.

Covington leaned forward in his seat. "Forgive me, I don't mean to mislead you. It's not something you've already done...." then he paused as if choosing his words carefully. "It's something you might do.... and might regret later."

Browne wasn't quite sure if this was meant as a threat, or simply sage advice. Not knowing, he remained quiet.

"There is a certain story one of your Midwestern newspapers is working on," Covington continued. "It's one without merit and I'd appreciate if you would... well, deal with the matter. In a fair manner, of course."

Browne had worn enough masks in his professional life to disguise his initial reactions to his guest's remarks. But remaining impassive now face-to-face was becoming increasingly more difficult. Thankfully, Covington's gaze moved from him to a slim file he had brought with him. Opening it, he took out several sheets of paper and slipped them across the table.

"These should be more than enough to ease your mind about the ethical nature of the request I am making," he said. "I don't think any responsible newspaper would base a story on what these two characters say, unless their editorial goal is merely to titillate readers. I think you and your colleagues have worked too hard to earn the respect you have to be remotely interested in that kind of thing."

Puzzled, Browne took the documents and glanced through them. One was a legal brief, a bizarre case of someone suing a cosmetic company for a lot of money over a suntan lotion. The second was a photocopy of a short article from a celebrity magazine, about a catwalk queen at an after-hours party crashing her car against a tree. An accompanying photo showing her with other revelers at a table on which a thin, chalk-white line of what seemed clearly to be cocaine was encircled.

"I understand it's a difficult call and you need to talk to your editor in Kansas City," his guest said as he finished reading. "But please keep in mind what's at stake. For everyone."

Browne let the comment ride. Instead, he said, "I'm confused. What exactly is the issue here and why is it so important?"

The response was a classic lesson in avoidance. "I don't want to show bias here so maybe its best you hear about it directly from your editor. But let me assure you, it will only give credence to persons who obviously don't deserve it." He pointed to the documents. "You can see for yourself. Two dubious characters at best."

Browne persisted. "But what has this to with new nano technology you mentioned?"

His guest seemed to consider an explanation. Instead, he said, "It's complicated science, it would take us hours to discuss."

His answer made Browne more suspicious than ever. "Okay, let me ask you this then. Do you intend to launch such a product soon?"

Browne's directness was met in equal measure by Covington's evasiveness. "Believe me, there's nothing more I'd like to talk about, but as you know, new products are the lifeblood of any company. That's all I can say at the moment."

"I see."

With that, his guest rose as if to leave. "It has been a pleasure to meet with you. Thank you for your time. I'd appreciate if our discussion remains confidential. All will be revealed, I promise. I will make sure your reporters are the first to receive information and I'll make sure my guys are available to answer any questions they might have."

Then, infusing his words with a show of corporate camaraderie, he added, "We all have tough decisions to make. It's unavoidable, part and parcel of the unfortunate financial times we find ourselves in right now. But I do emphasize, I'd like to work very closely with you and I think my colleagues in the cosmetic industry would also. You can be sure I'll do my very best to encourage them through our association."

Browne was smiling graciously as his guest disappeared behind the elevator doors, but as he returned to his office his mind was spinning. Such a peculiar meeting but what was he to make of it?

***

He needed to talk to Kansas City quickly but before doing so he ran over in his head the pros and cons of his visitor's offer - the damage, the gain, the maybes, the what-ifs. Sitting down at his computer, he accessed monthly P&L figures and calculated year-end predictions. Wasn't it just yesterday, and the day before, and the day before that, he'd done the very same thing? With disturbing results. This time, however, he added in Covington's number. Then he clicked on the review button. And waited while the computer re-configured.

A few seconds later he sat back. And marveled. He knew it'd make a big difference but seeing the numerical picture before him was truly uplifting. It was as if he'd waved a magic wand in front of the screen. Like seeing three plums come up on a Las Vegas slot machine. To verify further, he reverted to graphics software and watched bar charts transform under the new inputs, black ones shooting upwards like miniature skyscrapers, red ones shrinking to low-rise apartments. And that was without taking into account ad deals other cosmetic companies Covington indicated might sign up.

The sweet taste of success lingered. Succulent images swept through him. Of Kemp at the next board meeting, as taunting and unflappable as ever, reading the end-of-year financials, his face crumpling into a ball of paper. Of *The Kansas City Guardian*'s upcoming centennial celebrations. Of the congratulations he'd receive, the tinkling of champagne glasses preceding his keynote speech, the swell of applause that would follow his triumphant presentation.

And all he had to do to turn fanciful notions into simple reality was make a single long-distance telephone call. He stretched out his hand.

Chapter thirty-one

McCarthy couldn't believe his ears. He tried to interject but couldn't make himself heard over the words rushing at him from the other end of the line. Becoming more frustrated by the minute, he came close to slamming down the phone and ending the conversation pronto. But wisdom told that was the worst thing he could have done. Few in their right minds do that to their bosses and continue picking up a paycheck.

He'd been standing in the middle of the newsroom talking to the picture desk editor about illustrations for a full-length feature on city re-zoning when his assistant tapped him on the shoulder and whispered he had an urgent call from New York. He didn't need to be told who it was.

He hadn't spoken to Browne since they'd discussed Colm's story idea. That conversation had ended upbeat, his publisher's tone being as close to excited as McCarthy had ever heard it. "That's perfect, just the kind of thing I was hoping for," he'd said then. "It'll rouse the troops to find better stories. Better stories means more readers. More readers means more advertising. They'll feed off each other. The greater the budget, the more enterprising stories we can do."

To say McCarthy was pleased by his words was a severe understatement.

But now this. How could things have changed so quickly, and why?

It wasn't that Browne was angry at anything in particular. His voice, while assertive, was calm, controlled, a tone that made it even more difficult for McCarthy to accept his words: "....take Heaney off the assignment."

By the time McCarthy managed to get a word in, he was seething inside, but calmed himself sufficiently to respond somewhat diplomatically. "He's only just arrived over there and now you're telling me you might recall him? Because of a change in policy? What policy?

What change? I don't understand."

McCarthy listened for a few minutes until he reached the limit of his patience. "I'm quite aware the unfortunate financial difficulties the company's facing, the whole industry's in the same boat," he said, his voice restrained. "What I don't understand is what that has got to do with Colm being in Ireland, unless you mean the expenses of sending him there. It's very little and we already discussed it and you agreed. In fact, you more than agreed, you were very enthusiastic. Only then did I give the reporter the go-ahead..."

He was forced to listen again as Browne interrupted. "Potential lawsuit?" McCarthy looked down the earpiece of the phone incredulously as if he'd find an answer hiding there. "For what? We don't even have a story yet so how could we possibly be sued? And by whom?"

Again the other voice took over.

"I've never even heard of this company. And I'm sure Colm doesn't know either otherwise he'd have mentioned it to me. Anyway, isn't the whole idea not to shy away from sensitive stories as we've been doing? I thought we'd decided to go at it full-force, find stronger stories to revive our brand. Reclaim some of our former glory and prestige. You said that was important to get into the international digital media consortium. That's why we met. That's why I took the job. That's why I've made all the staff changes I've made around here."

The conversation went on for another five minutes. McCarthy wanted it to go on longer. He had a lot to say and even more to find out. But Browne said he had an important business meeting.

"Look Richard, from where you're sitting, this may seem simple," McCarthy said. "But it's not. I can order the reporter back. Sure, that's easy. We can change his airline ticket within the hour. That's easy also. What's not easy, however, is guaranteeing he'll be on that plane."

He stopped as Browne spoke into the phone, then continued.

"I may be his editor but knowing him as I do, I can almost guarantee he'll not agree," he said. "And that'd leave us in a quandary. If Colm finds the woman and gets the exclusive - and if anyone can, it'll be him – and we refuse to publish, he might go to another newspaper or magazine, and to hell with the consequences. He's hot-headed that way. He'll find a job elsewhere. In fact, this story will probably help him find a better one than the one he has right here. So, we'll lose twice - a very good story and a very good reporter. And when word leaks out, which it will, we'll be back to square one, or worse. With egg on our faces."

A few minutes later, the call over, McCarthy rammed the phone down. Leaning back in his chair, he raised his eyes to the ceiling and ran his hands slowly through his thick mop of hair. Then he banged his fist down on the desk, so hard the metal in-tray bounced in the air and fell off the edge, sending sheets of documents floating like so many square snowflakes in a wide arc across the floor. Stunned by the noise, his young assistant outside the glass-paneled office almost fell out of her chair. Catching her breath, she shot a glance at him nervously. Seeing the look of apprehension on her face, he shook his hand peremptorily, "I'm fine, I'm fine," he said brusquely.

Standing up quickly, he began marching slowly around the room, trying to rein in his thoughts. Then he began randomly gathering up the documents scattered all over the floor. That's when he noticed it. His eyes narrowed with interest. Picking it up, he brought it to his desk and sat down.

Embarrassed by her own reaction earlier, the assistant had turned sheepishly back to her computer screen. A few minutes later, however, the sudden stillness in her boss's office made it impossible to concentrate. She glanced up again. The metal tray that had crashed remained upside down on the floor, its contents still scattered about. But her boss now sat motionless in his chair seemingly oblivious to the mess. She wondered what was going on, but couldn't even see his face to form an impression. It was hidden behind a document he held tightly in his hands.

Chapter thirty-two

Browne was pleased his conversation with McCarthy had gone as planned. Now all he needed was to get the ad contract signed.

But something niggled at him. Sitting at his desk mulling over the situation, his gaze drifted around the office settling upon the porcelain cups behind the glass case. 19th century, gilded in gold leaf, custom-made to commemorate the first official commercial printing press in the United States. Funny, he never used them. For vanity sake mainly, reminding him – and others - of the status he'd acquired after years in the newspaper industry.

His eyes moved from the glass case, slowly surveying the rest of the office, as if meaning lingered among the furniture. In one corner stood the walnut Aubusson Louis Seize writing desk, reportedly used by Benjamin Franklin in completing his autobiography. On the wall opposite, his favorite watercolor - naturally – his wife's work, painted during a vacation in Hawaii paid by the company for exceeding sales targets. It showed a boat gliding on azure-blue waters, its sails unfurled, two slim figures on deck manning the ropes. Meant to be metaphorical, she'd said, depicting their future together after he retired. *'Exploring the world'* was how she'd described it. He smiled, remembering her words, but his smile slowly faded. Work hadn't left much time for exploring anything.

His gaze moved on. To the trophy shelves at the far end of the room. Polished to a shine under the strict supervision of 'Field Marshall' Martha, they marked his meteoric rise within the industry. Titles launched, circulation figures reached. Admiring their elegant designs, Browne's eyes rested upon a framed photograph with a small, velvet case beside it, an incongruous item among all the silverware. He ambled over for a closer look.

The face of a young man, an awkward smile upon his lips, looked up at him, a black mortarboard askew on his head barely defying gravity. Draped in a flowing gown falling just above well-polished shoes, the figure clutched a rolled parchment in one hand, an even more slender item in the other, holding them both high, the latter thrust forward as if worried the camera might not capture the metallic-looking object clearly enough. Leaning over, Browne lifted the velvet box and opened it. An ornate pen nestled inside sent Browne's mind wheeling back through time. He could almost feel the muscles in his right hand tighten as he remembered the familiar feel of it between finger and thumb.

Columbia Journalism School. Class of '60, though the word 'class' was, he recollected, a most inappropriate term. If truth be known, he'd spent hardly any little time in classrooms, preferring the hubbub of the college newspaper office than boring tutorials on the theory of communications. Nights spent stretched across a typewriter catching forty winks during tight weekly deadlines were too many to remember. While barely managing academically, he was deliriously happy when selected news editor of the *Columbia Daily Spectator* as a junior, a rare occurrence in the paper's illustrious history. Those were the days. Of civil rights and Martin Luther King and Nixon and Watergate and Deep Throat.

That experience had launched his career - a trainee post on a weekly in Vermont, the latest acquisition for the Leland Group; then a general assignment position at a small daily in New Hampshire. By 29, he was news editor; by 32, in the editor's chair. Then the call came. The Group was experiencing exponential growth. Hadn't enough trusted managers to put into the business side of things at HQ. How would he like to move to New York, from the practice of journalism to the practice of publishing? Strange. Up until then, he'd thought they were one and the same. He'd learned quickly they weren't. That's when counting stories began to count for less than counting money. And there was lots of it. The newspaper industry was booming and Leland was in rapacious take-over mode. Moving up the corporate ladder was smooth, from weeklies to dailies, with *The Kansas City Guardian* being cream on his already-rich cake. Profits soared as *The Guardian's* circulation doubled in just three years.

That's how he ended up in an office overlooking Central Park with porcelain cups and a row of silverware, not to mention a house in the Hamptons. Journalism didn't get him here. Publishing did.

Had he ever looked back? Regretted '*his move across the newsroom floor*? Sometimes, but not often. More so recently. Could he have become the next Carl Bernstein? Who knows? Too late now to even consider.

He lifted the pen from the box. Graduation day. He'd left the conferring ceremony quickly, hurrying across campus to have a last lingering look around the newsroom he'd probably never see again. It was dark and empty, all lights out. That left him with a hollow feeling. He didn't want to remember it that way. It had always been a place ringing with voices. Ideas and ideals sweeping around like flocks of birds in noisy flight. He remembered regretting coming over and was turning to leave when they'd all popped out. From all corners, all his colleagues, all shouting his name, all regaling him, mocking him for being so easily fooled, an editor caught off-guard on his own turf, they taunted. That's when they'd presented him with the pen. He held it up to the light now and read the inscription though he knew it off by heart, *'Keep writing. We'll see you at the top.'* Yes, he probably would have made it there.

Thinking of newsrooms made him think of McCarthy. A younger version of what he'd been, maybe the reason he'd chosen him. And now? Was he corrupting the man? For a moment he felt dismayed, then he reminded himself. He was a publisher now. His job one of saving jobs, not saving stories. There would always be more stories. There may not be more money. The offer was just too good to turn down.

Chapter thirty-three

Colm stood still, the saltiness of the night air biting on his tongue, his car keys gathered loosely in his hand. A thousand stars winked down at him, a dizzying pattern of sparkling gems spread across the firmament. He couldn't remember the sky ever being so alive with light, urban America's endless neons having eclipsed nature's electrical system.

He was tired. It had been a long, four-hour drive here with so many twists and turns he'd wondered if he was simply going in ever-widening circles.

He'd passed the town of Letterkenny, only pale penumbra from scattered shopfronts indicating a few souls might still be awake, then down a steep road to Kilmacrennan. That's near where he'd made a sharp left turn, beyond a sign saying '*Doon Well,*' a Pagan place of worship he'd read about, and towards Glenveagh, a wide expanse of raw, national park. That's when the standard elements of modern life ceased to be – traffic lights, houses, cars, even people. It was late, but still. It seemed he'd entered a time portal to another world. Aside from whispered words of the wind, all around him was silence. Shadows crowded in on him, making the landscape seem alien and unwelcoming. He could make out clumps of reeds and heather either side as he drove, but the road was deserted, no movement at all. Not a deer or a fox. Not even a wayward field mouse crossing the road. Then, further along, mountain ranges suddenly rose majestically, menacingly - he wasn't quite sure which - out of the gloom, their dense sides blacker than the night. He half-expected to hear the howling of a lone wolf from a rocky shelf high above warning the rest of its pack of an approaching intruder, but knew they'd been long driven out of Ireland.

As the landscape grew ever more desolate, Colm feared he'd made a mapping error but then the moon emerged momentarily from behind clouds and he saw the glistening white shale of pyramid-shaped Mount Errigal and far below him the dull gleam of lake water, the *Poisoned Glen*' where in a mystic past the ancient one-eyed giant, Balor, had been killed by his grandson, Lughaidh, the poison from his eye spilling across the land, destroying all vegetation before it.

A half-hour later and here he was, in the middle of sleepy Bunbeg, a few miles from Bloody Foreland, Cnoc Fola in Gaeilge, his final destination. The street ahead of him, deep in shadow and empty of people, meandered gently past a small café, a pharmacy, a grocery store, then disappeared into the dark void beyond.

He could hear the sea somewhere close by, slipping and sliding across stones with a soft, rhythmic swishing sound. The vague outline of hills lay in the distance. A broken telephone line above him swung loose like a child's skipping rope, causing a group of crows to flutter their wings frantically to maintain their precarious hold. Hearing a sharp cracking sound like shots fired from a gun, unwanted reminders from a past he had tried to bury, he glanced apprehensively around. It came from a plastic bag trapped under a large granite stone, the wind tugging at it relentlessly.

It was just after ten. Intuition told him where to go. Unlike America, rural Irish pubs were not loud places for a cold pitcher and Monday night football on a giant plasma screen. Here they were largely unchanged for generations, filled with ruddy-faces straight from the boat or the field, men occupying the same stools their fathers' fathers occupied before them; nondescript places that harbored shady nooks, petri dishes of local intrigue where gossip simmered tantalizingly like fragrant broth; quaint places that sheltered the lonely and the lost, the dreamer, the depressed and the damned. A place to stay for a drink or ten and hear tales of joy and woe; a hot tip for the next day's races; precise predictions of weather yet to come. Maybe even, with luck, the whereabouts of a mysterious woman and details of her comings and goings.

Such a place wasn't difficult to find. Any self-respecting Irish town had rows of them. He glanced around him. Light streamed from a large window further along the street. A sign across the front read simply, '*Teach Hiudai Beag's.*' It was Gaeilge, for what he wasn't sure, perhaps 'small musical instrument' but he knew an Irish pub when he saw one. As he pulled open the door, conversation rushed out as a gust of cold air rushed in. Everyone noticed everyone notice him, yet not a single eye turned in his direction. There might have been an imperceptible lull in conversation as the door closed behind him, but he couldn't even be sure of that.

Dimly lit, compact, and as wide as it was long, knots of people there, mainly older men, talked animatedly. Talk flowed swift and easy from one to another, a melodic seesaw of voices jostling for space in the rush of words. A framed multicolor poster, probably brought home by one of the thousand and one emigrants taking the 747 westward from Shannon was taped to a wooden pillar announcing in bold, flowery lettering, 'Celtic Music & Arts Festival, Boston.' A striking photo of a lone fiddle resting ghost-like on a bare wooden chair, the phrase, 'Echoes of Erin,' was inscribed beneath. Both subtle reminders of Ireland's bittersweet legacy of empty hearths and long goodbyes.

Colm made for the bar, across a floor of worn wood, its natural grain speckled black with shoe leather, indelible imprints of the past.

"Rough night, eh," a pot-bellied barman said smiling as he approached the counter. "What'll it be?"

"Pint of Murphys," said Colm, returning his smile.

He watched as the barman filled a glass slowly with the brown creamy liquid. Lifting it, admiring its soup-like thickness, he took a deep mouthful, feeling the smooth foam lick his dry lips, relishing the cool, bitter taste of roasted hops that slid slowly down his throat. After paying and seeing a vacant corner couched in shadow, he headed there, a quiet place to watch unnoticed those around him and best decide on a strategy to obtain quick, valuable information.

He was barely seated when suddenly, a high-pitched screeching rushed at him almost tearing out his eardrums. The howl of a banshee? The squeal of a donkey in labor? Momentarily startled, his eyes scanned the room searching where on earth the unholy sound was coming from before finally his gaze settling upon a burly man on a stool holding tight to what resembled a small octopus, its head sticking out of his armpit, its tentacles dangling loosely across his knee. Bearded and big-joweled, the man with shoulders on him as broad as a bull's back was squeezing the poor creature's head repeatedly against his side with his elbow like a blacksmith working a set of bellows while simultaneously blowing air into one of its tentacles, causing it to screech ever more loudly in a merciless cacophony of sound. The man's face, bloated and red from exertion, resembled a birthday balloon ready to pop.

Colm sat mesmerized, the sound soaring above the silence that had fallen upon the room. Then, much to his surprise, the beginnings of a melody began slowly emerging from the tangle of notes. Within seconds, an ever-more complex rhythm, primordial in nature, was playing sweetly on his ears. The uilleann pipes, one of the most ancient musical instruments in Ireland. As if on cue, other instruments appeared magically from nowhere. A young woman drew a flute out of her handbag; an elderly man, his nose long, red and boney, produced a tin whistle from a most incongruous hiding place, a battered felt hat on top of his head. Another pulled out a small hand-drum from under his chair.

"What about a few wee tunes ta warm us up," one man said, his fiddle resting upright on his knee.

"What about '*I Buried My Wife and Danced On The Top of Her*,' " someone close by replied.

"Aye, in your dreams ye did, in your case more like '*An Phis Fhiluch*,'" put in another, causing those all around to burst into laughter.

"What about '*Drowsy Maggie*' followed by '*The King of the Fairies*'?"

"I prefer '*The Farting Badger*' or '*The Cow that Ate the Blanket*,'" chimed in another.

"Are ye sure ya don' mean '*The Cat that Ate the Candle*'? The one on John Carty's first album," said the man beside him.

"Oh for crying out loud, ye pile o' gobshites," shouted the older man with the uileann pipes. "You're a gaggle o' old geese. Will ye houl yer whists. Are ye here to play music or ta jabber all night? Let's warm up the place with '*The Mullingar Lighthouse*,' then '*Granny Does your Dog Bite*' '*The Mason's Apron*,' '*Toss the Feathers*' and finish up with '*The Rambling Pitchfork*.' "

With that, all talk stopped. Fiddles slipped under chins. Bows skimmed across strings, jumping and leaping like their handlers were puppeteers high on cocaine, creating a dizzying pattern of twirls and whirls. Flute and tin whistle came rushing in behind one after the other, then the man with the hand-drum - Colm recognized it as a traditional bodhran made from stretched goat skin - began sweeping the side of it with the nob of a stick, weaving a haunting rhythm with swift gliding movements of his wrist.

Before the rising musical grandeur of what he was hearing could fully register in Colm's mind, as if they had all been waiting for a pre-agreed signal, those around him started bouncing their feet off floorboards, like they were frantically padding down fresh cement. Hands hoisted into the air, palms beating furiously on palms. As the tempo quickened, Colm's own feet began beating a lively rhythm along with the rest. Melodies leaped around the room like gusts of wind coming in through the open door, licking, looping and lapping in and around the furniture this way and that. And just when it seemed it had reached its climax in a thundering finale with one instrument sending its storm of notes surging across another, a second flourish would begin, rising like the sea itself pouring over rocks, surging into every crack and cranny, sending musical waves hurtling into the darkening world outside.

After many minutes, without warning, the music, at first brash and raucous, slowed its frantic pace, its volume falling. The resounding sounds of the uileann pipes faded as the gentle rhythms of strings took up the flow. A ballroom of romance began, a waltz tempo so sweet and gentle and silky that Colm imagined the rough wood floor beneath him transformed into a gleaming marble ballroom with sparkling champagne on silver trays and chandeliers shimmering in a golden light. Within minutes, this too dissipated, as the plaintive notes of a tin-whistle fluttered like falling feathers in the air and a lone voice, rusty and forlorn, sang about love lost, the last snows of winter and how only rivers run free and the image of a woman standing alone on a windswept pier, her clothes soaked, her eyes wet with tears as she stared out to the raging sea as a ship sailed into the far horizon, its ghostlike form fading from view. The lament caused a sudden stabbing feeling in Colm's chest. Images from the past rushed at him which he tried to quell. As the singer's voice hovered over the room, others joined in the chorus, slowly, awkwardly at first as if afraid to be heard above the rest, the volume gradually gathering strength until the whole room was swaying as one, including that of the pot-bellied barman who leaned across the counter, his eyes misty. Rising in unison to the climactic last verse, they then slipped into silence, leaving behind a collective sadness, a weary sense of despair.

As the last notes of the tin whistle ended, muffled conversation resumed around the room. Still feeling an emptiness inside, Colm lifted his glass and drank deeply for comfort. Then felt a soft touch on his shoulder.

"Oiche mhaith, a chara. Cad e mar ata tu?"

Colm turned, knowing enough Irish to understand the simple greeting. A leathery, weather-beaten face with flint fragments for eyes beamed unblinkingly mere inches from his own. The head to which the face belonged was nodding up and down like on a string, a few feathers of white hair fluttering across the brow. Before he had time to take in what had been said, the voice continued.

"An bhfuil Gaeilge ata agat ar chor ar bith?"

Asked if he knew Irish , Colm's brain went into overdrive. He fought to find the few words he learned at school long ago. "Tá beagán... Gaeilge... agam," he said, hesitatingly. "I know a little.'

"Maithu. Ca bhfuil tú ag dul?"

Perplexed, Colm searched frantically for the right words, but his memory failed him. Seeing the struggle in his face, the man promptly switched to English.

"If we speak at this rate, lad, the pub'll be closed afore we even know each other's names." He leaned across, stretching out a thick, calloused hand.

"Ernie. Ernie McMahon."

The man's grip was strong. Plenty of turf cutting in that, thought Colm.

"Colm. Colm Heaney."

Introductions completed, an awkward silence sat between them.

"Great music," Colm said breaking it.

"Tis so. Sure aren't we the home of Enya, Altan, Ian Smith, Pat Gallagher and Goats Don't Shave? If ya don't know that, ya must be new here."

The way it was spoken, Colm wasn't sure if it was a question or a statement. He answered anyway.

"Yes. Just arrived. A short visit. A few days only."

"A few days is it? It's an outa-the-way-place to be just for a few days. What brings ya this road?"

Colm hesitated. He took a sip of beer to disguise his indecision. He wasn't sure how much he should say. He decided half-truth was best.

"I'm a journalist. Here to interview someone called Ivan. He has a lab on the island."

"Which one? We have five of them."

"Five labs?" Colm's voice was filled with incredulity.

The man looked at him, his eyes twinkling with mirth.

"No. Five Ivans."

Colm stared back blankly. The man chuckled, a twinkle in his eye. "Slainte," he said, holding up his glass. "Is fearr Gaeilge briste ná Bearla cliste."

Colm hadn't the faintest idea what the man had said but he clinked his glass anyway.

"So you're here to talk to a man called Ivan, eh," the man said finishing his drink in one long swallow. "Not many with that name 'roun here. Should be aisy findin' 'im, I'd say." He paused, wiping froth from his lips. "But reachin' him might be hard."

Colm's eyebrows knitted with concern.

"Hard? Why?"

"Well, you say he's on an island. If ah'm thinkin' correctly, that's a piece o' land surrounded be' water, right?"

Colm nodded, feeling as if he was back in high school geography class.

"So, less you've a boat and a pair of oars in your pocket, it might be hard ta reach 'im is all ahm sayin'."

Colm sat silent, even more confounded. "Well, yes, of course, right," he spluttered.

"So, you'll be needin' a boat, I 'spect, right?"

"Yes, yes, I will," said Colm, hoping there were no more trick questions to answer. He felt foolish enough.

The man leaned back and adjusted himself on the stool. Silence followed. Colm filled it.

"Do you know where I might get one?" he ventured.

"A hard thing to find on the longest coast of Ireland. But sure ah'll give it ma best shot fer ye."

***

Time passed quickly and Ernie certainly needed no coaching in the art of conversation. While Colm had learned nothing about Patricia, though he had broached the subject several times, he had learned a lot about the history of the area, why it was called Gaoth Dobhair, meaning 'inlet of the sea' and, of utmost importance, how to tell the sex of a lobster. Sensing quiet around him, he glanced over his shoulder. The pub was empty except for the barman squatting, half-hidden, his back arched under the counter, stacking beer bottles on shelves. Broad shoulders and a large fuzz of ginger hair were all that remained visible of his tall and gangly frame. His head popped up momentarily. "Time please," he shouted. "The guards'll have me scalp if you stay any longer."

Colm and Ernie glanced at each other and nodded in acquiescence. By Colm's watch, they'd been there three hours. A stack of empty glasses showed they'd been valuable clients. They disengaged carefully from their stools. Feeling the room sway, Colm leaned his hands on the wall for support. Then they both shuffled unsteadily across the floor.

"Slan abhaile, safe home," the barman said, coming around behind them to unlock the front door for them.

Outside, the sky was a gray-black veil. A fine mist of rain settled on their shoulders.

"Raining again," murmured Colm.

154

"Not again," Ernie cut in. "Only the once. But then it never stops."

"I'm sure it's not that bad," Colm said. "The sun must come out some time."

"D'ya know how we know whether its winter or summer aroun' 'ere?" asked Ernie, turning.

Colm shook his head.

"The temperature of the rain."

Colm smiled. Ernie – he had found out over the last few hours – was, in Irish slang, 'a quare fella.'

"The faeries'll be ou' tonight," Ernie said, gazing up at the Heavens. "There's notin' they like better than a wee bit o' mist ta hide their mischief."

Colm turned to face him. "Faeries? You must be joking. That's just old wives' tales."

"Not 'roun 'ere. Strange things right at ye're doorstep 'ere. We call it ceo draiochta. The fairy fog."

He put his hand on Colm's shoulder, stumbling as he did so. "Ha' you never been somewhere when a rush o' air comes outa nowhere rustling your hair and bendin' the bushes 'roundya and then tis gone?"

Colm shrugged his shoulders. "Maybe."

"I was passin' an old cillin near here one night - a children's graveyard lying in a cleft between the mountains. Suddenly there was a strong gust o' wind, from nowhere, but was everywhere. Twas the sighs of faery children turnin' over in the col' ground."

Colm shivered, whether because of the image Ernie had conjured up or the effect of the damp air he wasn't sure. He pulled his coat collar higher. Ernie had told him about a small hotel not far away, he was glad he wasn't walking there.

"Listen now," Ernie said, pointing down the street. "Remember what ah said. Ye can't miss Mary's place. She'll take care o' ye. And stay inside when ye get there. The bog people'll be about too."

Faeries and bog people? What sort of a crazy place had he come to? Colm was about to ask Ernie what he meant but the old man had turned quickly and was already headed off in the opposite direction. "Do you need a lift anywhere?" Colm shouted out but the figure was fast disappearing into the mist. Colm thought he saw a dismissive wave of a hand, and that was that. The lights inside the pub went out. All around him was dark.

155

Chapter thirty-four

Being a Lirin, a humanoid species of skilled pyrotechnics, he could mentally generate fires at will. Became a member of the Starfleet crew in the year 2251, exploring unknown territory in the universe as communications officer on the USS Enterprise alongside Lieutenant Spock, a Vulcan. Among his many exploits, he helped fight off the Ngultors, a green-colored, four-armed insectoid race, and the Klingons from the planet Qo'noS who had eight-chambered hearts, two livers, multiple stomachs, twenty-three ribs and three testicles. His name was Nano and everyone feared him.

Chris turned away from the computer screen and gazed out the window into a black sky speckled with stars. His nostalgic journey back to childhood - as an ambitious six-year-old armed with a USS Enterprise membership card he'd found inside a breakfast cereal with new galaxies to conquer - was a well-earned reprieve from the hard research and plethora of meetings he'd been involved in since he'd stepped out of the elevator with the Senator a few days before. Nano, after all, had been one of his favorite characters, he recalled. A bit like himself, a loner, someone keen on details.

Yet here he was. Again on a mission. On a search for nano. Okay, finding his old colleague from Lirin during on an Internet search might not be described as particularly central to the task at hand, but he enjoyed the nostalgia. A little levity was welcome after three full days of exhaustive document searching and interviews with key people in science, medicine and industry. He patted the thick vanilla folder beside him with satisfaction. He'd more information than his boss could ever wish for.

To his great surprise, he'd learned that nanoscale materials had been used for over a millennium - nanoscale gold in stained glass in Medieval

Europe and nanotubes in blades of swords in Damascus. However, only with the invention of high-powered microscopes were researchers able to see things at the nanoscale. Over the last thirty years, nanotechnology had transformed almost every major industry.

"You name a product and it's probably got them," a specialist told him. "DaimlerChrysler's uses them for chip resistant paint for cars. Burlington Industries for a water-repellent cotton material. GE to improve its water filtration systems. They're used in pharmaceuticals, medical equipment, sporting goods, electronics, computers, imaging technology. The list is endless."

Chris had looked up the stats. Revenues worldwide from nanotechnology, known as the new industrial revolution, was estimated at over one trillion dollars. The US alone held almost tens of thousands of nanotechnology-related patents.

But his focus was the cosmetics sector and the sheer amount of money expended there left him shocked. Around three billion dollars on nano research, with even more in the pipeline over the next five years. A report by one environmental group identified more than one hundred cosmetic products containing nanomaterials including toothpaste, shampoo, lipstick and perfume.

"Without doubt, it's the largest single investment in product development the industry has ever made in its entire history," a public relations spokesperson for a cosmetics company told him. "So much is at stake, some execs are frightened. Depending on R&D outcomes, the results could change the entire sector, not just in terms of product scope, but who will be tomorrow's leaders. Remember, we're talking about an annual sixty billion dollar cosmetics business in the US, with much of that earned from products containing nanomaterials. Brand recognition or brand collapse, either could happen overnight, all because of these tiny particles."

The more Chris burrowed his way through materials, the more people he interviewed, the more a key problem asserted itself - while a huge amount of money had gone into development, very little had gone into efficacy. *'Get the product to market'* not *'make sure the product is safe'* was the entrepreneurial catchphrase. Even more dismaying was the federal government's response. The latest budget proposed spending $1.8 billion on nanotechnology, but just 6.6 per cent, was earmarked for studying safety issues.

"There's literally thousands of nano products out there, and there's no proper regulations in place," Rick Mooney with Consumer First told him. "These things we're rubbing in our skin, spraying on our faces, may be dangerous but government regulators are behind the curve. They're still trying to figure out what to do and, as an easy option, have adopted a wait-and-see approach. This attitude puts lives at risk."

Medical experts said they feared a repeat of a pattern played out with breakthroughs such as asbestos, DDT and PCBs - government authorities, wary of getting in the way of innovation, ignoring warning signs until a full-blown public health problem hits.

Chris had called the Environmental Working Group, which had created what it called a '*Skin Deep*' database, listing chemicals in everyday cosmetics. "Must we have body bags before the government does anything?" one scientist told him passionately.

Asked why there wasn't a public outcry for more money to investigate safety issues, he was told: "The yuck factor. There isn't one."

"Yuck factor?" he'd asked, confused.

"Public-perception research shows people are less concerned with nanotechnology than with, for example, genetically modified foods," Professor Jennifer Kuzma of the Humphrey Institute of Public Affairs told him. "People don't see nano as having quite the same yuck factor. This has led to collective Washington indifference."

Chris smiled at the irony. Is there anything yuckier than dead bodies?

Politicians hadn't become involved in the issue yet because voters hadn't demanded it. But consumer groups were mobilizing. Like football, it was the first huddle after the opening punt. But Chris knew. It wouldn't be long before major headline articles appeared in the mainstream press, on television news, on cable talk shows. The perfect opportunity for his boss to paint Barden and his ilk as '*Beltway Bandits*' lobbying on behalf of special interests at the expense of peoples' health. The perfect opportunity to show he was not a man indifferent about Washington status and membership of the capital's social and political hierarchy, but rather a man of the people, elected to look after their needs, protect their rights and warn them in advance of threats coming their way.

Yes, tacking nano concerns on to his boss's broad anti-chemical swing at the cosmetic industry was a natural move, one that could pay big dividends. The professor's parting words to him echoed in his ears. "The yuck factor is the key. One highly publicized incident or exposé, then things would change instantly."

That's why he was sitting here now at the restaurant table waiting for Cathy. They'd met at a Public Relations Society of America soiree at the

Smithsonian where she'd told him she worked in marketing, in cosmetics. Nano had been the perfect reason to call her. Would also give him something to talk about if he got tongue-tied, which inevitably happened where members of the opposite sex were concerned. Glancing up, seeing her standing beside the maître d, he hurriedly closed his laptop.

***

"Oh, ok, I suppose. I mean, what woman doesn't like cosmetics..." she was saying as her rigatoni with grilled peppers arrived at the table. They'd been talking for a good half-hour, mainly personal stuff, growing up, family background, vacation plans. Only now had the subject of work been broached and being more a listener than a talker, Chris had popped the question.

"It's just that, well at the moment... things aren't too..." She looked down at her wine glass as if the right word she was searching for was floating there. "...rosy."

"Why?" the word was out before he realized it, sounding way too abrupt. But she didn't seem to notice.

"Oh, probably me making something out of nothing. But let's talk about something else. I don't want to dampen this lovely evening."

"No, it's fine, really, it's very fine," Chris cut in, trying to be reassuring.

Her eyes rested momentarily on his. They stayed that way a while. He wished it could have been longer.

"My boss brought in a high-paid public relations consultant. Don't ask me why. I don't get it. The company's doing well, everything's going smooth..." She hesitated. "Are you sure you're alright with this? I mean, don't you want to talk about... well, something more upbeat."

"Not at all," he replied hurriedly. "If I wasn't doing what I'm doing now, I'd probably be a therapist. A good listening post."

"You're too hard on yourself, that's your problem," she said warmly. "I find it easy being with you."

Chris felt he was about to self-detonate with pleasure. "Thank you," he managed to mumble. "But please. Go on."

"Well, I'm being left out of the loop on something, some issue this consultant has been brought in on. I don't like that. Whatever it is, given the chance, I'm sure I could handle it just as well, if not better."

"I'm sure you could also," Chris replied automatically. A broad smile from across the table was his just reward. It lit a fuse making self-detonation inevitable. "What do you think it is?"

"I really don't know. We're developing a nano product…"

Chris froze. It was almost as if she'd read his mind. Now he was in a predicament. He'd wanted to talk about nano, of course, but he was leaving that topic for dessert and coffee. In truth, he wasn't sure if he was using it as an excuse to see her, not vice-versa. If he told her now he was deeply interested, might she think that was the only reason he'd asked her to dinner? Cathy was speaking more rapidly now, not giving him a chance to say anything even if he'd wanted to. Her voice rose in intensity.

"…it could be a major breakthrough for us but as with all new products about to go to market, we're being extra careful. Can't let rivals get wind of what we're doing. About the product, or the launch plan. And let me tell you, keeping secrets in this industry is almost impossible. And, of course, we need to make sure there are no teething problems."

"And are there?" Chris couldn't help himself.

"Well, none that I know of. We've gone through the usual battery of tests. But my boss and this consultant are very tight-lipped about something. They won't tell me what it is though I overheard them mention some doctor in Kansas City by the name of Gray but I don't know much more than that. From my research, he's a skin specialist at the main hospital there and is involved in consumer affairs but there's no link whatsoever I can see between him and us."

"Can you not simply call the doctor and find out?"

"I could but I'd be crossing swords. It would be considered an official company call and that could cause problems for me upstairs."

Chris sat bolt upright, an idea having struck him. One that would not only ease his rising guilt about not telling her his own interest in nano but help Cathy out of a bind. Who knows, even though he'd talked to more than enough experts, maybe he'd learn a bit more."

"Why don't I call?" he said enthusiastically.

Cathy's eyes widened. "You?

"Yes."

"Why you?"

"Well, I'm not linked in any way to your company for one so I'd be merely a neutral observer interested in the subject."

"But what makes you think he'd tell you?"

"Well, I do work for a prominent Senator." He pushed on. "Worth a try, isn't?"

"Maybe." He saw doubt – or was it the beginning of suspicion – in her eyes. But he pushed on.

"I'll call first thing tomorrow morning. Without mentioning your name, of course. How's that? And I'll report back to you if I find out anything that might be of help." It was more of a statement of intent than a request for permission and it was accepted as such.

The rest of the evening went smoothly. They even caught a late movie, shared a bag of popcorn. After driving her home, she leaned over and gave him a peck on the cheek for his gallantry, an action that set off fireworks in his belly. And other nether regions. He promised to call later in the week.

Gazing through his passenger window he watched as she fumbled in her handbag for her key, then inserted it in the lock. Her back was to him. That's why he didn't hear what she muttered under her breath, "Now Mister Know-it-All Larry, let's see if your Daddy can get you out of this one."

Chapter thirty-five

Blinding light pouring in through the window meant he'd overslept. Not surprising considering the flight from New York, the long drive up from Dublin and one, or five, drinks too many the previous night. If the sun had not stayed so long staring at him, he'd have gladly woken even later.

And finding Teach Jack's in the wee hours of the morning hadn't been easy either. '*Straight ahead, ye can't miss it,*' Ernie had told him. But Donegal roads, Colm had learned, were anything but straight. More like long curled lengths of rope, and almost as thin, looping this way and that, most of them leading him up rutted laneways to open fields where sheep and cows shifted uneasily when his headlights settled on them. Finally, overjoyed at finding the place and buoyed by a liter of Murphys, he vaguely remembered singing a snatch of '*My Way*' unSinatra-like to the night receptionist, then stumbling upstairs and collapsing into bed.

Now, sitting up, rubbing dregs of sleep from his eyes, he gazed around his spacious room. A sofa with thick padded shoulders sat against a nearby wall with a varnished wooden table in front, a lamp standing on it decorated with idyllic rural images of horses pulling carts laden with hay and ducks waddling merrily along the side of a pond. A large bay window its heavy curtains wide open was the reason he was bathed in sunshine.

Standing up, he felt his back as tight as a drum. A jog in the sunshine would loosen him up, clear the ale-fed fog from his head. Padding slowly across the plush-carpeted floor, he opened his suitcase and pulled out socks, shorts, runners and a '*Show-Me State Games*' T-shirt he'd picked up at a soccer tournament in Columbia. He slipped out of the room, skirted along a corridor, then down a half dozen steps to the reception area. He heard voices ahead but as he turned a corner, the muffled conversation stopped. Two plump middle-aged women were staring at him as if he was an alien just arrived from Pluto.

"Good morning," Colm said cheerily, breaking the silence.

The women remained speechless, their gazes lingering on his shorts and bare legs, as if ascertaining whether the alien species was dangerous or not.

"Nice morning for a run," he added quickly, encouraging conversation. From the looks he received, he felt he'd just asked for a pint of blood in a breakfast bowl.

"Run ya say," the older one said. "We don' do much of that roun' here." She paused as if to let him speak, but he didn't, not knowing what to say. "If ye're short o' transport, we can always call 'round and get a donkey fer ye," she continued. Colm blinked in surprise, a thought crossing his mind. If last night's transport nightmare was anything to go by, it wasn't such a bad idea.

"And I guess ye'll be having the raw egg and oyster breakfast special for your voice, Mister Sinatra," one of women added, nudging her companion.

"Actually, I was thinking of skinning a cow and eating it on the run with a dozen fresh mussels instead," said Colm sending the two into another bout of laughter. Pulling tea towels from off their shoulders, they shooed him out the door like an unruly rooster.

Outside, Colm thought he'd walked on to a giant movie set. The sky was a cloudless blue and gently rolling fields and dark bog stretched below him to a smooth, sandy shoreline, a glistening stretch of water and beyond it a series of rocky, hump-backed islands. The sea shuffled this way and that, as if it were a body in bed seeking the most comfortable sleeping position. Surf-capped waves flowed landward as if an unseen hand was unrolling layers of cotton wool. The little clutch of tiny houses on one of the islands, their whitewashed gables gleaming in the sunlight, resembled a flotilla of sailing ships, their anchors firmly attached to the ground. Seeing the fine tapestry of land and water, a sense of wellbeing coursed through Colm. If he had to go hunting for a fugitive, he thought, this was certainly the prettiest of places to do it.

Less than an hour later, however, the scene had changed dramatically. Instead of sandy seashores, the barren landscape around him reminded Colm of stark World War One images he'd seen in movies and magazines, the classic no-man's land of anti-war poets, Siegfried Sassoon and Wilfred Owen. Trenches lined flat, dark terrain as far as the eye could see. Gouged deep into the earth, their smooth sides glistened as they crisscrossed each other at oblique angles. Jogging alongside a shallow tawny moat where underground rainwater had collected, he half-expected bayonets and tear-gas, and men in metal helmets to rush over the top and lunge at him.

On the rim of a hill, he could make out moving dots, black ants in motion, but as he drew near he saw they were small groups of men, scattered here and there, moving up and down in a rhythmic motion. Their bodies tense with effort, some dug into the entrails of the damp, dense earth with long, curved wood-handled spades. Others lifted thick oblong black bricks and flung them into wicker baskets which they swung on to their backs, before plodding slowly along the slippery surface to the lane along which Colm was running, there adding them to an already impressive stack.

Colm realized with surprise what they were doing, the first time he had ever actually witnessed such a scene. For hundreds of years, turf bogs such as these had covered much of Ireland, providing life-giving fuel for warmth on freezing winter nights, keeping the phantom of death away from damp, draughty cottages. He had seen scores of tourism postcards and brochures featuring images of what he was now looking at, but they belied the harsh reality. The slow, backbreaking work he saw before him was evidence of that.

As Colm drew close, the men – dressed in hefty boots, thick pants, their sleeves rolled-up tightly on their arms - lifted their heads to gaze at him. Dressed as he was in shorts and the latest brand of Nike running shoes, daintily making his way along the muddy lane, swerving to avoid black pools left by overnight rain, he felt self-conscious. Out of sheer embarrassment, he waved as he passed, receiving waves of acknowledgment in return.

Soon he was leaving the bog behind, heading down towards the shoreline again. Patches of stunted gorse and rough-angled stones lined a steep path along which he gingerly picked his way. Finally, reaching the level of the beach and nearly out of breath, he slipped off his shoes and walked into the water, feeling its coolness refresh his tired feet. Steeped in thought, he sensed a movement out of the corner of his eye. Glancing to the far end of the beach, all he could see were tall rocks rising perpendicular out of the water, their sharp spines piercing the sand hills behind before burrowing themselves under the thick reeds there. He scrutinized them closely. Nothing. A pair of seagulls swept across his vision, gliding effortlessly on gentle air currents, then swerving downward, landing sharply with a gentle plop on the water where they bobbed like gray-white corks. Then he saw it. A split-second blur of movement behind the farthest rock. Curious, he started towards it. Then, just as he drew level, he heard a soft hissing sound. Pebbles landed at his feet. A skittish sheep? A frightened rabbit? He jumped back quickly and looked up. A figure, slender, moving fast, a woman, her body rustling the reeds. She gave a fleeting glance backwards as if checking for pursuit. One glimpse, an instant, no more. But that's all he needed.

The eyes, the face. His heart leapt in his chest. He started shouting, "Hello, hello, Patricia, wait, wait." But his words faded into the vast expanse of land and sea. He rushed to the rock, began climbing feverishly, but his bare feet failed to find a grip. He stumbled and fell back. He tried again but shells encrusted on the rock's side like jewels tore skin from his hands. He looked around for his shoes, saw them, a hundred feet away. He ran across the sand, jabbed his feet into them. Rushing back, he clamored up again, finding precarious footing in shallow dimples. He reached the top, breathless. His eyes swept desperately across the sand-hills and fields beyond. There was nothing, nobody. A burst of seagulls cackled overhead as if mocking him. She was gone.

For an instant he wondered if it was pure imagination, that his mind focusing so much on her had conjured her up for him, a gift of fantasy. Or, even stranger. Was someone playing a bizarre game of cat and mouse? This was the second time he'd seen her and each time it was a mere momentary glimpse, and each time she was rushing away from him. To see, but not to catch. What kind of a game was that?

Chapter thirty-six

"I'll be doin' a spot o' fishin' roun' the back o' Inismeain for a wee while. High tide's at six, so ah'll pick ye up in a coupla hours. Don' be late or ye'll be stranded on the island."

"Okay Ernie, thanks, I'll see you then."

Colm stepped from the boat on to a narrow pier built of rough concrete poured over pebbles that led to a wooden shed, weathered paint peeling off in strips along its sides. Lobster pots with green and orange netting were scattered about in no particular order as if someone in a hurry had dropped them carelessly.

Ahead of him a low wall ran as far as he could see, bordering rolling fields of wild heather and tumbling grass and reeds. Beyond was a line of striated cliffs, then a broad backdrop of concrete-colored sky. He gazed to his left. A clutch of stone houses, deserted, most in ruins, stood clumped together at the top of a rise. Standing ominous, they reminded him of specters waiting menacingly for unwary travelers to intrude upon their sacred ground. Taking a deep breath, he began slowly walking in their direction, passing a boat anchor, rusty and worn, that lay across a rock at the side of the path, its seafaring days long gone. Further on a washing-line drooped between two long makeshift wooden poles stuck in the ground.

While the houses resembled a motley collection of collapsed doors, roofs and walls, one - a spacious, whitewashed single-story building – stood out from the rest. As he approached, he recognized the heavy door of thick wood with horizontal reinforced iron bars across it that Ernie had mentioned. Hardly a necessary precaution on a remote island like this, he thought. Unless sheep had turned to killing their owners and stealing their belongings. But steal what? There was nothing but stone and grass here. Reaching the door, he raised his hand to knock when it burst open and a beefy man with a mop of thick unruly hair on his head and face stood there. Stood there isn't perhaps the best depiction of what he did. Planted his feet more like it. For the man, Colm could see, jumping back in surprise, had legs like sturdy oaks and a body that reminded Colm of wine barrels in a Tuscany vineyard he'd once visited. The image of Harry Potter's bearded mentor, Rubeus Hagrid, sprang to mind.

"So you're the fella, eh?" the man said curtly.

"Sorry?" Colm replied sheepishly.

"The reporter. The one I've heard so much about."

Colm hesitated for a second.

"You must be, there's not many come here pen and paper at the ready," the man continued, looking down. Colm followed his gaze, seeing the top of the notebook sticking out of his pocket.

"Guilty as charged," he ventured.

"Well then, what are we waiting for? You guys still work on deadlines, don't you? I'm Ivan by the way. Though you probably know that already from the good doctor. Named after Ivan the Terrible. Some say I look like him."

The man turned sideways, adopting the pose of a bodybuilder, hands clenched together in the air. "Whadaya think?"

"Ivan the Terrible, hmm," Colm muttered. "Russian history's not really my forte so can't really say for sure."

"History? I'm talking wrestling, man. Ivan's number one. From the Ukraine. Won the world heavyweight championship at Madison Square last year. A nasty bruiser. Flattened Big Bad Bob in the first. Not a man to cross on a dark night."

"Oh, I thought …" Colm stopped mid-sentence. "Never mind."

"I like the nickname," Ivan continued. "Gives me a sense of power. King of the island you might say." He grinned widely, evidently chuffed at the notion.

Must be the fresh sea air bringing out the humor in people, thought Colm. First those two women at Teach Jack's talking about donkeys and raw eggs, and now this. Feeling the need to continue the levity, he added, "I'm Colm, by the way. Not Colm the Conqueror or Colm the Cantankerous. Just plain old Colm."

Ivan laughed, a deep bellowing sort of laugh that reminded Colm of a hungry bear finding a hidden store of honey. "Pleased to meet you," he said, jabbing out a giant of a hand. Colm looked down at it, an image of bone-crunching machines in meatpacking plants rushing instantly to mind, his hand ending up in a dog-food can if he put it there. Not to take it, however, might mean worse. With some apprehension, he reciprocated. To his relief, the man's grasp was softer than he anticipated.

"The good doctor speaks highly of you," Ivan re-joined.

"I'm glad to hear that."

"Well, come on in then. We'll have a cup of tea together."

Shoving open the door with a flourish, Ivan ushered Colm through. At first, all he could see were boxes. Everywhere. Stacked recklessly in a pile. He almost tumbled over them as he stepped into the room. They seemed to cover every available space. Scattered on the floor. Blocking the door of a refrigerator. Perched on an armchair. Some were wood, some carton, some glass-fronted.

"Sorry about the mess," Ivan said apologetically, making a path through the debris.

"But as you're here, let me show you something," he said, pride in his voice. Puzzled, Colm followed as his host inched his way forward.

"Meet my companions, my miniature menagerie," he announced, indicating a box opposite. "But be careful. Don't go stepping on one. Sometimes they escape. Not often but when they do, they're impossible to find. Usually end up getting squashed underfoot."

Uncomprehending, Colm stared ahead unblinking. All he could see through the transparent glass sides of the box was a thin layer of sawdust along the base. Nothing more. He glanced disconcertingly at his host who was staring intensely at it too, furrows of concern wrinkling his brow.

"Breeding's inhibited, may have to adjust the temperature," he muttered under his breath. He put his hand into the box through the open top, softly flicking away loose particles. Then it happened. A puff of dust. Colm blinked, not knowing quite what he'd seen.

"Come closer, they won't bite," his host encouraged.

Colm leaned slowly forward, putting his face close to the glass. "There's nothing there."

"Of course there is, they're as plain as daylight."

Colm narrowed his eyes. Another puff of dust startled him. Then he saw it. Tiny. Pale. Almost the same color as the sawdust around it. A perfect camouflage. But what?

"Always showing off," Ivan said, as if referring to an unruly child.

"What is?"

"Rhinotia hemistictus."

Colm shot a glance from Ivan to the box and back.

"Huh?"

"A long-nosed weevil."

Colm stared at him skeptically. "Oh of course, of course. What am I thinking?"

His attempt at sarcasm was ignored. He tried a more serious approach.

"And what may I ask is a long-nosed weevil doing here?"

"Relaxing mostly, I'd guess."

"No, I mean what are YOU doing with it here?"

Ivan turned, surprised.

"You mean the good doctor didn't tell you?"

"Tell me? Tell me what?"

"What I'm doing here, of course."

"He said you were involved in fascinating experiments related to human skin but that I should get more details directly from you."

Ivan shook his head, disbelievingly. "So you've come all the way here from America to interview me without even knowing what I'm doing?"

"Actually, I came all the way here to interview…" Colm hesitated, deciding not to continue. If the Ivan the Terrible was in any way ego-sensitive he'd end up as dog-food, "….well, you're part of the reason I'm here, but not the whole reason."

Ivan smiled wryly.

"I see."

Before Colm could explain, a soft scratching sound made them both swing round. There was commotion going on in one of the other boxes.

"My subjects cry for attention," Ivan said. "We have much to talk about, my friend, but first it's feeding time. If we don't do their bidding forthwith, they might suck out our eyeballs and turn them into jelly."

Colm shuddered. What on earth had he got himself into?

***

"Experiments in biological warfare? Russian military intelligence? Are you pulling my leg?" Colm asked, incredulous.

"Not at all, that's how it all began. With a doctorate in applied biology, they needed me. Insects and the viruses that kill 'em. That was my thing. Still is. Until bog mud came along."

They'd been sitting for over an hour on simple wooden chairs at a small table. The room featured basic furnishings, a small black stove in the corner with a wicker basket beside it and makeshift shelves attached to one wall with steel brackets, all lined with books. Ivan was refilling two large mugs with tea, Colm eyeing him with curiosity.

"But what's killing thousands of people in a subway station got to do with skin preservation?" he asked. "Unless you skin them afterwards and hang them up like cow hides in a tannery."

"The good doctor was right," replied Ivan. "You are a man of imagination. I like that. We need more like you in research. You'd make even me seem sane."

"Well, isn't that what you said?"

"Not exactly. In fact, no. Producing biological germs is the single greatest deterrent to actually using them. Like nuclear weapons, if you're enemy knows you have them also, it won't use them either. Russia has enough bio-warhead material on hand to knock out the top one hundred cities in Europe, and Europe has even more, and the US probably more than both together. That's why relative peace reigns in this supposedly free world of ours."

"Yes, but…"

"You've been watching too many Hollywood movies. Biological warfare is quite a well-respected profession in Russia I'll have you know. Such jobs are much sought after. Well-paid. Secure tenure. Ample promotional opportunities. Generous pension. Good perks, including two weeks free use of a government Dacia during your vacation. And a brand new Trabant after ten years in the lab. What more could a person ask?"

"Okay, if it was such a good life why did you leave?"

"Gorbachev, perestroika, glasnost. The fall of the wall. End of the Cold War. Freedom, democracy. Take your pick."

"I see."

Ivan sipped on his tea. "Actually, none of those things."

"No? What then?"

"Boredom."

"Boredom?"

"Yes, plain old boredom"

"Making biological weapons, boring? Hardly."

Ivan ran his hand across his chin, ruminating. "The lab was on Vozrozhdeniye Island in the Aral Sea," he said. "If you can avoid it, you don't do biological warfare experiments near people. We'd hibernate there. Summer, winter, all year, didn't really matter. We'd sit around, play cards, talk about our work. Nothing else to do. Drink bottles of vodka, the real stuff, none of this watery commercial pea soup. By the liter. Kept us going as we devised formulae, revised formulae, updated formulae. Anthrax, smallpox, bubonic plague, brucellosis, tularemia. Then after a few years, we'd finalize the product. But then, we couldn't use them. Remember, they're produced as deterrents, not for real use. The spores would simply be put away in containers, until Armageddon day."

Colm nodded. "Which hasn't come. Yet."

"Exactly, and let me tell you, waiting for something to come that doesn't come is awfully boring."

"So what did you do?"

"I moved into agriculture. Still investigating insect viruses. Their composition, their activities, their feeding habits. Greedy locusts devouring the corn crop. Caterpillars deftly destroying oak trees. That sort of thing."

"But what's that got to do with human skin?" said Colm feeling a little exasperated.

"Well, by studying the relationships between the viruses and their host bodies, I discovered certain biologically active substances – BAS for short - that can be used to heal damaged skin."

"Interesting but before asking about that, how did you end up here of all places? You're Russian."

"Funding."

"Funding? Here on this remote little island?"

"Yes, a rare species called a research grant. Lean pickings these days, even leaner in Russia."

"I see."

"Also, having a research facility on an island entitles you to a little bit more, especially if it's an Irish-speaking one. Being a minority language, Brussels and the Irish government put extra money into preserving what they call the 'teanga.' The tongue."

"But Russia isn't even an EU country."

"Ah, but I was born in Romania."

"Doesn't matter. You don't speak Irish."

"I know, I know, but do you think they'd listen to me when I tried to explain that?" That mischievous grin Colm was beginning to like spread across Ivan's face. "No sir. They said, 'cupla focal?' And I said 'cupla focal' right back and that was that."

Colm shook his head in disbelief. "Cupla focal, a couple of words. You said a couple of words in the Irish language and you ended up with millions of Euro and an idyllic island life in the sun.'"

"Sun? Obviously, my friend, your time away has erased much of your memory circuit. There's so much rain here in Donegal, they've thirty different words in Irish for it. As for millions, I've barely enough for equipment, supplies and a small salary. And to hire a couple of local people sometimes when I need them. That and a promise to include turf in my studies was enough for the funding board. As they say around here, *'May the Lord in his Mercy bless the European Union.'"*

Ivan spread his hands in the air, "And that, my friend, is why I'm here."

Colm shook his head. He felt a sneaking admiration for this strange fellow from eastern Europe.

"Turf? Dr. Gray told me it was an integral part of your research."

Ivan didn't respond immediately.

"So…" Colm said encouragingly. "Tell me how it works."

"Now if I told you that, you might go off and sell it to some big multinational corporation and become an extremely wealthy man."

Colm wasn't sure if he was joking or not. Just in case, he added.

"Then again, I might be just the best man to publicize it for you. Then you'd be the wealthy one."

Ivan eyed him. "Hmmm, maybe."

"So now. Insects? Turf? Heal skin? More like making a person's skin crawl. It reminds me of leeches I watched sucking blood from an old woman's face back in Kansas City."

"Oh, yes, the good doctor sent me that story. I enjoyed reading it. One of the reasons I agreed to see you. Plus the other thing, of course."

"Other thing?" Colm sat up, his antennae rising.

Ivan waved his hand dismissively. "We can talk about the situation facing our lady friend later." He lifted his mug and took a long, slow sup of tea. Recognizing the sign for what it was – Doctor Gray having done exactly the same thing before entering into a convoluted explanation of his work - Colm shuffled himself into a more comfortable position. Listening, he knew, was the price he'd have to pay to get to Patricia.

"There are more than one and a half million different types of insects," the Man Giant began. "And from being a simple killer of them I now turn them into miraculous medical applications that heal damaged skin. Put plainly, through laboratory techniques such as centrifugal separation, I extract various elements, mainly proteins, enzymes and lipids, from the insects. These substances support cellular rejuvenation, keeping the skin's natural tone and preventing collapse of collagen, the substance that helps maintain elasticity. They also increase the skin's ability to deal with cold, warmth, pollution and free radicals. In other words, they're wonderful anti-ageing products."

"But insects? Why insects? Colm asked. "Surely there are easier and better ways to heal skin."

"Easier, maybe; better, hardly. Synthetic products are certainly easier to manufacture en masse but their use is worrisome. We don't understand their side effects. They're simply not natural. And I'm a natural kind of guy." He did his grin thing again. "Nature's been around for millions of years, fixing this, fixing that. It knows a thing or two about healing. Why not use what it offers?"

"You speak like a doctor we both know. Who's whose disciple?"

"Neither, we're both true believers. That's how we met. An international conference on skin transplantation. He entertained me with stories about cutting up cadavers and I him about cutting up creepy crawlies."

"A match made in heaven. But believers? In what?"

"In a nutshell - a more thoughtful approach to medical applications, and an end to the blind rush to cater to what some number cruncher somewhere decides is market demand."

"So you're on a mission, right here on this little island. To protect people from medical mishaps and bring natural revolutionary skin products to the world."

"Well, I don't know if I'd be that melodramatic but if you say so, then, of course, I'll be glad to accept the Nobel Prize, the Order of Lenin, the Legion of Honor, and whatever other illustrious medallion you wish to pin on me for my life's work."

"You talk about insects, but what about turf? Are you rejuvenating skin with thick, oozing black goo that's been around since the Dark Ages?"

"Such a delicate way with words, my man. You should try writing. You make it seem so delectable I want to run up there right now and guzzle down a gallon of it."

"Speaking of running," Colm said, trying to shortcut the conversation back to Patricia. "I was up earlier today doing exactly that."

"You were? What a peculiar man you are. It's a strange bipedal activity, the understanding of which I've never fully grasped. As you can see. In fact, you're only the second person I know in this whole area who does it. No coincidence you're both Yanks I suppose. But she's much more fun to watch do it than you."

"She?" Colm's pulse leapt.

"The lady you came to see. It's a wonder you two didn't crash into each other rounding a corner. As there's no shortage of them around here, I'd have thought that'd be a strong likelihood."

"You mean Patricia? The American woman?" Colm could barely contain himself.

"Why, do you see a hundred other Yanks hanging around the place? In case you haven't noticed, there's isn't a McDonald's for fifty miles."

Colm tried again. "I've come a long way, it'd be nice to at least say hello to her."

"You could try."

"How? Where can I find her?"

"The house on the hill. The big hill. The whitewashed one. The house, I mean, not the hill. Nice garden. Full of cabbages and potatoes. And a mountain of turf by the door. Ernie delivered a load there the other day."

"Ernie knows her?"

"Of course he does. He's her uncle, her guardian you could say. This ain't New York where no neighbor knows another. Everyone knows everything here. Sometimes, too much, if you know what I mean." He winked knowingly. Colm smiled, in part at the likeable nature of this fellow in front of him, but mostly at his good fortune. Only one day here and he'd already almost bumped into her, literally, and now had found out where she lived. An idea popped into his head. Why not go there right now and introduce himself? Because, a voice answered, what happened to her at the hands of the paparazzi back in the US would mean she'd probably slam the door straight in your face. How do I get over that scenario? His brain was sifting for ways when Ivan interrupted, as if reading his thoughts.

"Daylight's safe enough to go up. Not when night falls. Got to be careful then."

"Careful?" Colm was momentarily confused. "About what? Does she have armed guards posted at her door?"

"The bog, of course. You could end up at the bottom of it. Become one of the 'corp portaigh.' The bog people."

"Bog people? What the hell were bog people?"

Chapter thirty-seven

Bog people? Even the sound of it sent shivers through Colm that evening as he sat in his hotel room lingering over the day's events. Ivan had proved a most intriguing character, his stories the stuff of adventure novels. Biological weapons. Fragments of insects for treating skin. And bog bodies floating in soil, trapped in time.

"How far back do you want me to go?" he'd replied when Colm had asked him to explain over on the island.

"How far back?" the question puzzling him.

"Yes, so I know how much to tell you."

"Well, everything, so as far back as…well… as the beginning," Colm replied, not knowing what else to say.

"Okay, if you say so." Ivan filled his mug with tea, a singular act that should have been Colm's first clue.

"About a million years ago …"

Colm eyes snapped open as if he'd been hit with a brick. "I said I wanted to hear everything but I didn't mean literally everything. Could you not start a bit, well… a bit closer?" he asked, his voice that of a child urging a parent to skip to the best part of the story.

"Mister health-science-whatever writer, the very spot where we stand was tossed up out of the belly of the Earth about three hundred million years ago," Ivan replied. "You're just getting the last page. Anyway, I thought you'd be enthralled to learn from a soon-to-be Nobel laureate. Then my talks will be booked solid, years in advance. And you'll be but a particle of dust in my past."

Colm let out a sigh and stretched across the table for the teapot.

"Okay, okay, but remember. Your loss. Let's start five thousand years ago. Great elks with antlers nine feet long roamed the forests here, the land one of sweeping mists, gentle rains, soft sunlight. A place of pagan carvings and secret rituals, where the soothing lilt of the harp floated over clear crystal lakes and rivers. A time of Cu Chulainn, Queen Maeve and the Knights of the Red Branch, legendary figures of the Celtic Twilight." He paused, his face taking on a softer expression, "In fact, strange to say, if you stay around here long enough you begin to sense it still."

Colm cocked his head sideways, shooting his host a puzzled look. "I thought cold, clinical rationale was the language of the scientist. You're going all fuzzy on me. You've been listening to the song of the Sirens out here too long."

He expected a snappy response and got one, "Are you finished with the interruptions?"

Colm covered his mouth with his hand intimating he was done talking.

"With Ireland having no natural coal reserves and with ten per cent of the country covered in bog, turf became an invaluable source of fuel," Ivan said, unfazed. "When large-scale mechanization came into play, large tracts were carved out."

He hesitated, gauging Colm's reaction.

"How's that for cold, clinical rationale?" he queried.

"Like a polar ice cap. Now can we get back to the bog bodies?"

"I thought that's what you'd want. Makes for a better headline, eh?"

"Even you have to admit, 'Human skeletons found in ancient bog' sounds a tad more interesting than 'Turf contributes to electricity needs.'"

"Human cadavers."

"What?"

"It's physiologically imprecise to call them skeletons. They're cadavers."

"Is there a difference?"

"Yes, a big one."

"You mean a bog one."

Ivan ignored Colm's perky attempt at humor. "Skeletons – I'm sure even an excuse for a science-medical-whatever writer like you would know - does not have any skin. Human cadavers do. And these ones did. Lots of it and hair and nails also."

"I see. So who were they, and why were they there?" Colm was enjoying this bit of repartee and, so he sensed, was Ivan, as perhaps anyone alone on a deserted island might. The big man was smiling, a teacher delighted at finding an attentive student.

"Back then this whole area was covered in deep lakes," he continued.

"But gradually they filled up. Layer upon layer of compost formed from the bodies of animals and birds, all clamped together with grass, sedge and tree stumps. In a word, turf. That silent brown, seemingly lifeless landscape you see out there is a rich tapestry of life. And death. A most peculiar place."

"Peculiar?"

"Well yes, aside from being home to such a varied flora and fauna – sphagnum moss, bog cotton, water spiders, beetles, dragon flies, slugs, not to mention mallards, snipes and curlews - where else would you find bog bodies?"

"Bodies, as in human? With arms and legs and things? You're joking, right?"

"Not at all. Thousands of years old, some of them. Well preserved. Lying there underground. The Irish equivalent of Egyptian mummies. And - by the way - I didn't say they all had arms and legs. And things."

"But how? I mean, they weren't smeared with embalming fluids and wrapped in bandages, were they?"

"No, no need. Au natural."

"Au natural?"

"Yep, just as nature intended."

"Hold on now," Colm protested. "You're losing me."

"It's simple. Turf bogs are unique in one key respect. Microorganisms can't survive there."

"So?"

"So? Those busy miniscule things are what causes you and I to decay and disappear. But because they're not around..... voila."

"Our body parts stay together."

"Mostly."

"Oh, come on."

"It's true. These bogs developed after flooding. Waterlogging prevents decomposition, a process carried out by micro-organisms which require oxygen to do so. There's very little if any oxygen in turf bogs. That's why organic material – which is really all we humans are, though we harbor ridiculous aspirations that we're more - survives for a very long time. Such anaerobic conditions make for excellent preservation fluid."

"Fleshy bodies trapped in time," Colm said, imagining a pile of them floating to the surface where he had just been jogging that morning. That the workmen shoveling away there might at any minute poke their spades into ancient human heads, eyeballs popping out all over the place.

"Bog vampires. That's probably how Bram Stoker got his inspiration for Dracula."

"Your imagination is going into overdrive again."

"Well, we are in an Irish-speaking area after all and *'droch-fhoula'* does mean *'bad blood,'* " Colm replied. "But what have ancient bodies in a bog got to do with your work here?"

"Take it easy. I'm coming to that. Didn't I skip a few million years for you? You can at least be patient. You reporters are all the same, especially you Yanks. You want it all, and you want it now."

"You got it buddy." Colm smiled wickedly.

Ivan ignored the taunt, asking, "Which country has the largest tracts of turf in the world, eh? Right here, the Emerald Isle's full of them and they've found bog bodies all over the place, many of them thousands of years old. Meath, Kildare, Galway, Offaly, but also right here in little old Donegal. International specialists worked with the Irish Antiquities and the National Museum's Conservation Department analyzing them, then they organized a special exhibit of these preserved body parts. One of the most popular events the museum has ever hosted."

"And you being a certified bog body hunter went along?"

"Being a man who makes a living out of preserving skin, of course."

"And what did you find out? Why are there so many dead bodies in Irish bogs?"

"Various reasons. Accidents, a simple slip and down they went, never to rise again. Murder, no more convenient place to hide the most important piece of evidence. But my favorite - sacrifice and punishment. Long ago it was believed bogs were places between ground and air, between heaven and hell. By putting them there, souls were trapped. They couldn't join their ancestors or their Gods and they couldn't return to the land of the living."

"Morbid but fascinating," mused Colm. "But I still don't get it. How is your research connected to bodies in turf bogs?" Then, seeing his chance to steer the conversation in a certain direction, he added, "You said you're treating Patricia, the American lady. You're not intending to submerge her in a bog so someone can pluck her out a few hundred years from now as a well- preserved cadaver are you?"

"With that kind of imagination, you should be a murder writer, not a medical one," Ivan said lightly, before turning serious again. "Folklore has it that after battle Celtic warriors retired to the bogs to treat their wounds. They would coat themselves in peat and crawl into a sweathouse, essentially a hole in the ground. Being great believers in the importance of solitude, they'd take this time to rest, to be and to heal. It was a time for contemplation and reflection. You could say that under my guidance, Patricia's following this same ancient tradition."

Turning in his seat, he lifted something from a nearby wicker basket, then continued, "High-pressure liquid chromatography analysis has revealed that this...," he handed a lump of turf to Colm. "...contains up to two hundred organic ingredients including a whole range of medicinal plants such as sundew, heath, crowberry, and bog whortleberry that help heal damage skin and preserve its natural beauty. It also has plenty of sterols, molecules vital to cell membrane. They help skin retain moisture, improve elasticity and strengthen its protective barrier."

Having been handed a lumpy bit of turf for the second time in as many weeks by two health experts, Colm gazed at it with newfound respect. Until now, he saw it merely as simple fuel for the fire. Now it was a sparkling emerald of many colors.

"Turf also contains an abundance of humic and fulvic acids, antioxidants produced by biodegradation of dead organic matter - in effect, turf - which help regenerate skin," Ivan continued, gliding effortlessly into lecture mode. "Interestingly, their use dates back to ancient times when Egyptians used straw and mud to make building bricks. Scientists found these acids released from straw and mixed with the mud, strengthened the material, producing bricks less likely to lose their shape, or break. You can but imagine the immense benefits for damaged skin."

"Quite a strange correlation," said Colm.

"Indeed, but logical. Anyway, because of their mild astringent and anti-inflammatory properties, these substances are useful in the topical therapy of skin diseases such as atopic dermatitis, cheiropodopompholyx, psoriasis and mild focal hyperhidrosis." Ivan was warming to his subject. "The compounds can be made into gels, creams or ointments and used on the body and scalp. They are also antibacterial, antifungal and photo-protective."

"The first two I understand," Colm interjected. "But photo-protective?"

"It's a complex process nature has developed to minimize damage to the human body - mainly the skin - from exposure to ultra violet radiation," replied Ivan. "It transforms the energy of a UV photon into small amounts of heat that are harmless. If the energy was not transformed, free radicals and other harmful chemicals would generate."

"Cells would function poorly or simply die and life as we know it would be impossible," Colm intercepted, remembering a pre-summer feature article he'd written on the dangers of excessive sunbathing. "We'd all suffer from severe melanomas and other cancers."

"Now you're talking like a true medical writer," Ivan said, pleased by his contribution. "The substance, melanin, is very important in this whole process. It dissipates more than ninety-nine per cent of the absorbed UV radiation as heat, so only a tiny number of molecules undergo harmful chemical reactions."

"And that's why we use sunscreen lotions," Colm added.

"Yes, but don't be fooled by blurbs on bottles," countered Ivan, a shadow crossing his face. "Cosmetic companies use hefty doses of poetic license to boost sales. They say the UV filter in their lotions acts as 'artificial melanin.' That's misleading. Synthetic substances in sunscreens do not dissipate the energy of UV photons as heat as efficiently as real melanin. In fact, penetration of sunscreen ingredients into lower layers of the skin can be dangerous as parabens and preservative chemicals used in sunscreens, are also absorbed into the skin."

"Are you saying in a nutshell that everyday sunscreen lotions can actually cause skin cancer?" Colm asked disbelieving.

"Epidemiologic studies are on-going but yes, some investigators suggest sunscreen lotions are a risk rather than a protection, and a cause of malignant melanoma."

"Surely, simple tests show if there is a danger and from what," Colm asked.

"Yes, but that brings us to the big issue. Quantitative composition of cosmetic products can't be assessed properly because companies that make them won't provide a detailed breakdown of ingredients or their concentrations. They simply don't want outside quality control. And with the introduction of nanoparticles, the situation has become even more menacing..."

He paused mid-sentence, "But I won't go into all that. I'm sure the good doctor has told you more about sunscreen lotions and nanoparticles than you ever wanted to know."

Colm was taken aback. "Actually, he hasn't mentioned them at all."

"Really?" Ivan's knitted eyebrows displayed a surprise bordering on shock.

"Why?" Colm asked. "Should he have?"

"Well, after what happened... I thought..." Ivan hesitated. Not a man short of words as Colm had learned, he seemed now to struggle over what to say.

"Is there something I should know?" Colm asked bluntly, seeing his hesitation.

Without answering, Ivan stood up quickly from the table. "I think I heard Ernie's boat in the harbor," he said over his shoulder as he made for the door. "You'd better hurry or you'll miss it."

Then he was gone, leaving Colm alone, a shapeless lump of turf resting in his hands.

Chapter thirty-eight

They were sitting in the corner snug in Teach Hiúdaí Beag. It being midweek, not many people were around. Though warm inside, Ernie wore a thick coat and a blue balaclava pulled well down over his ears, "Ahm keepin' as much of the heat inside me as ah can so ahl have a full reserve tank ta keep me goin' til ah reach home," he'd explained earlier when Colm pointed out the discrepancy between his indoor attire and the temperature.

"Bog people, that's fer sure, plenty of 'em too, their bodies all floating aroun' up there," he'd said when Colm mentioned what Ivan had told him.

"Bodies floating around in bogs? Are you all nuts around here, or what?" Colm exclaimed, incredulously. "Is there something in the potatoes you're all eating?"

Ernie ignored the remark. "Sure haven' we got more roun' here than any other part 'o the country," he replied, pride in his voice. "Plenty o' open spaces for 'em to float 'bout in, ya see. But now the two in the one bog, now that's an entirely differen' matter." He stopped and pondered in silence for a moment, then resumed. "Ah but then again, wi' all tha' happened to 'em, why wouldn't it be so?"

"Happened?" Colm said intrigued. "What happened? To whom?"

"To Oisín and Niamh, o' course," Ernie looked askance at him. "For a man born in Ireland, ye don't seem to know much 'bout tha legends o' your own country,"

"Maybe I've been away too long," Colm replied quickly. "But anyway, go on, tell me the whole story. I only remember bits of it."

"Tell ye what?"

"About the two in the bog."

Ernie took a long, slow swallow from his glass – merely medicinal, to oil his vocal cords, he'd explained earlier, but before he could continue, a voice behind them intervened.

"Well, well, is it yourselves then?"

Colm turned in surprise. A diminutive man barely up to his shoulders, with a large veined nose and cabbage-like ears, stared intently at him, a beaming smile on his face.

"Ah, for the love o' Jaysus," Ernie exclaimed, his rising voice filled with exasperation. "Would you get away outa here and gi' me 'ead peace. Sure isn't there enough trouble in the world without ye adding to 'em wi' your weedlin' presence."

"What unChristian language to be usin', a chara, and me on me best behavior," the newcomer shot back. "I just popped in for a quick wan and who did I spy but ye're good selves and thinkin' ye could do with some fine company, here ah am. But if ahm not wanted, sure the road is long and wide and ah can go anywhere ah plese, buíochas le dia." Then, not waiting for a response, the man hefted himself up on to the high stool right next to them.

"I don't think ahve had the pleasure." A bony hand stretched across the table to Colm. "Séamas. Séamas Mac Giolla Bhrighde, eldest son o' Máire Rua – that's Red-haired Mary in the Queen's own. Here in person and at your service."

Colm, momentarily taken aback, mumbled. "Colm Heaney."

"There's a bit of the Yank about ye, methinks" the man said, his eyes narrowing in rumination. Colm opened his mouth to explain, but before he could do so, Ernie spoke up.

"Now Seamie, it's wan thing fer ya ta sit down wi'us, but tis quite another ta have ta listen ta'ya all ni', so don' be goin' askin' a millin questions," he said. "We were 'avin a quiet enough conversation until ye appeared outa nowhere. Ye'll not go startin' interrogatin' the poor man or ahll have ye kicked out tha' door."

"Now would ah do such a thing, Ernie? And me as shy as a silver sixpence. Sure don't ah keep meself ta meself mos' o' the time?"

"It's not the times yer keep yerself to yerself ahm worried about, tis the rest o' the time. And ahm after thinking this might be one o' them times. So le do thoil, dún do bheal, a chara."

Sensing this verbal tussle could go on indefinitely, Colm stepped in. "We were just taking about bog bodies. And the two up above. Oisín and Niamh"

"Aghh, them two, sure tis only poetic tales to be told roun' the hearth by a seanchaí on a winter's night," Seamie said dismissively.

"Ah, Sweet Mary, Joseph and all the saints above," Ernie exclaimed, almost knocking over his pint as he swung round abruptly. "Ye canne just come dancin' in here like a dandy and say a ting like that."

"Why, sure tis true," Seamus replied, indignant.

"Tis not."

"Tis so."

"Agh, you're as useless as tits on a bull."

Seeing them eye-to-eye, fearing this might erupt into an endless to and fro, Colm took hold of Ernie's shoulders and settled him back in his seat.

"Easy now gentlemen, easy," he said. "Let's hear the story first. Then we can all fight afterwards."

"The story is…" Ernie shot a warning glance at Seamie. … "now don' ye go interrupin' me, ye amadan."

The little man didn't seem to hear the words of admonishment. He sat staring at the wall, slowly sipping his drink, the face of an angel on him. Colm sensed the two had battled like this since they were sucking on their mothers' milk yet would probably die of loneliness if the other wasn't around.

"Long ago, there was a fella by the name o' Oisín, the son o' a great chieftain," Ernie began, raising the glass to his lips and pausing for another swallow. "One sunny mornin' he was out huntin' when he saw a pure white horse gallopin' toward him. On it was the most beautiful girl he had ever set eyes on. Her name was Niamh, wi' hair as gold as the sun and her dress the palest of blue, all studded wi' stars."

Colm cast a quick glance from Seamie to Ernie. Their leathery faces - raw and hardened by years working the land and fishing the sea – had softened. Like innocent children, not grumpy old men, one listened intently, the other caught up in the act of storytelling.

"When Oisín asked who she was and where she'd come fro', the woman said, '*I'm Niamh from Tír Na nÓg, me father is King there.*' They sat down on a grassy hill and talked all day abou' all kinds o' things. Finally, Niamh asked Oisín to go wi' her but he wanted to know what sorta place *Tír Na nÓg* was. '*It's the land o' eternal youth,*' she said. '*A happy place with no pain or sorrow, a place where no-one grows old.*' So, with that, Oisín said goodbye to his family and friends, got on her white horse and off they went galloping across the land." Ernie paused, savoring the attention he was getting.

"Time passed easily in *Tír Na nÓg*," he continued, wiping his mouth with the back of his hand. "Oisín didn't know how long he had been away, but he began ta miss friends 'n family back home so he decided ta go back on a wee visit. Niamh pleaded wi' him not ta go but he was plenty determined. *'Take me white horse then,'* she said. *'But whatever you do, don' touch the soil of Ireland. If you do, you'll never be able to return to me again.'* When Oisín reached home he saw an old man strugglin' wi' a large cut of turf in the bog up above by Bloody Foreland. He leaned over to help, and with tha' didn't he fall off his horse and his feet hit the soil. In a second sure he was transformed inta an ol' man, his skin all wrinkled and cracked. A lot a time had passed, ye see. He'd been away a hundred years n' more. And when he asked, he was told all his family and friends were long since dead and gone. And so he died too, right there in the middle o' the bog."

Colm leaned closer, captivated by the tale.

"Worried sick at not hearin' news o' Oisín, Niamh rode like the wind n' searched the bog up and down for any sign of him," Ernie went on. "She found none, but never gave up. In point a' fact, the only thing she did gi' up was her own life, cos being away from Tír Na nÓg she too grew ol' and lonely and died. And they say her ghost still searches up there inta bog fer the body o' the only man she ever loved."

As Ernie finished his story, quiet settled around the table like a thick layer of fine dust, each listener in his own world of thought. Then Seamie placed his hand gently on his friend's shoulder. "Ah, tis a bittersweet story, sweetly told, a chara," he said. Ernie nodded, his eyes swimming. The two men shook their heads sadly as if the young couple had been members of their own family. And that it had all happened just yesterday not hundreds of years before. If at all.

"People 'roun here say when the mist's settled on ta bog they sometimes see out o' the corner of their eye the vague shape of sometin' movin'," added Ernie. "But when they turn, they're not sure if it's just a trick o' the light or a passin' shada'."

"Or maybe Oisín and Niamh tryin' ta find e'ch other," put in Seamie.

"I think we're all in need of a stiff drink," Colm said, breaking the silence. "Either that or we'll slit our throats to put us out of our misery."

"Well, don't be relyin' on this oul gobshite ta get us one," said Ernie, a big grin breaking out on his face. "Sure's he's of Cavan stock, a miserable sod o' a man who'd rather peel an orange in his pocket than share a slice." Seamie tut-tutted, continuing to stare with an air of moral superiority at the wall ahead. After ordering another round, Colm judged the time right to switch talk to Patricia.

"I was surprised to see a woman out jogging today," he ventured,

185

gazing at each in turn, gauging their reaction. Neither responded but their silence seemed forced, as if they were feigning disinterest.

"Probably American," he continued. "Couldn't imagine many women around here going out running. Not according to what cleaners at my hotel made of me this morning when I came down."

Still nothing. He pushed on.

"Unusual to see a woman like that alone out here, isn't it?"

This time Colm fixed his gaze firmly on Ernie, remembering full well what Ivan had told him. The ploy worked. "I wouldna say she's alone now," came the reply. "Ah mean, we're all here watching o'er her. Did ye not get a chance to talk to her?"

"Didn't have the chance. Was too fast for me."

"She is that, keeps a trim figure that lady. Not like some wimen 'roun 'ere. As wide as milk cows, some o' 'em."

"Aye, but on cold, winter nights tha' can be mighty comforting..." Seamie's voice trailed off when he saw the sharp look Ernie give him.

"I'd like to get to know her," Colm continued. Then took the plunge. "Will you help me?"

The question scampered like a rabbit across the table. Seamie and he shot sidelong glances at Ernie, who sensing their stares, blurted out, "Well... ah'm not sure... ah suppose ah could try."

"I'm counting on you then, right?"

Ernie glanced up at him. "Gi' me a day or two."

Colm couldn't tell if he meant it, or it was just a polite brush-off. But there was nothing more he could do. He knew Ernie would be talking to her, if he hadn't done so already, and he hoped he'd spoken well of him. That would make meeting her easier, and more productive.

Outside, the air was cool, damp with rain. With mumbled goodbyes, the three men parted, each going their separate ways.

Up ahead, the road lay empty, mist billowing in from the sea. Colm had just reached his car and was bent over fiddling with the key in the lock when he heard footsteps. He swung round quickly. Ernie was standing right behind him.

Chapter thirty-nine

Doctor Gray sat staring at the wall putting his thoughts in order. Over the last few hours, he'd gone from utter despondency to something better. Having verified the most valuable piece of evidence was safe, happy he'd taken the added precaution of not leaving it in his office desk, he'd tried again to reach Patricia in Ireland. A sleepy voice answered on the sixth try, perking up when she recognized his. He told her about the theft of the documents and about Colm's arrival. A long silence ensued.

"Hello? Hello?" he said, trying to control rising panic. "Patricia?"

"I'm still here," she replied finally. Then paused. "Look, we knew this might happen. We both decided it was a risk worth taking. I still believe that. Anyway, it fits with what we'd planned, doesn't it? I'm a decoy, and that's what decoys do. They take attention away."

The even-handed way she accepted his news eased Doctor Gray's growing apprehension, but didn't eradicate it. Knowing where she was, they might come after her. Whoever they were. He didn't even know who'd stolen the materials never mind what they might try. Though he could make an educated guess. But try what? That was the unknown that worried him most. Maybe he should just persuade her to come back. He was about to do so when she started speaking again.

"Anyway, don't worry, doctor. It's amazing what a thousand miles of water can do. I feel much safer here than I ever did over there. And aren't Ernie and Ivan here to look after me?"

"Yes, but…"

"No buts, doctor, let's stick to our plan. It's our best….. our only, chance. We've come too far to go back now."

She was right, of course, but his mind kept repeating the same question that had been revolving in it from the very beginning: was the price too high?

"How's Christine?"

He was hoping she wouldn't ask but knew she would. Truth, though uncomfortable, was best.

"No change. Still being monitored round-the-clock."

"I see." He could hear dejection creep into her voice.

"But we remain hopeful," he said encouragingly. "Many patients emerge from comas with all their faculties intact. Rest assured, she's been well looked after." That seemed to buoy her spirits and they moved on to other things.

Remembering his therapeutic advice, he asked.

"How's your gardening skills coming along?"

"I think I can add Miss Greenfingers to my list of beauty titles," she replied, a bounce of pride in her voice. "Flowers blooming on my potatoes. Roosters. Not the feathered kind. The tastiest, Ernie tells me. And parsnips, carrots and some garlic. All thriving."

"As are you it seems," he said, feeling a paternal warmth flow through him.

"Yes indeed, I'm learning a lot about Mother Nature here. You'll be interested to know many of her creations here are medicinal. The saltmarshes down below me at Magheragallon are scattered with beautiful creamy-white flowers of Grass-of-Parnassus. I pick them and distill with water. They're a wonderful eye lotion. Did you know they date back to the first century to the slopes of Mount Parnassus in Greece, sacred to the God Apollo?"

"No, I didn't know that, but remember, my dear, I live in Kansas City, a long way from the nearest saltmarsh."

"That's why you must come over. There are also lovely spreads of Devil's-bit Scabious, so dense they form a misty layer above the other vegetation. They've got violet-colored flowers, like small pompoms. The story goes that the devil was so angry at the plant's amazing healing powers he bit the end of."

"You'll be writing your own botany ..."

"They're coming under close scrutiny these days as it's the only caterpillar food-plant of the Marsh fritillary butterfly and these beautiful insects are disappearing fast all over Europe," she continued.

"As I was saying, you'll be writing your own..."

Suddenly, realizing they were talking across each other, they both stopped, bursting into laughter. Feeling the moment ripe, he asked, "Have you given any more thought about testifying if I find a way for us to do so?"

A short silence ensued. "We had an agreement, doctor, remember?"

He said nothing. It would be wrong to push her now. She had more than enough stress to deal with. And anyway, he still hadn't found a way to get his information heard by the committee. They hung up agreeing to talk more that weekend.

An hour later, he was still trying to work out what was the best way forward when his office phone rang. A call from Washington, his secretary announced. As he was due to deliver a paper at the annual meeting of the American Association of Dermatology there, it was probably someone verifying attendance and schedules. A young man's voice, his tone formal, came on the line.

"Good afternoon Doctor Gray, my name's Chris Harris. I'm public affairs assistant to Senator Edward Clarke here in Washington. I'm sorry to bother you."

Gray's eyes narrowed. Senator Clarke? Why would... he didn't have time to think further for the man was speaking and what he was saying sent his mind into overdrive.

"I'm conducting some research for the Senator on nano use in cosmetics. Your name was passed on to me as someone I should talk to and I wondered if you could enlighten me."

He could scarcely believe what he was hearing. Was this Jack's idea? Yesterday, after the theft, they'd talked about telling someone in authority about the whole situation but couldn't think of anyone suitable. And now this. Then a shadowy thought lunged at him. First, the stolen documents. Then this phone call. Could it be a trick to get him to reveal more?

Wary, he told the man he was busy, saying he could call him back. The man seemed fine with that, giving him a number and an extension. Gray mulled over what to do. He contacted director enquiries. It was Senator Clarke's office. Within seconds, he had dialed the number. Soon he was listening intently to the same voice.

The man talked about the committee hearings, how important it would be to know more about nano, how complex the subject was, how he'd value his input, and so on. Gray felt himself relax. The man seemed genuine, doing his best to do his job well. He answered some basic questions, promising to send further documentation as background. Then out of the blue.

"We'd be particularly interested to know about the situation at Bellus."

The statement came as a bombshell, leaving Gray lost for words. How could they know? It was impossible. So few people knew and none of them would ever speak out without his say so.

"How did you get my name?" he asked, realizing he'd not asked the most obvious of questions. There was a momentary silence on the other end of the line.

"That's not really important at this point," the man said simply. "What is, however, is that we're on the same side and can help each other. That's why it's important this conversation should remain confidential."

"But how did you ..." Gray stopped, recognizing the truth of what the man had said. He faced a dilemma. But while this call might be a Godsend, he couldn't risk divulging sensitive information to a man he'd never met. Then an idea came to him. Suddenly, the dermatological association conference took on new significance.

"I'm sure Senator Clarke would welcome that very much," was the man's response to his proposal a few minutes later. "When do you arrive?"

Setting down the phone, Gray turned to the framed photo on his desk. His daughter looked as pretty as ever, a beaming smile lighting up her face, her university scroll clutched tightly in her hands. Summa cum laude, the beginning of what was supposed to be a glittering academic career. "This is for you," he murmured, blinking back tears.

Chapter forty

The tough tone was hard to overlook, but Senator Barden subdued the urge to strike back.

Donors rarely asked for an urgent meeting when they were happy so he knew the appearance of one of his biggest contributors meant trouble. He braced himself for an uncomfortable meeting.

"I don't mean to be disrespectful, after all he wasn't one of ours, but still, even you have to admit, Truman had a point when he said, '*The buck stops here.*' And may I suggest, there's no place it applies more than right here, right now, in this very office." Dick Covington looked stern, a one-hundred-thousand-dollar-campaign-contribution-a-year stern. He'd have to lighten him up a little.

"I'm just wild about Harry," the Senator quipped, hoping a touch of Broadway music hall levity might take the sting out of the man's tail. He could see at a glance it didn't, so he decided to acquiesce. "Nuking the Japanese, pushing the Marshall Plan, ridding us of Commies, facing down the Bear, the Berlin Airlift, the Cold War. The list is impressive. How he was ever a Democrat is beyond me. But, granted, he was a true man of action."

"Exactly, and that's precisely what I've come here for." His guest was obviously in no mood for small talk.

Just then, his assistant entered with coffee, giving Barden a chance to re-group his thoughts. "Dick, let's start over, shall we?" He paused momentarily. " It's always good to see you, we don't see each other often enough. I was just telling Mary here that she should call your office to set up a lunch between us."

He waited for a similarly conciliatory response but, getting none, continued, growing more irritated at the business leader's arrogance. He may have financed a chunk of his political campaigns, but it was he, at endless hustings, who'd brought in the votes.

"With your hectic schedule, I'm sure you're not here to discuss the merits of Truman's dropping the bomb or his economic policies in post-war America," he continued, swallowing his pride. "Let's get down to business. What can I do for you?"

"You can start by telling me what you have been doing for me."

Barden felt his face redden, his anger barely under control. His bulldog nature was legendary, but, like vintage wine, he reserved it for special occasions, mainly on-camera performances in the chamber. Not that he wouldn't relish the opportunity to put this fellow in his place. He didn't like Dick Covington one bit, never had; probably never would. In fact, he quietly hoped he would retire soon so he could deal with someone more personable, someone not averse to the finer things in life – a fragrant oscuro cigar, a dry-aged rib eye - not someone so drily obsessed with profit margins and market expansion. But he knew he also had to be thankful. Covington's business acumen, bereft of sentiment, meant they both did well off each other. '*Parasitic*,' envious observers might term it. '*Practical*' others might say. They'd skirted the rules, they'd won their battles, had done so for two decades, end of story. Bellus, and companies like it in the cosmetic sector, enjoyed elevated '*don't touch*' status in the eyes of federal legislators and he'd enjoyed long tenure as a card-carrying member of the nation's political elite.

And more.

Bellus had not only generously funded the super PACs that kept annoying political whippersnappers at bay through every election cycle with character-destroying ad campaigns but also provided him a lucrative living far beyond the piscatorial entrees and Senate Bean Soup in the members' private dining room.

Like many of his colleagues, Barden had never formally registered as a lobbyist – people of his stature never did, preferring the euphemism, '*public policy activist*.' Instead, in the age-old tradition of Washington, he '*developed strategies*,' using his contacts to open doors. By trading on his political connections, he'd built up sizeable revenue through his non-profit consulting business. His '*Center for Health Renewal*' drew in over three million last year for services, its glossy brochure described as, '*advising clients how to reach the gilt-edged leaders that matter across industry and government*.' Hadn't he helped create a strong national osteoporosis campaign by shaping government policies toward the disease? Of course with a client that happened to manufacture calcium products. "I provide guidance and strategic advice on the best way to inform policy makers to achieve the optimum outcome for the people of this nation," was the pat response he'd settled on for interviews.

With all this in mind, he needed to tread carefully. His visitor was here not so much to lambast him - though whatever was nettling him, he seemed more than ready to do so – but, he sensed, because he was scared of something. Barden needed to handle him gently.

"How can I help?" he said calmly.

His mollifying tone worked its magic. Covington's facial features - taut to the extent of making his rather oversized lips seem peculiarly sausage-like – began to soften.

"These committee hearings, Senator, they're worrisome," he said. "I – we, – I think I speak for the rest of my colleagues in the sector - we thought it would be long over. You assured us in previous meetings it would be. In the past, it's been a routine affair, a blip on the screen, lost amidst the plethora of such hearings you guys seem to give birth to endlessly on the Hill. But this one's taking an inordinate amount of time."

His guest stopped speaking as if expecting an answer. An answer to what Barden wasn't sure, as he hadn't actually been asked a question. As for the committee, what could one expect when a group of powerful people with extremely large egos and an innate need for their voices to rise above others were corralled in the same room together? But he couldn't say that. Businessmen like Covington were like infants in prams with rattles. Now silent, he seemed to have momentarily grown tired of shaking his. Perhaps a bit of mollycoddling was in order.

"We live in changed political times," he began slowly. "We don't rule the roost as we once did and we have to take account of that fact. The other side want to have their say and it's understandable. After all, you have to admit, they haven't had many opportunities recently. Together we've done an excellent job of maintaining the status quo. Self-regulation fully intact. How many industries can boast that these days? The FDA's power pared back severely. A switchover of specialized personnel from them to us. Even favorable tax rates and financial incentives."

"Yes, of course, I'm aware of all that. But these hearings, better they're over quickly than we being caught by surprise."

"Surprise?" Barden's eyes narrowed suspiciously. "Is there something I need to know?"

"No, nothing relevant."

The vagueness of the term 'relevant,' Barden had learned, meant it's importance was lost in a maze of its own making. But from the firm set of Covington's jaw, he could see that demanding a more precise definition right now probably wouldn't work. The best approach was to use the kind of language people like Covington liked to hear and to indicate that if there was something important it's repercussions could go far beyond them both and the individual fiefdoms they'd carved out for themselves.

"I understand your business perspective, Dick, but you should also understand my political one," he began. "Our specific battle has become part of a larger war, a war we're fighting on all fronts, especially in healthcare. The Democrats have hoisted their adolescent populist banner *'fairness for all and responsibility from all.'* Of course, as always, equitable taxing policies is their war-cry and they've selected healthcare to symbolize what they perceive as the differences between rich and poor, between them and us. If this thing that's bothering you impinges on peoples' health, we'll lose further ground."

Enjoying the attention he was getting, he hoisted his sentiments on to the platform of patriotism. "Populism only goes so far then it becomes dangerous, by encroaching on the normal workings of the free enterprise system, the very system this nation is built on. The Democrats are dividing Americans with the bitter politics of envy. They're undercutting free-market capitalism and amplifying class-warfare arguments. People need to be lifted up by a desire to succeed, not dragged down by a resentment of success. We need unity, and we need it now. That's why voters need to be suspicious of big-government activism."

Was that the thin crack of a smile breaking through the stony features of the beak-nosed man across the table from him? Confident he was speaking the right language, he pushed on.

"We may hold an advantage in money and mechanics, Dick, but we don't want to give them the edge in message and momentum. So if you have something to tell me that could be key to the outcome of this particular committee battle, I need to know, and I need to know now. Otherwise we could have an almighty avalanche of regulations on our hands from one end from the country to the other. And I don't need to point out what that means - both for you and for me."

"Senator, your words, as you know fine well, are music to my ears, but let's talk bluntly. We want this committee thing over and we don't really care how that's achieved. We're paying hefty amounts into the American Legislative Exchange Council to get bills passed in dozens of states, and now we need to make sure there's no change in federal policy."

Barden, fuming inside that his little monologue had had so little effect, remained silent.

"What about a moratorium on future speakers, you've had enough already anyway?" Covington added quickly. "Surely you can bring the whole shebang to an end that way and draw up a final report that changes nothing."

Not for the first time, Barden was irritated by his visitor's shortsightedness, but remained calm.

"Even if we could, Dick, it wouldn't look good. Would come across like we're hiding something. Maybe bring even more attention on the issue. Anyway, we don't have the power or the numbers. Remember, the committee's led by one of them."

"Shift it to another committee then?"

He took a deep breath. What a pitiful understanding this man had of the political process.

"Or finger the main man?"

"Finger the main man?" He sounded like a mafia boss in a gangster movie.

"Yes, you know what I mean. Focus on Clarke . He's the main man pushing this whole thing. Pork bellies. Surely there's something you can offer him that'll make him back off. All politicians want to come bearing gifts to their people."

Barden shook his head slowly. "Healthcare is Clarke's bailiwick. He's built his reputation on it, he's not about to throw it all away now. Media hounds would be sniffing all over him if he did."

"What about some dirt?"

"Dirt?"

"Yeah, find something in his closet. Something we can hang him with."

Hang him? From gangsters to cowboys. His visitor's growing desperation was worrisome. What was he hiding that he was so keen to keep under wraps?

"My goodness Dick, you're talking about a man who has spent decades on the Hill, not some greenhorn, first-term Senator we can just sweep under the carpet. Finding dirt isn't easy. And using it well, even if you do find it, is equally as difficult. It's not the first time such attempts have backfired badly. It's a high-risk game and we're not ready to play it yet. I'm not saying we won't look for 'dirt.' My staff is always looking. But we can't produce a white rabbit, or a black one for that matter, out of a hat just like that."

"For God's sake, he's not a saint. Surely you can find something on him."

Mention of the word '*saint*' reminded Barden of something. He hadn't thought much of it at the time, but maybe… Seeing Clarke slip into the chapel, during the middle of a working day. Maybe nothing strange. But he'd have it checked it out all the same.

Then a thought struck him, annoying him greatly. This nervous numbskull across the desk from him was making him clutch at straws. He didn't like that. And he certainly didn't like the fact the arrogant son-of-a-bitch was withholding something. Obeying the rules of their unwritten agreement was vital. Had he gone and broken one?

Chapter forty-one

Turning a corner, Colm spied the white cottage way up ahead with a mountain of turf by the door just as Ivan had described.

He reduced speed to a crawl until the engine purred softly. The sea behind him lapping loudly on the shore helped muffle the sound. He could see someone in the garden, their back to him, spreading soil with a rake. Stopping under the cover of a sycamore tree, he opened the car door gently. Taking out the binoculars he'd borrowed from Teach Jack's, he slowly adjusted the focus. Yes, it was her. No doubt. Even clad in dungarees, he'd have recognized her attractive figure anywhere. How could he not? Slim body, long slender legs, unruly strands of thick auburn hair escaping from under the brim of a peaked cap.

Her slow, methodical movements whipped up feelings he'd rather not have right now. He decided to walk the rest. That way maybe she wouldn't see or hear him. Even if she did, what could she do? Run and lock herself in the house. That would be ridiculous. A scene out of a movie. Still, not wanting that to happen, he left his car door ajar, afraid closing it might spook her. The word – and now seeing her up ahead - made him think of a beautiful wild stallion on a vast open landscape, an image not too far from the truth.

He felt a twinge of guilt as he drew nearer, a predator sneaking up on a victim. He tossed the thought from his mind. It might seep through into his face and give the impression he was dangerous when what he wanted to convey was of someone new to the area who lost his bearings and was looking for directions. But would she remember him from the gift store in the hospital? Strangely, her back had been to him, just like now. Then, outside the hospital, when he'd chased after her car. He could have sworn she'd glanced through the rear view mirror and saw him. But again, he wasn't certain. She might have just been pulling away, the way his imagination was pulling away at him.

Yes, posing as someone lost was a risky strategy here but what alternative did he have? He'd asked Ernie but hadn't heard back from him and didn't know where he was. If he said he was a journalist, she'd probably turn on her heels. Maybe call the police. Yes, it would be a lie. But then again, not really. He was new to the area. At least it might give him a few minutes to talk to her. That alone was worth the ruse.

Walking softly, delicately avoiding a few broken twigs, it donned on him – and he found this hard to believe – he had never actually met this woman, hadn't spoken as much as a single word to her. How could that be when her face, her body, her imagined voice, had already suffused so much of his waking and sleeping moments, thrilling him no end?

He had reached the edge of the narrow driveway. The garden was but ten paces away. Across a narrow driveway of loose gravel. She was working in the section nearest the house, her back still to him. Any second now his movements were bound to attract her attention. If they didn't, what should he do? If he touched her on the shoulder she'd surely jump with fright. Anyone would, especially up here, away from everything, not a soul around. He wondered if he should say something or make a sound so she wouldn't be so shocked. Not wanting a hysterical woman on his hands, he decided yes, he should. After all, this meeting should be pleasant, one showing him to be a decent sort, amiable, intelligent, trustworthy. Who knows, maybe she'd see him as Prince Charming come to rescue her and rush into his arms for protection. More likely though she'd whack him over the head with the spade and bury him and he'd become one of Ivan's bog bodies. Then, he'd be the story, not her. He shuffled off these crazy notions, swallowed hard and gave a light cough.

"Espresso or cappuccino?"

Her back to him, the voice seemed to spring out of thin air. From some angelic waitress in the sky?

"I can make both," the voice continued in a level tone. "Your choice."

She spoke softly, still rummaging in the soil. He remained motionless, taken completely by surprise.

"Cat got your tongue?" She turned slowly, her face expressionless, not warm and welcoming, not cold and cruel. Neutral. Was that the beginnings of a sneer or a smile at the corner of her mouth? For some reason, the image of Kathy Bates from 'Misery' entered his mind, though being belted over the head with a spade by this beautiful woman might involve a modicum of pleasure.

"You must have come a long way, it's the least I can do," she

198

continued, looking at him closely, appraising him.

"Ah... well... thanks...that'd be great," his mumbled words matched his thoughts, all scattered around like the seeds on the soil before him.

While his mind registered he was staring at her, he found it impossible to avert his eyes. Her face was more than he had imagined. All its parts aligned in perfect proportion. Nose, lips, eyes, mouth all neatly linked to each other, smooth as glass, no jagged edges. And the whole better than the sum of its individual parts. If there was anything awry, it was her hair. On one side, cascading over her neck and shoulder. On the other, tamed, tucked above the band of the hat, revealing a shapely ear. Lopsided maybe, but perfect in its imperfection. Little or no make-up made her less glamorous, less unreachable than the magazine covers he'd seen her in. Comely. That was the word that came to mind. Maid of the mountain kinda. Oddly, as if hiding something, her neck was wrapped loosely in a scarf. The very same one she'd worn in the hospital store. Lime green with an intricate black pattern across it. What was behind it?

"I'll just finish up here first, why don't you take a seat, enjoy the view." She indicated a small wooden bench nearby. He walked over and sat down, feeling like a scolded schoolchild. He didn't know what else to do. He was only there for a second or two when he stood up again, suddenly agitated, nervous, feeling his plan of surprise was ruined.

"Can I help?" he blurted out, simply for something to say, his arms hanging limply by his side.

"No, my hands are used to it now, yours will blister," she said, matter-of-factly. She spread loose soil carefully around a potato plant.

He sat down again, his mind racing, staring into the distance. Over rolling hills with a bright purple veneer of heather bushes, then the layered chocolate, both light and dark, of the bog, and on to the open sea, spread before him, a shimmering silk cloak in the mid-afternoon sunshine. Her reaction to his arrival had put his conversational gambit into a tailspin. His coughing making her aware someone was behind her should have surprised, if not alarmed, her. But it did neither. Had she been expecting him and that accounted for her calmness? He was bemused. But what should he say now? Go on with 'the visitor lost' routine?' Also, she'd said, 'you've come a long way.' What did she mean? She'd also said his hands would blister. Insult maybe, truth absolutely. He hadn't used a spade in years. A pen was hardly good practice. Did she know who he was then? The lost visitor strategy didn't seem like such a good idea after all.

"Lovely spot," he said for something to say.

"My favorite," she replied. She bent down to pick up a small stone among the soil and tossed it through the air towards the hedges. It sailed gracefully, fluttered the leaves and landing out of harm's way. She leaned on the spade, surveying the garden one last time.

"Ancient Celts believed we all belong to the land rather than the land belonging to us," she said turning slowly to him. "And as such we're unlikely to damage something we belong to."

Colm sensed there was hidden meaning behind her words, something far beyond simply the culture of the Celts, but he had no time to think about what it might have been.

"In addition, Ireland's Gaelige name 'Éire' is derived from a Celtic Goddess Éru who was considered to be the Mother Protector of the land of Ireland," she continued.

Then, without another word, she set the spade down and walked towards him, holding out her hand as she approached. She smiled and Colm thought the brightest sun he had ever known had suddenly appeared from behind a cloud.

"Nice to meet you," she said.

He took her hand in his. It didn't fit like a glove – their thumbs got a bit tangled. If she'd had blisters, he didn't notice, nor would he have minded. Its softness made him think of the commercial she'd featured in that he'd seen on the Internet. He had felt a bit weird watching it. No wonder. He'd watched it seventeen times. She squeezing moisturizing cream from a tiny bottle, smiling confidently into the camera. '*Your hands are important, treat them well,*' she's said into the camera. To him. Seventeen times.

"What can I do for you?" she said abruptly, shattering his reverie. He studied her eyes, trying not to but failing badly. From the hospital photos, the magazines, his passing glimpses of her, he had thought them dark brown. Now he'd have to say nutmeg. They narrowed as she spoke. A hint of suspicion? Knowing?

He played for time. He was in no hurry. After all, he'd found her. And she hadn't run away.

"You mentioned coffee?" he said hopefully.

"Yes, of course, what kind do you take?"

"Espresso," he said, smiling as best he could.

"I'll just be a minute." She turned towards the house. He watched her lean, lithe body. Her movements easy and fluid. He'd probably have guessed 'model' if asked. She'd not invited him in. Understandable.

200

Unknown man? Known man? Same thing really. He sat down, pondering his next move.

She emerged into the light a few moments later, two espressos in delicate porcelain cups on a tray. She set them down on the bench between them. He lifted one and sipped from it. Deliciously fragrant.

"So?" She gazed across at him expectantly.

"Well, I'm new to this area, never been here before," he began, feeling cowardly as he spoke. Then he stopped. Perhaps it was a subtle movement of hers. Perhaps it was just his imagination. Perhaps nothing at all.

"Sorry, I can't do it," the words came out in a mumble. So low, she inadvertently leaned forward to catch them.

"I'm sorry, what did you say?" she asked, her face a puzzle.

Colm took a deep breath. "I said, 'I can't do it'."

"Do it? Do what?"

Colm put his cup down on the tray. "I can't do what I was going to do."

"Which is what?" her voice sounded as if she knew exactly what, but wanted to hear it from him.

"I think you know who I am and why I'm here," he said, gazing fixedly at her. They both sat silent each in their own world of thought.

"You get extra points," she said pointedly after a moment. "But nothing else. I'm done talking. It's all squeezed out of me. I've no more to give."

She took a sip of her coffee. They both sat gazing over the islands below, as if waiting for a ship to appear on the horizon with a secret cargo they'd both been waiting a very long time for.

"See that island down there, the one to the left, with the few small houses on it," she asked.

He nodded.

"That's Gola. No-one lives there anymore. They abandoned it fifty years ago. But their dinner plates are still on the tables. Just as if it was yesterday."

She stopped as if to gauge his reaction. Silence ensued.

"Toto," he said finally. "I've a feeling we're not in Kansas anymore."

She smiled broadly. "But maybe we're over the rainbow."

They stayed staring down at the sparkling sea. Neither knowing what more to say. Both thinking they'd said enough. For now.

Chapter forty-two

"Hello, Mister Atkins, Mary at reception here. I'm sorry for interruptin' ye but there's a telephone call from America for ye. Would you like ta take it?"

"Yeh, thanks," the man said gruffly, tossing his wet coat on to the bed and throwing his shoes across the floor.

"Jimmy?" a voice asked.

"Yeh, that's me," he answered pressing the phone between shoulder and ear while he pulled off his sodden socks.

"Joe here at the picture desk. How's it goin?"

"Fine, fine, got caught walking in the rain, whatdaya want?" Jimmy was impatient to take a whisky from the mini-fridge and get under a hot shower.

"Head honchos here are thinkin' of running this on the front cover so we're gonna need a bunch of close-ups to look at."

"Okay."

"Readers will wanna see her face and neck. We hear there might be something wrong with her. Scars maybe. Get some detail."

"Okay, Joe, okay. I know what I'm doin.' What dya think I am? A photographer on a high-school year book for Chrissakes."

Holding the earpiece close, Mary sucked in her breath and made a hurried sign of the cross. A ball of wool and a pair of knitting needles lay on her lap forgotten as she listened intently. Bingo was tomorrow night, she'd have a few good stories to tell the girls between numbers.

"Any chance of nudes?"

Mary raised her eyes to heaven, blessed herself again twice over.

"Nudes?"

"Yeh, like outside her cottage, sunbathing topless on the grass, or some such thing. As a former beauty queen, she must have a helluva body so would be good to see as much of it as we can."

"Are yeh crazy, Joe? Where dya think we are? Coney Island in August? South Padre during Spring break? Chicks lining' the boardwalk posing for Playboy? Noah's ark's beached here for Chrissakes. It never stops fuckin' rainin.'"

"Well, do your best anyway."

"Do ma best? Of course, I'll do my best. Don't I always. But I can't perform miracles, especially not on the skimpy pay you give us freelancers."

"What about in a bikini then?"

"Joe, are you goin' deaf? Or have you got a banana for a telephone there? Didn't I say it's wet here? And you want her prancing around buck naked like some garden gnome dancing the samba dressed only in a piece of dental floss."

"There's an idea. A wet T-shirt shot. Talk to her about it. Say it'll kick-start her career no end. That'll help."

"Ah, for cryin' out loud."

"We're brainstormin' here, Jimmy. Ya gotta work with me. And by the way, a bit of respect wouldn't go amiss."

"Respect, Joe? You're in the wrong business. We don't do that, remember? Her wrapped head to toe in a big raincoat and a pair of rubber boots with a thick woolly hat on is the best you're gonna get. Be happy with that."

He paused, there was no response, "Listen, pal, I gotta go or I'll catch ma death of cold. I'm soaked through."

Hanging up the phone, he turned to Chuck. "You'll never believe this...." But Chuck wasn't paying any heed. He was under the covers, snoring. Jimmy walked around the room looking for the mini-fridge. There was none.

"Ah, for Chrissakes, I'm surrounded by a bunch of idiots."

Chapter forty-three

When Colm entered the lobby of Teach Jack's, it was veiled in darkness except for a dim light over the reception desk. So thick was the silence around him he felt like a thief in the night. His shoes made a squeaking sound on the wood floor so he went on tip-toe.

As he approached, he saw a woman asleep there, her head resting on the counter, strands of loose hair falling across her cheek. She looked cute in that innocent, vulnerable sort of way, an infant lost in dreams, far removed from the mundane cares of the world. He felt like putting a soft cushion under her to make her celestial travels all the more comfortable. The stairs up to his room were thickly carpet. There'd be no sound to wake her.

Night-lights guided his way along the narrow hallway. Nearing his room, he noticed something white and flat sticking out from under the doorway. He bent down, pulling it out. It was an envelope, his name scrawled along the front in a lazy hand. Inserting his key in the lock, he quickly switched on the wall-light, tossed his coat on the bed and tore the envelope open. It was a short, abrupt message, as if the author had been busy or sleepy. The image of prostrate prettiness below made him think the latter.

Mister Paul Vickers called from the US, please call him at Tel. 212-646-2353.

His eyes widened with surprise. He knew nobody by that name. Even more of surprise, the area code was New York. He hadn't been there for years.

There was no time on the note. But it had to have been within the last three hours, since he'd left for Hiudai's. He resisted the urge to go down stairs and ask for more information. He'd check in the morning. Glancing at his watch, he realized it was early evening in Manhattan, plenty of time to call himself. Then all would be revealed.

He grabbed the phone and leaned his back against the bed-board, stretching out his tired legs. The call was picked up on the first ring.

"Celebrity News, may I help you?" a chirpy woman's voice said down the line.

The name momentarily stunned Colm into silence. His mind began racing.

"Hello," the voice repeated. "May I connect you?"

A few seconds later, still shaken, Colm found his voice.

"Hello, I was wondering if you could tell me the formal title of Paul Vickers please," he said, trying to sound calm.

"Would you like me to put you through to his extension?" the woman replied helpfully.

"No," Colm replied, quickly concocting a reason. "I just need to send him a document and wasn't sure of his position."

"Mister Vickers is photo editor," the young woman said. "Do you need our address also?"

"Yes please, thank you."

Colm noted down the information and hung up, his mind in a whirl. What the hell? How did they know he was here? And what were they after? He'd done some freelance work on the side for a few extra dollars, but mainly health stuff, for *American Medical News* in Chicago, *American Nurse* in Washington. Not for any publication in New York, and certainly never for a glossy celeb mag. He'd have remembered that. The only celebrity story he had ever written about was while on general assignment covering the launch of Michael Jackson's Victory Tour at Arrowhead Stadium and a U2 concert. Though, remembering with a smile, he'd also written an obituary on the dentist of former President Harry S. Truman. Did they count?

But what was going on here? The only way *Celebrity News* could have found out about him was by calling his newspaper in Kansas City and if they did, it would get to McCarthy as editor and he'd not tell anyone his whereabouts or what he was doing here. There was no reason for him to do that. Or was there? Why give their exclusive to a celebrity magazine?

He lay back, eyes narrowed, brow furrowed. Then he stood up. Sleep, which a few minutes ago had surreptitiously slipped into his senses, had vanished. He needed to walk this through before talking it through.

From the top of the stairs, he gazed down into the lobby area below. All was as before. Darkness, utter silence, the woman on the reception desk still asleep. Suddenly her arms stretched out, her head lifting slowly.

He padded softly down the stairs. She was brushing back strands of unruly hair with her hands when he reached the lobby. He coughed lightly. She spun round, giving an involuntarily gasp.

"Oh am so sorry, ya scared the daylights outa me," she said, her face reddening. "Ah was away with the fairies."

"I'm the one who should be sorry," he said. "It's an ungodly hour to be walking around. I went to Hiudai's for a few pints and just got back late. They locked the doors and dimmed the lights so the Gardaí couldn't see in."

"Well so, I'm sure the craic was mighty."

"It was, at least what I can remember of it."

He drew closer, showing her the piece of paper.

"I wondered if…" he began.

He hadn't a chance to say more for the woman interrupted in a rush of words.

"Oh, my dear Lord. Ah'm real sorry Mister Heaney, it's ma fault. Ah don' know what ah was thinking. Kevin, ma youngest, came down with a high temperature and a fit o' coughin' and ah've been worried sick. Got no sleep at all last night but couldn't take time off. And it's not often we get a bunch of Yanks here, most of our visitors being Nordies, from Belfast and Derry and such. Anyhow's when ah took the message, ah must ha' sent it up to your room withou' thinkin, and forgot it was for the other Yankee fellas that came after ye."

Colm's heart skipped a beat.

"Yankee fellas?"

"The two men who arrived late this evenin'. Said they got no sleep on the plane over then 'ad a long wait in Dublin airport for the connection 'ere to Carrickfin. Dog-tired, like mysel'. Not to be disturbed for any reason til mid mornin', they said. Oh dear, ah hope ah didn't inconvenience ye too much."

"No, not all," Colm replied quickly, putting her at ease. "I was a bit surprised, that's all." Then, changing tone, he asked, "Who are the two new guests?"

"Young fellas, mid-twenties, 30s" she said, keen to help, relieved there'd be no formal complaint. "One had a big camera bag over his shoulder. Said he'd put me picture in the paper." She blushed. "Not much luggage between 'em. They're only booked in for a cupla days. Left this for me." She pulled open a drawer.

"Ah was readin' 'bout the shannigans twixt Brad and yer woman Angelina," she continued, lifting out a glossy magazine. "Ah mean, have they notin' better ta do with their time than talk about whether he's more into Jennifer or her?" The cover photo was of the celebrity duo arm in arm at a gala. A 32-font headline blurted out, *'Together, or just holding on?'*

"Did they say why they were here, these two fellas?" he asked, affecting as light an interest as possible in the subject.

"Said they were on some kinda mission. Reminded me o' tha' film, *'Mission Impossible.'* But it wasn't mission, now I think of it. Was another word, one just like it. Ah yeah, assignment, that was it. Said they were on assignment, looking for a celebrity of some kind. Kinda like Julia Roberts when she run away here ta Ireland from Hollywood, after her break-up with whatsname Sutherland all those years ago."

"Did they say who?"

"Never heard o' the person. Wasn't Jennifer anyway. Or Angelina fer tha' matter. And definitely wasn't that *'Sex in the City'* lady, Sarah Jessica Parker, who has a wee house down the road in Kilcar. With her twins 'n all, she's well settled with Mathew Broderick right now." Then she paused, her eyes brightening. "Ah, now, I remember. It was someone by the name of Patricia."

While her answer merely confirmed Colm's suspicions, mention of Patricia's name made his heart jump. One thought rolled around his head. To get to her before they did. If he didn't, all would be lost. Both for him and for her.

Chapter forty-four

He sat gazing out his bedroom window, the sky as black as pitch, reflecting his mood.

He couldn't sleep, his mind heaving with questions. He'd tried McCarthy but his secretary said he was out of the office. How did these guys find out about him? Patricia's mother? No, she'd never speak to a celebrity magazine. Unless they posed as someone else, as he had done. Gray? Brown? McCarthy? Everything to lose, nothing to gain. At least, nothing he could imagine.

He stopped, realizing how unimportant the answer was right now. They were here and he knew what they were here for. Time was running out. He had to act fast. But how? The simplest way was to drive to her house immediately and warn her. But she'd made it more than obvious when he'd gone there that she didn't want to talk to him. Anyway, it wasn't even morning yet. She was probably asleep. And even if she wasn't, she wouldn't open the door. What single woman would? Colm was still wrestling over what to do when the first dull rays of daylight slipped gently over the ocean outside. He watched as a bruise of reddish-orange light seeped its way across the horizon, turning black to gray.

Then he remembered. She was an early-morning jogger He might catch her on the beach again like last time. He'd go there first and if he didn't see her, he'd head straight for the house. He still had time. After such a long flight, the paparazzi wouldn't be awake for hours. Pulling on shorts and a T-shirt, he quickly made his way downstairs, through an empty lobby. Then he was out the front door into the crisp air. He had a plan.

The narrow road he'd run on before lay directly opposite. He could see it wind its way snakelike down a gentle slope towards the sea, disappearing in places, behind a clump of trees, a flurry of rhododendrons, over some gentle rises, to reappear a few hundred yards further on. All about him was stillness, a magnificent landscape empty of human presence. A flock of hooded crows, dark and shapeless, were perched on an overhead power line like so many crumpled plastic bags. They seemed unwilling to wake from slumber and greet the new day.

He started running, turned a sharp bend and there was the beach and the sea in front of him, the water spread out, a silk curtain rippling in the breeze. Twisted fingers of jagged rock stretched out into it, striated as if a giant cat had scratched madly at them. Their color and texture reminded him of dried skin, dull, smooth and cracked.

He looked around. No-one. Either he was too early, or too late. Or maybe, after seeing him yesterday morning here, she'd changed her route. He paused, breathing hard, then started again, jogging towards a large outcrop of rock that he could climb to get a clear view.

A sharp squeaking beside him made him jump. He jerked his head round fearing he was being attacked by some animal he'd disturbed, then felt ridiculous. A small bird, its size out of all proportion to the loudness of the 'birrrrrrrrr beek-beek' sound it made, was burrowing furiously into a pile of seaweed. Black and white, it reminded him of a raffish little character in coat and tails, a long, pointed beak, bright red at the tip, like it had a lit cigar in its mouth.

"Don't worry, it won't bite." A voice said out of the blue. "It prefers seafood to human flesh."

Before he knew it, the person had glided past him effortlessly, a slender figure he recognized instantly. As if verifying what had been said, the little bird emerged from the sinewy wet pile, a small crab pinched in its beak. It gazed up at him with disdain, shook its head vigorously, then rose in the air and wheeled out of sight beyond the rocks.

"An oystercatcher. Lot of them around. They mix with the plovers and sandpipers. Gulls, of course. And corncrakes in the fields beyond, though their numbers are sadly declining."

Colm's somber mood lifted instantly. She was talkative. Maybe his task would be easier than he'd thought. Maybe this was her way of reaching out to him. But just as hope fluttered its wings, she was gone. Or at least going, fast. Already three steps ahead and accelerating, her feet shooting tiny sprays of sand back at him. With effort, he increased his pace to keep up.

"Didn't know you were an ornithologist," he muttered into her back, unable to think of anything better as an opener.

"Unavoidable, more birds than people here. And they keep to

209

themselves, which is refreshing. They value privacy."

Ignoring the notion this was a put-down, or maybe because of it, Colm blurted out what was on his mind. "Speaking of privacy. I'm sorry to tell you but yours is about to be shattered."

Her pace slowed almost imperceptibly. He was now only a pace behind. "I thought it had already," she shot back, cold formality edging her voice.

"The paparazzi are here," he said.

The effect of his words was immediate. She stopped so abruptly he crashed right into her, knocking her over, she a pin and he a bowling ball. They both tumbled off-balance and fell to the ground, spread-eagled, their hands almost touching, sand spraying all over their hair and clothes. Picking himself up, he turned to help. But Patricia was already on her feet, glaring at him with such intensity, he was afraid to say anything, a self-survival instinct kicking in.

"You guys never know when to stop, do you?" she said, her words wrapped in bitterness. "You're like spiders. You stalk, strike, sting, then record the agonizing death scene. All in the name of news."

Colm stood motionless, taken aback by the ferocity of her words. His mind a blank, he stared open-mouthed.

"At least, the others don't pretend," she continued, not stopping for breath. "They're just paparazzi, paid well to get a compromising picture of some unfortunate victim. Button pushers, the lot of them, and they know it. But you, you're worse. You pretend to be better. But you're no different, really, are you?"

Colm could feel the skin of his face prickle as if someone had dragged it across a cactus frond. Then something inside him snapped.

"Who the hell do you think you are?" he shot back equally strongly.

His words rushed out harsh and clear, stopping her in her tracks. "I came here to warn you about two lowlifes who've just arrived to plaster your face across a celebrity magazine cover and this is the thanks I get. You don't deserve to be helped. You don't appreciate it. You can't see beyond your own self-pity as you wither away here behind a mask of cynicism. A condition I should add, according to you, is only reserved for those in my profession."

"Don't give me that nonsense," she shot back. "Who do you think I am? Some stupid airhead." Her eyes glinted in the early morning light. "You'll try anything to preserve your precious story. Then cajole me into going back there to speak to the high and mighty in Washington and you taking credit for persuading me to do so. Well, to hell with the committee. I'm sick of all this duplicity. To hell with nano."

Colm stood transfixed, utterly lost. Nano? Where had he heard that word before?

"Or is it maybe that you need a few sexy shots to illustrate your story, close-ups of my brain," her voice was shrill with indignation. "What about going in through the hole in my neck, then you can really show where those tiny things have traveled to in my body. You've taken me from every other angle, why not that one? It's the only one left."

Colm's face was blank. Hole in her neck? What was she rambling on about, this woman with fire blazing in her eyes and grains of sand clinging to her tousled hair and body giving her beauty a raw, almost primordial dimension. Was she delirious?

"I have no idea what you're talking about," he said.

But she seemed not to have heard for she was now staring beyond him out to sea. He followed her gaze, but all he could see were the hump-backed islands like a pod of whales at rest; the abandoned, derelict cottages with their whitewashed walls like so many flags of surrender on the horizon.

Then she was gone, accelerating fast, her feet kicking up sand as she ran. He shouted after her but she didn't look back. He tried to catch up but even if he'd known she was going to take off like a rabbit, he'd never have been able to keep up. After a few hundred yards, his chest heaving, he stopped, feeling empty, except for a flurry of unanswered questions rushing around in his head.

What under God's earth had she been on about? Hole in her neck? Nano? Committee? Washington? When he thought of that city, the only people he thought of were politi... His mind whirred trying to make sense of it all, but failed. He wasn't sure what this was all about, but there was one thing he was sure of – whatever it was, it was much bigger than he'd been led to believe. And there was only one way to find out more.

Retracing his steps, he glanced down at the sand, seeing the vague shapes of their bodies where they'd fallen over. They merged as one. For a second, he wondered if it meant anything. Then decided it meant nothing. Or everything.

Chapter forty-five

"I'm very sorry to hear about your daughter, Doctor Gray."

"How did you know?"

"Your assistant told me you were at the graveyard when I called earlier."

"Thank you, Colm, I appreciate your concern. It's been a year now but it's never easy. With time, you think it will be. Everyone says so. But it's not." His words trailed off into silence.

Hearing the raw emotion in the doctor's voice made Colm reluctant to pursue the tough questions he needed answers to. "I'm sure you did everything possible," he said, sympathy in his voice. "Some things are simply beyond our understanding."

"Yes, sometimes I think that. Other times I think I could have, should have… If I'd known then what I know now…" The voice trailed off again. Then it returned, stronger, renewed by a sense of determination. "What killed my daughter, Colm, could end up killing many more people. That's why it's so important we stop it."

Following his argument with Patricia on the beach and her mention of nano and a Washington committee, Colm had been left utterly confused. Only the doctor could clear things up. That's why he'd called him immediately he'd got back to his room at Teach Jack's. Instead, right now, he was feeling even more confused.

"I think now's the time to explain everything," Gray said as if reading his thoughts. Colm sat in a chair overlooking the sea, waiting. "Patricia phoned me, upset at what happened between you on the beach. She's been through a lot but I managed to calm her down and persuaded her to stop considering you an enemy just because you're a journalist. With a woman's intuition, she said you'd probably have found out everything anyway soon enough. Her final words were, *'Better the devil we know'* but I don't think she really meant it that way. Believe me. Her bark is worse than her bite. Considering where you are right now and the arrival of the paparazzi, perhaps 'between the Devil and the deep blue sea' is more appropriate."

The doctor's attempt at levity made Colm smile, "I'll take her words as an indirect compliment and trust things get better between us," he said. "To be honest, after our little tête-à-tête on the beach this morning, they couldn't get much worse."

"I told her I trusted you. I always have. I know that sounds hypocritical to you right now but please believe me. I couldn't tell you more. I'd have been breaking doctor-patient confidentiality. Please bear with me. I've got a lot to explain. Let me start at the beginning... with my daughter Claire. She died from melanoma. She was only twenty-one."

Colm listened in silence.

"What is important is not so much the final diagnosis, as what caused it," the doctor said tersely. "Sunscreen lotion. That ordinary everyday product millions of people pluck from store shelves up and down the country every summer. A basic, inexpensive cosmetic meant to protect our skin from the sun's harmful ultraviolet rays."

This was too much for Colm to comprehend. "Surely that's impossible," he said. "How could a simple lotion cause someone's death?"

"Chemicals. Metal oxides. Titanium dioxide to be precise. Odorless, absorbent. Used in a variety of products, from paint to food to cosmetics. In sunscreens, it's a white pigment, an opacifier. But it's also a carcinogen and a photocatalyst."

"But..."

"I know it sounds crazy. But I'm far from crazy, though sometimes I've been made to feel that way by those trying to hide the truth. Let me explain as simply as I can."

Colm heard passion rise in the other man's voice. It surprised him. Until now, he had been the outward personification of calm. It was hard to imagine what he'd had to endure inside himself all this time, a skin specialist unable to save his own daughter from skin cancer.

"No matter what manufacturers claim, sunscreens cannot dissipate energy as fast as melanin, the natural brown pigment the body produces to shield itself against ultraviolet light by protecting the skin through absorbing UV radiation and dispersing its energy as harmless heat," the doctor said. "Worse, chemical ingredients in sunscreen lotions can

213

penetrate to lower layers of the skin, causing cellular malfunction. The cells become cancerous, lethal to surrounding tissue."

"But how?" Colm asked, incredulous.

"They can increase the amount of free radicals and reactive oxygen species. These atoms, once formed, start a chain reaction, the chief danger being the damage they do when they react with important cellular components such as DNA or the cell membrane."

"Are you saying the very products meant to protect us can actually harm us?"

"Exactly. And even though research results now emerging show they may be dangerous, these very same rogue chemicals are labeled safe to use by regulatory bodies charged with protecting our health, including the FDA."

"Safe to use? Yet they kill?" Colm queried, flabbergasted. "Is that how your daughter died?"

"From chemicals entering her cells, yes. She was the victim of a technological breakthrough that has raised the level of potential danger even more. New generation cosmetic products, including sunscreens, made of tiny particles can now cause worse damage than the larger molecular counterparts of their predecessors."

"You mean nano."

"Exactly. Cytotoxicity – the level of toxicity in cells - is dependent on particle size. The smaller they are, the more chance they can enter the cell, the greater the damage they can do. We call them nanoparticles."

As he absorbed this new information, a light suddenly flashed inside Colm's head. "You set this whole thing up, didn't you?" he exclaimed. "The leech story. It was just a ruse to get me to the hospital, so we could meet, so you could check me out in person, right?"

There was no immediate response. "In my defense," the doctor said finally, his tone measured. "I had already read your stories and admired you very much. Meeting you and seeing how seriously you took your work as a medical journalist was no surprise."

Colm barely registered the compliment. His mind was a fast-moving stream picking up flotsam and jetsam as it went, bits and pieces of information that helped him put the whole story together in an instant. "Me seeing those photographs of Patricia in that file in your room was no accident."

Silence.

"In the hospital lobby back there in Kansas City. You knew she might be there. That I might see her. Maybe even speak to her."

Colm stopped. He was unsure whether to be upset he'd been so easily duped, or full of praise for this elderly doctor who'd manipulated him so well without breaking his medical code of conduct.

Before he could decide either way, Gray spoke again. "It's not over yet," he said softly. "Patricia's a victim of these nanoparticles."

Colm felt a sudden emptiness inside. "What do you mean victim?" Then he asked the question whose answer he dreaded. "Is she dying?"

"We're doing everything possible."

Colm realized he had been holding his breath. "That's... that's... good," was all he could manage.

"You being there is also good, Colm. I know Patricia's initial negative reaction to you hardly merits this, but it's true. In fact, what happens now rests squarely with you both. What you both decide to do or not depends on the level of trust between you... which brings me to Washington. Let me explain the whole story."

Chapter forty-six

"Do you want the good news or the not so good news?"

"The good news. If it's good enough, I can hang up the phone happy."

"It's sunny with blue skies here in Kansas City."

Colm was puzzled. It wasn't that McCarthy didn't have a quirky sense of humor, but he also knew him well enough to know that's how he dealt with stress. He wrapped up difficulties in light-hearted abstractions, then came at them from oblique angles to find his way to understanding. A bit like interpreting a Picasso.

"And the not-so-good news?"

"You can come back and enjoy it."

"I will, believe me, I will. In a little while... I've found her."

He paused so McCarthy could take in the momentous news. "She's nice enough, bit of a tiger, but reluctant to talk. Can understand why after what's she been through with the tabloids, but I'm hoping she'll...."

"Browne wants you back."

For a moment there was silence, then Colm spoke, confusion in his voice. "Did you hear what I just said?"

"I heard," McCarthy said, flat-toned. "Did you hear me?"

There was another, longer, silence.

"Okay, okay, this is some kind of joke, right?"

"No, I wish it was. Browne says..."

For the next five minutes Colm listened, the room phone pressed tight to his ear. This was supposed to be a story update, not the nonsense he was hearing.

"Well, he can go fuck himself," he said abruptly. "Who does he think he is?"

"It's not who he thinks he is, it's who he actually is. He's your boss, my boss. Boss to us all. He's the man paying the bills."

"I don't give a damn. I'm here and I'm staying until I wrap up this story."

"He'll fire you."

"Tell him to go right ahead. Then try explaining it to everyone else there in the newsroom. And beyond. The only thing it'll please will be Pratt and his cohorts, no-one else. And I don't think either he or you want that. Morale will slump below the radar." Colm paused for breath, a conciliatory tone creeping into his voice, "I thought we had a new beginning going here. That we were going to go after bigger and better stories."

Colm was right, of course, McCarthy knew that. Every journalistic bone in his body told him so. Huge swathes of anger and guilt had torn him apart since his conversation with Brown. Placed in a no-win situation, he'd been skulking around his office like a caged cougar clutching in his hands the single piece of paper that offered the only remote hope out of this mess. But deep down, he knew. While intriguing, a feature story about a beautiful model hiding in rural Ireland involved in an experimental skin treatment was not Pulitzer-prize winning material. He needed something bigger, better.

"Now it's my turn," Colm spoke, nudging him out of his dark hole of rumination. "I've given you the bad news - I'm not coming back. Now the good news. And there's a lot of it. I just talked to Doctor Gray and you'll never guess."

Chapter forty-seven

"Some people are unhappy, Dick."

"Unhappy? About what?"

"The ways things are going, the way they're being handled."

"Things?"

"You know what I mean."

"It's my company. I should know. The question is how do you?"

"The cosmetic business is as porous as chalk. There aren't any secrets anymore, we both know that. Only better marketing, more colorful packaging, stronger distribution. And, of course, pricing. So let's not beat about the bush. Word's out something's wrong. People are getting nervous. It could affect them all. Virus-like."

Covington leveled his eyes at the man opposite, a man he both disliked and admired in equal measure. He wasn't too surprised when he'd gotten the call earlier to meet. A former detective, Bill Garner's no-nonsense approach had earned him the nickname 'the Minder" and the job of prime troubleshooter for the Cosmetic Association when it was first launched to fend off unwanted government interference in the industry, the premise being that a national association gave the perceived alternative of self-regulation, without actually having to do it.

"Look, send word back, things are under control. No need to worry. We've got it covered. We've got some people working on it."

"That's the problem. They're worried about what kind of people you might have working on this. Pardon my French, but if this bit of trouble is serious and leaks out, we're all in deep shit."

Dick didn't reply. Sometimes it was best not to. Give less away that way, especially to a detective.

"It's not as if you have exclusive property rights on nano, Dick," Bill continued. "We're all in this together, remember. It's the biggest thing to come the industry's way in decades. Hundreds of millions pouring into it. I'm no expert but I'm told it's the bees-knees though I suppose that's not the key biological ingredient." He smiled at his little joke, but he was the only one.

Covington sighed, impatient, irritated by the man's condescension. He was being softened up, he knew, but sensed the pressure hose was ready to be turned on if necessary.

"Also, we've agreements overseas to be concerned about," Bill continued. "With other associations representing other companies developing other products. If something goes wrong with one product the effects won't be just local or national. They'll be global. We'd be faced with a financial tsunami. And with Democrats pushing their consumer protection agenda real hard, our self-regulatory status could go up in smoke."

Covington could contain his patience no longer.

"Bill," he snapped. "Tell me something I don't know."

"So?"

"So what?"

"How are you handling this?"

"Private and confidential. You don't need to know the details."

"That's exactly why they sent me, Dick. To find out details."

They sat silent for a while.

When he spoke again, Bill's voice was more mollifying. "As a member in good standing, Dick, you know you've certain responsibilities, certain rules to follow. Rest assured, the association will do all it can to support you, but they need to know. They want to be in the loop. No surprises. They've all got products ready to launch. If this blows, well... who knows? Let's face it, if the tables were turned, you'd feel the same way."

The two men sat eyeing each other across the table in a quiet corner of the restaurant.

"It's not like tobacco, Dick. They muddied the relationship between smoking and cancer for decades, but it's not like that anymore. The Internet has changed everything. It's the great communication leveler. Industry no longer has a one-way conduit of information to consumers."

"C'mon Bill. I'm sitting right here in front of you. Don't talk down to me."

"I'm not, believe me. I'm just saying... look, we still can use some of the old weapons, I'm not saying we can't. We can fund skeptics to research alternative explanations, just like the tobacco lobby did."

He paused, as if realizing he was taking the wrong tack. "For

Chrissakes, Dick, we all knew it could come to this at some point. We're not ostriches. Perhaps not as quickly as this, granted, and not you guys at Bellus. And certainly not with a hall full of Senators gathered in committee on the Hill analyzing the situation. But it's never too late to mount a good PR campaign, to manufacture doubt about science."

"Do you not think I've been trying that?"

"How?"

"There's a saying in the PR business."

Bill's eyes widened with interest. "Yeah?"

"That for every PhD, there's an equal and opposite one..."

"...and if there's not, you create one." Bill finished his colleague's sentence.

"Exactly."

"So?"

"We're working on that. At the university in Kansas City where this interfering nuisance of a doctor works…"

"And?" Bill was obviously impatient. His taskmasters wanted answers fast.

"We've approached certain members of the Board of Regents about setting up a designated center on skin research, with an emphasis, of course, on the potential benefits of nano. With our name on it. Would keep this self-serving snoop under control. Then push him out of the system altogether. Early retirement or some such excuse."

"And?"

"They're still considering our offer."

"Why? You'd think they'd jump at the money. There aren't many grants around anymore."

"The doctor's been there a long time. Part of the furniture. May have turned over the first sod on ground-breaking day for all I know." He smiled sardonically. "Just when you think loyalty has gone the way of the dinosaurs, the dinosaurs raise their heads."

"How much did you offer?"

"Three mill start-up. Plus annual contributions."

"Pretty generous."

"You'd think. Said they'd bring it up at a future board meeting. But you could tell. They knew what we were up to, the old fogies. You could see it in their rheumy eyes. Anyway, these doddering old farts aren't rabbits. They don't move too fast. And certainly not fast enough for us."

"What about the consumer non-profits?"

"What about them?"

"Isn't he getting help from them?" Bill queried. "We've already put word out they're extremists, activist fearmongers. We're labeling them the *'Toxic Ingredients Movement,'* saying they're cherry-picking chemicals to make it seem there's a problem. We can spin some more, push 'the bored, lonely people fiddling with unreliable Internet info' message. The old 'earning money by selling fear' trick. They survive on motivated donors. Maybe it's time to demotivate them."

"We run the risk of shooting ourselves in the foot if we push too hard. We might just highlight exactly what we're trying to hide."

"And the media? I hear on the rumor mill you've hired a couple of shutterbugs for a character assassination job."

"Where you getting all this information?"

"You share with me. I'll share with you."

Covington said nothing. Being an association member was one thing, divulging sensitive information with fellow members was quite another. "Look, Bill, we're not doing this just to get a stupid story in the tabloids. She's vulnerable, maybe at breaking point. If we push a bit she might crash and burn. Prime witness gone. End of affair."

Bill pursed his lips, trying to decide on something.

"If you don't mind me asking," he said finally. "Why didn't you wait?"

"Wait?"

"Until you were sure."

"Sure about what?"

"That these things, these nanoparticles you're using don't do any harm."

Dick stared across the table. For a troubleshooter, his naivety was boundless.

"You can't say they do harm, no-one can. At least, not for certain. Anyway, do any of us know anything for certain, ever?" His response drew silence. "Most things in the world are made of chemicals. We just made them skin deep. There's only so many tests you can do, and sometimes when competitors are breathing down your neck you haven't much time to do them properly. It happens."

Bill nodded. He knew the mantra. He'd heard it from enough clients. Get product to market pronto. Sometimes, his years in homicide seemed a doddle compared to this. There the task was crystal clear: separate goodies from baddies. Here, it was more difficult. Here, they dressed in silk clothes, rubbed shoulders with lawmakers, ate in swanky restaurants, drank together at the 19th hole. At least the pay here was better. But sometimes, he wondered. That's when his conscience pricked him. So he didn't do it often. He stood up. "I'll see what I can do to calm the horses," he said, stretching out his hand. "But I'll be back again. You know they'll want regular updates."

He turned to go, then remembered something.

"I presume you've cancelled her contract."

"Lawyers found an out clause. The party, the photo, the drugs. Plenty enough to cause harm to our reputation. They're confident we're on solid ground."

"But there's no proof she took cocaine. In fact, plenty she didn't."

"I'm sure we can fix that. Anyway it's perception."

"Bet she's as angry as hell."

"Doesn't know yet. Don't want to rouse her. Anyway, I don't give a shit if she does. What's important is that the link's broken. Anyway, she signed a confidential agreement. If she spoke out, she'd be dust and she knows it. No-one would hire her."

"I see."

A few minutes later, Covington watched as the broad-shouldered man crossed the street to the parking lot opposite and got into a black Lincoln Continental. He breathed easier. But it was far from over. In fact, it was just beginning. If his plan failed, there'd be no help coming. Promises meant nothing. Bellus'd be hung out to dry. And he'd be the sacrificial lamb.

He lifted his cell phone. He needed to know. Right now.

Chapter forty-eight

If it hadn't been for a hometown rally on farm subsidies Chris attended as a high-school senior, mainly to avoid the tedium of '*Introduction to Art*,' he might have ended up as a doctor or a lab researcher. His grades in biology, physics and chemistry meant he'd have had a good shot at either. But the main speaker that particular day, a state representative with a flair for rhetoric, waxed poetic about the overriding importance of what he called 'open discourse' with such fiery passion that the soul of the timid, young teenager was stirred beyond measure. His choice of university major changed radically to public administration. His fate was sealed.

That's why an added sense of pride surged through him now, sitting as he was between two prominent leaders in heated debate. Having brought them both together, he imagined himself the pivotal cog in the wheel, the irreplaceable communication link between consumer advocate with almost four decades of health experience, Doctor E. Gray, and veteran politician, with a similar number of years in the nation's highest debating chamber, Senator Edward Clarke .

For either, it hadn't taken much persuasion. Following his telephone conversation with the doctor about nano cosmetics, he realized this would be a match made in Heaven. Aside from freeing time in their busy schedules, the main challenge was doing it with the utmost discretion, avoiding the attention of the all-seeing, all-hearing '*Prying People on the Hill*' as he collectively termed all those working inside the beltway. A medical file stolen in Kansas City, which the doctor mentioned, and the suspicious behavior of some of Barden's people during the '*Fragrance Day*' event, meant this meeting had to be as secretive as possible. If the opposition got wind of what was going on, they'd move into action instantly, upending that invaluable of all weaponry in the armory of political activism - surprise.

While Doctor Gray's lecture at the American Society of Dermatology provided convenient cover, it in itself didn't provide an adequate disguise for a one-on-one meeting with the Senator. A brainstorming session had come up with a relatively easy solution.

That's why Chris was sitting, notebook and pen in hand, in his cramped third floor Georgetown apartment a pot of coffee brewing behind him sending a wave of bitter aroma into the living room. That's why a muscular, plain-clothes guard stood outside in the corridor, observing passers-by with a casual, but expert eye. And that's why the two stalwart leaders faced each other across a small table and, understanding fully the limitations of time, grappled with the question of how best to work together towards a common goal – persuading a Senate committee that stronger regulations were necessary to rein in the cosmetics industry to better protect consumers.

"Tiny particles, huge data gaps," Doctor Gray was saying. "That's the problem in a nutshell. Federal agencies have earmarked a lot of money to uncover the potential benefits of nano, but little to uncover potential adverse health outcomes."

The Senator sat attentive, his gaze unwavering. "Is our knowledge of nano that limited?"

"So limited they're still doing tests on leaf-eating caterpillars," the doctor replied.

The Senator shook his head in disbelief.

"Not only don't we know what health hazards workers producing nanomaterials on the factory floor are facing, we don't even know what harm silver nanoparticles used as antimicrobial agents in everyday socks could do when they leach out into household washing machines and flow into wastewater treatment plants. With that in mind, consider how much greater the danger for people applying nanomaterials directly to their skin every day. When we talk about high-risk categories, nano-cosmetics is a list-topper."

Chris was finding it hard to keep up in his note-taking but there was no stopping the doctor. He was on a roll.

"It's not simply the level of toxic chemicals in nano-cosmetics we should be worried about, but also their modus operandi, how they move, how they change," he said. "As they can travel under the epidermis, the body's outer layer, and as they can aggregate in clusters, where do they go, what damage can they cause? We also know very little about what they might morph into from their original manufactured state once

224

inside our bodies. Can they interfere perversely with key biological activities that keep us alive?"

The doctor paused, as if allowing his listeners to absorb what he was saying, then continued.

"We desperately need a roadmap around what must surely rank as the largest unknown territory science and medicine has entered into during our lifetime. That means....." he stopped and began counting off on his fingers... "A taxonomy of nanoparticles. Protocols for assessing exposure through recognized national and international bodies including the Society of Toxicology, the International Society of Exposure Science and the Society for Risk Analysis. An exposure assessment toolkit. A minimum data set and standardized format to facilitate surveillance studies. A system akin to REACH. Exposure registries - lists of specific users who may be prone to nanoparticle exposure in cosmetics and other substances."

Chris had heard of REACH, an acronym for 'registration, evaluation, authorization and restriction of chemical substances,' the European Union's regulation on the safe use of chemicals. He knew the cosmetic industry would scream loud and hard to prevent its passage this side of the Atlantic. He also knew it would scream even more against the idea of a registry. 'A lawsuit just waiting to happen,' he imagined them saying.

"Who does your washing, Doctor Gray?" Clarke asked out of the blue. Chris' face shot up from his notebook. What a bizarre question?

"I beg your pardon," the doctor stammered, his face the epitome of astonishment.

"Who does your washing?" the Senator repeated deadpan.

"Well..." Doctor Gray started, uncertainty in his voice. "...there's a nice lady who does household tasks at my home... but... why do you ask?"

Clarke smiled warmly. "Because you have a helluva long laundry list."

For a few seconds, the doctor's face was a blank, then a broad smile swept across it. He chuckled, as did the Senator. Chris joined in, tickled pink his plan was working.

"Having told me - and to quote old Blue Eyes, my favorite crooner, not in a shy way - what you would like," the Senator continued, settling back to the business at hand. "How do you propose I am to extract it from my colleagues in the committee room?"

"An unusual case can sometimes trigger added interest and extensive investigation, right?" the doctor replied without hesitation, as if expecting that very question.

225

"Sometimes, not always." Hard-won experience had taught the Senator to avoid simple yes/no answers.

His answer didn't seem to faze the doctor. "And if such a case happened to be quite a well-known face, even better still, right? Especially for attracting all-important media attention."

Clarke again nodded realizing full well how esteemed colleagues in the Senate and the House had acquired a reputation, indeed a propensity, for organizing timely high-profile personality visits to attract the spotlight. It had become part and parcel of dog-and-pony public relations campaigns, feeding a popular media increasingly dominated by a menu of quick sound bites, celebrity gossip and infotainment. It wasn't his cup of tea and was frowned upon on The Hill when he was a freshman Senator, but times had changed. If it worked, if it helped keep one in office, highlighted an issue, why not. That's why he leaned forward ever so slightly now and listened even more intently.

"Such a celebrity figure could create a domino effect," the doctor continued confidently. "It could forge a favorable vote not only for greater regulation of nano but also for increased funding into researching its potential health hazards. That would mean a higher caliber of government researchers in this highly-specialized field, which, in turn, would help provide better training ground for students, the nation's future generation researchers. Ultimately leading to the saving of lives."

Clarke's mind raced. For decades Barden and his cohorts, with their vast reservoir of money, for lobbying and advertising, had toyed with him, cat with mouse, mocking his efforts for greater transparency in the cosmetic sector. Did the doctor have the silver bullet he so desperately needed to affix his name to a hallmark bill in an area he'd branded his own? A bill that would raise his political star a notch or two. Though distasteful, if it took a cause célèbre to accomplish these objectives, he'd willingly endure the inevitable media circus. But an annoying thought occurred bringing him back to earth with a thud. If the road ahead proved to be a long, drawn-out one, exhausting tests of endurance might drain whatever precious time and energy he had left to him. But that was a private matter to be dealt with another day, in another place.

"Not to sound heartless, but are you saying you've found such a person?" he asked pointedly.

"Yes."

"Please continue," the Senator said.

"A cosmetic product almost blinded a patient of mine, and put her

226

friend in a coma," the doctor replied. "Worse, I think the manufacturer was aware of the danger."

Clarke's brow furrowed, both with suspicion and interest. This was a helluva statement. But it wasn't the first time someone had exaggerated the truth simply to be heard above the din of myriad voices requesting help from him.

"Why are you so certain these problems were caused by cosmetics?" the Senator interjected. "Could it not have been a hundred other things?"

"Logic, deduction and considerable scientific probing," the doctor replied. "One of the people, free of drugs or alcohol of any kind, crashed her car on an empty road. Police officers on the scene reported her disoriented, unable to speak, rubbing her eyes frantically, complaining of severe eye irritation and vision problems. A battery of hospital tests eliminated other possible causes. And believe me, gentlemen...," he paused, looking intently at the two men..."the investigative medical team went through the entire alphabet. Blepharitis, blepharochalasis, conjunctival hyperemia, chemosis, dacryoadenitis, entropion, ectropion, ptosis - you probably know it as 'lazy eye.' You name it, the lab techs checked for it. They even stained blood samples with Giemsa looking for infective larvae of parasitic nematodes. Onchocerciasis, African worms that cause loa loa filariasis, more popularly known as river blindness. The parasite itself is transmitted through the bite of a black fly of the genus Simulium..."

He stopped. Chris and the Senator were looking at him as if he had sprouted wings.

Seeing their bewilderment, a faint blush spread across his face. "The person had been in Turkana, northwest Kenya shooting a commercial," he said quickly in explanation. "Actually, it was her mention of the commercial - for a face cream – that provided us our first clue. A bright young spark on the team hit upon the idea the problem might be cosmetic related."

"And?" the Senator asked.

"We ran tests on all of the cosmetic products she had been using. Had to search through her handbag to do it. Not surprisingly, we found the usual carcinogens – ethylacrylate, coal tar, phenylphenol, selenium sulphide, lead acetate. You're familiar with them, I'm sure."

Both men nodded. Their long battle with the cosmetic lobby meant they almost knew the toxic ingredients alphabetically off by heart.

"But the chances of chemicals in traditional face creams getting inside human cells to disturb their complex biological mechanism and cause the problems she suffered would be impossible," explained the doctor. "Our cells have a wondrous defense system, their membranes forming an ultra-protective cocoon around the inner machinery and its DNA blueprints."

"A fortress under siege with armed soldiers manning the battlements against unwanted invaders," said Chris, smiling, proud of his metaphor.

"Something like that," said the doctor, appreciating his layman's contribution. "And unless you have a passkey, the drawbridge remains firmly closed. And you certainly won't get in if you're too big, which molecules in normal creams are. Think mayonnaise and you get the idea."

"So how do you know nanoparticles were to blame?" said the Senator.

"We used optical recognition algorithms, mainly high-resolution transmission electron microscopy and in-vitro and ex-vivo studies to identify the NPs shape, size and counts in both product and patient."

"But how can you have found out so much if, as you say, very little is known about the effects of these nanoparticles?"

"While we know little about their effects on humans, we know a lot about their effects on other organisms. This provides the basis for our understanding."

"Such as?"

"Interaction of silver NPs on green algae. Metal NP studies on adult oysters and their embryos. Electrophysiological changes caused in earthworms. Aside from the normal lab species, mainly hamsters and rabbits, a variety of organisms have been used to test the efficacy of NPs. Zebrafish, rainbow trout, snails, Mediterranean mussels, Manila clams, fish…" the doctor's tone indicated he could go on ad infinitum.

"But still. Nothing on people?" the Senator queried.

"Very little. Until now. Scientists are forbidden from crossing certain ethical boundaries, which while welcome, limits research advances."

A knowing gleam sparkled in the Senator's eyes. "So this person you speak of – this cause célèbre – she's a …" he was reluctant to use the phrase, his acute political mind deeming it emotively overloaded, one that could easily be tossed back at him later. But unable to think of another, he bit the bullet. "…a human guinea pig."

The medical world being as politically explosive as the parliamentary one, the doctor took a more circuitous route in responding. "The young lady is, of course, aware of her condition and has been co-operating closely with my medical team."

Chris watched fascinated as these two titans sparred with each other,

228

testing each other's knowledge, commitment, honesty even. He noticed the corner of the Senator's mouth twitch. It was the sign he was looking for. It meant he was impressed. And if he was impressed, committee members certainly would be.

"Then we found something strange in cell cultures we'd taken. Something that confounded us."

"What?" the Senator asked, his eyes narrowing with interest.

"Botulin toxin."

"Botulin?"

"Yes, most commonly known by its trade name - Botox. The single most popular cosmetic procedure in the world today."

"You mean the problem resulted from botox injections?" exclaimed the Senator, his voice the epitome of disappointment.

"That's what was so peculiar. My patient has never had botox."

Clarke glanced quickly at Chris, then back at the doctor.

"Let me understand this right," the Senator said. "You found large quantities of botulin in her cells but you don't know where it came from?"

"Precisely," the doctor responded. "There was plenty there but it didn't come from an injection. And it didn't come from eating rotten food either, the other most common route. Otherwise, she'd have had severe stomach problems. But we had to find out where it came from, and fast. Before it paralyzed her."

"Paralyzed?" Chris asked, incredulous.

"Yes, botulism comes from the Latin word for sausage 'botulus,' the doctor answered. "First diagnosed as a food-borne disease associated with German sausages, it's a serious paralytic illness produced by the bacterium clostridium botulinum. Usually, weakness starts in facial muscles supplied by cranial nerves. Symptoms include double vision, drooping eyelids, loss of expression, as well as difficulty speaking and swallowing."

"You say you searched inside the woman's handbag. But what would be there that could cause so much difficulty...?" Chris said, rubbing his chin. Then realized, "Of course. A make-up bag, one of the most important items in there."

Doctor Gray smiled, "Precisely, and what's concealed in a make-up bag?" he asked, sounding like a lawyer leading a key witness.

A shadow clouded Chris's face, then, realizing the trick word clue, he exclaimed triumphantly, "Why concealer of course."

"Exactly, the common variety that millions of women keep in their handbags to hide blemishes," the doctor added. "The kind you see in the cosmetic aisles of countless stores up and down the country."

"But how could an innocuous thing like a concealer cause so much harm?" the Senator asked disbelieving. "For goodness sake, it's only a two-inch long thin tube, not an arrow carrying with a deadly dose of curare."

"Rogue molecules," said the doctor. "Remember, nanoparticles are infinitesimally small, thousands of times smaller than the diameter of a human hair. In cosmetics, when they cross the epidermis, they carry anti-aging ingredients deep into the dermis."

"So you think this botulin toxin infiltrated healthy cells?" asked the Senator.

"Cosmetic companies have spent much time and money finding better ways to get rid of wrinkles," the doctor replied. "Botox injections wear off so you need to keep having them to maintain the anti-aging effect. As this causes inconvenience, cosmetic companies have been falling over one another to find the best botox alternative."

"Specialized nanoparticles that deliver the goodies deep into the skin," muttered Chris.

"Buckyballs to be exact," the doctor added.

"Buckyballs? What a bizarre name?" Chris raised his hands in exasperation.

"Scientifically they're known as carbon-60 molecules formed naturally in minute quantities under extreme conditions such as lightning strikes, but they are also produced artificially as spheres or oblong-shaped balls, known as fullerenes, and are among the most common nanoparticles used in cosmetics. They carry the botulin – like a miniature donkey with a load on its back - deep into the skin to fulfill the mission they're made for. To block nerve impulses. The result - muscles that no longer contract. And wrinkles that relax and soften."

"So what's the problem?" asked Chris. "That's what botox injections have been doing for years with no major complications."

"That's not quite true actually – recent experiments have shown that the botulin - instead of dispersing into various harmless compounds as had been thought - can move beyond the injection site and into other cells, with potentially devastating consequences," the doctor said. "But we'll not go into that right now. Suffice it to say, if injections of botox could have such consequences, what could buckyballs - each carrying whole cargoes of botulin through cellular membranes right to their very core – be capable of. Unanticipated 'off-target' effects could be lethal.

And if they bioaccumulate, chronic poisoning could occur. "

"So when your patient applied the concealer, it released these botulin nanoparticles which burrowed below her skin, and did …what exactly?" asked Chris.

"In layman's terms, they attacked the optical nerve, just behind the retina, a cable carrying images of what we see to the brain. The botulin caused her vision momentarily to reduce, then dim. And finally cut out."

"But surely such a reaction would have been discovered in pre-clinical tests," said the Senator.

"Yes, but as we well know, cosmetic companies are not the most co-operative of entities. They won't reveal their testing procedures. And certainly not their results. And under present regulations, they don't have to."

"So how did you find out then?" the Senator asked.

"We conducted cell behavior simulations using high-powered computing resources."

"Which showed?"

"How buckyball particles can dissolve in cell membranes, pass into cells and re-form particles which cause damage."

"And how did you detect this toxin in your patient?"

"Enzyme-linked immunosorbent assays, known as ELISAs, a biochemical technique. Electrochemiluminescent tests, most commonly called ECLs, and mass spectrometry. We also used a nerve conduction method called electromyography, or EMG. To differentiate botulism from other diseases that manifest in the same way, we also conducted a tensilon test for myasthenia gravis, a neuromuscular disorder that involves the muscles and the nerves that control them."

"Very thorough research indeed, I'm impressed," said the Senator, his mind already focusing on how best to parlay the information he was hearing to committee members.

"We had to be," the doctor replied somberly. "Lives were, are, at stake."

"No disrespect intended, but you said this botulin could paralyze," Chris said. "As this patient could be very important to us if she agrees to testify, what's her condition?"

"Paralysis occurs if the toxin has made its way to the brain stem, using the nerve cells as stepping stones," the doctor replied. "We conducted brain scans and cerebrospinal fluid examinations, but found no evidence the toxin had gone that far. Yet."

"Hopefully, she will be fine, please keep us informed," said the

Senator leaning back in his seat, pondering. "The scientific data I presume you could provide us may persuade enough committee members to our way of thinking, but...." He hesitated. "Ultimately, it'd be a case of your evidence against that of the cosmetic reps. And let's be perfectly frank, they're rich and powerful, and they can bring in boatloads of experts. The only element that separates this particular lobbying effort from previous failed ones is if this woman you speak about creates a cause célèbre. If she can speak out publicly and attract widespread media attention it could create a whole new dynamic, give us the popular momentum to push through what we want, an historic, far-ranging bill."

Doctor Gray's eyes lit up with renewed hope. Before the telephone call from Chris, he had been under a dark cloud. Theft of the documents had led the paparazzi to Patricia's whereabouts, the last thing he'd wanted to happen. He feared for her sanity in face of such renewed publicity. He was sure the cosmetic company had tipped off the celebrity magazine and would control the tone of the story that would be published, a character assassination job. He'd also heard on the academic grapevine that Bellus had approached his university's Board of Regents with an enticing offer. He knew full well what that meant. He was running out of time and options. Support from the Senator was vital if he was to have any chance of succeeding. Now it seemed he was on the verge of getting it. The problem was the cause célèbre. With Christine in a coma and Patricia undecided about speaking publicly, he hadn't much to offer. Hopefully, this would change. Until then, he needed to make sure the Senator did not leave this meeting thinking he was simply an anti-nano doomsayer on an emotional crusade because of his daughter's untimely death.

"Let me just say that while I'm concerned about lack of proper regulations, some NP applications can be medically beneficial. They could transport drugs directly to damaged or malignant cells, providing much sought-after cures for deadly conditions. Brain cancer, for example."

The Senator shifted suddenly in his seat.

"That's because drugs are far more effective if they're delivered through the membrane, directly into the cell," Doctor Gray continued. "Viruses long ago developed ways of sneaking through cell walls but now scientists are using nanoparticles to mimic them to transport drugs to the right places, even inside the brain itself," he said. "By using non-toxic pieces of protein, and incorporating buckyballs as passkeys, they can zero in precisely and kill certain cancer cells. Imagine the drug carried by the buckyball to be the chocolate filling of an M&M and you'll have a better idea of what I'm saying."

"And it works?" the Senator exclaimed, his expression taking on added intensity.

"Well, it's at the experimental stage, but results are promising."

"How long before they'll know for sure?"

"Who knows? Could be months, could be years."

"What's the most likely of the two?"

"Hard to say," the doctor replied, surprised by the Senator's sudden rapid-fire questions. "It's not just the speed of research but the regulatory framework within which it must be conducted."

"I see," the Senator murmured as if to himself. "The perils of bio-ethics, eh? Regulations prevent people being harmed, but can also impede research that might save lives. A double-edged sword."

"I'm afraid so."

The Senator sat back, pensive, a sudden thought having entered his mind. In life, he'd learned, all things were possible and the possible became probable fast, especially if a lot was at stake. If his enemies suspected his secret, it would be perfectly natural for them to send in a doctor to tease it out of him. He scrutinized the doctor's face, searching for a glimmer in his eyes, a subtle clue all was not as it seemed. But he could detect nothing. The man had given a perfectly acceptable explanation why he was here. His tone was sincere and his mastery of scientific detail supported his narrative. Also, he hadn't asked a single question remotely connected to his health. Applying the brakes of reason to his racing mind, the Senator took a deep breath. He was on safe ground. His secret safe. For the moment.

But what he'd just learned placed him in a conundrum. Two opposing options, with himself a potential winner no matter which he chose. Regulate use of nanoparticles? And save others. Or accelerate it? And save himself. Which was of greater importance?

Chapter forty-nine

...would overshadow the Saint Louis Post Dispatch...
...presentation at Columbia University, your own alma mater...
...acceptance speech ...nation's elite... politicians, academics, fellow publishers...

McCarthy's words echoed in Browne's ears, sending him trawling 'Pulitzer' on the Internet to remind himself of the details.

'Two and three-quarter inches in diameter, one-quarter inch thick. Silver with 24-carat gold plate. On one side, Benjamin Franklin, based on the bust by French sculptor Jean-Antoine Houdon. The words 'Honoris Causa' inscribed there. On the flip side, a husky, bare-chested man, his shirt draped across the end of a printing press. Around him, the words: 'For disinterested and meritorious public service rendered by an American newspaper...'

Should he be delighted he'd chosen such a formidable person to lead the Kansas City paper or furious at him for putting him in such a dilemma? If Leland's finances were rosier, the decision would be easy. But advertising dollars were scarce these days and desperate times call for desperate measures. Covington had called personally to say the contract was on its way. The offer from Bellus was gilt-wrapped, one not to be refused.

Not that he wasn't tempted by McCarthy's idea. *'Fellow publishers...'* He imagined himself on the podium as applause faded saying the words, merely out of respect, but really it would be superiority draped in modesty. After thirty years in the business didn't he deserve such plaudits? Hadn't he taken his turn dutifully at the helm of the Newspaper Publishers Association during the most difficult of times, when profit margins had taken the first of many nose-dives, when others were too frightened to lead, acting like deer in the headlights. Accepting the most coveted of all media awards would be the sweetest of cherries on the cream cake of The Kansas City Tribune's centennial celebrations.

Ever since 1917 when first unveiled, it had become the most sought-after recognition in the print media industry. The crowning reward for painstaking hours, days, weeks, months, sometimes years, investigating the nation's myriad halls of power – from politics to medicine, from banking to education to industry. For journalists, it meant countless meetings, often listening to convoluted gobbledygook, and the slow, dissection of mountains of documents searching for scraps of incriminating evidence. For publishers, it meant daring, backbone, sheer determination, facing the inevitable wrath of the guilty and the powerful, more often than not the two being one and the same.

It had become a Spring ritual for him for the past two decades. Taking the day off – a rare occasion in itself – he'd make the short walk to Mario's for his usual wash and trim. Home, a leisurely shower, his best silk shirt from the walk-in closet where it hung under plastic ready for such an elevated occasion. Then, his wife checking his bow-tie wasn't askew, he'd step outside to a sleek limousine to take him to the lofty Doric columns fronted by Daniel Chester French's sculpture of the goddess Athena.

Inside the ornate Rotunda of Columbia University's most impressive building, topped by the largest all-granite dome in the country, he'd enjoyed the lively company of astute men and women of a similar ilk discussing over fine wine and fine food the latest twists and turns of the public – and sometimes private – lives of the high and the mighty.

Every year, seated at an elegant table among the nation's best and brightest he'd applauded achievements. Of others, however, never his own. With each succeeding year, the hard edge of disappointment, had softened, hut hadn't dissipated. The whiff of possibility lingered, keeping the annual Pulitzer Prize Awards ceremony at the Low Memorial Library on his list of 'must-go' events. Only once had he considered striking it off. The year the best feature story award eluded the 'big league' players and came to the Midwest - to Missouri, the Show-Me state, the place where his own career had flourished. That was the sweet part. The bitter was that it had gone, not to Kansas City, but to the east side of the state - to the man he himself had once hired as a mid-level manager.

He recalled the words of the Pulitzer chairman: "You and your staff have joined the highest American aristocracy of ideas and standards of excellence that others must follow. Your life's work has been accomplished and society is all the better for your efforts."

He remembered Bill Barlow, publisher of The St. Louis Post Dispatch, a man whose career he had launched, returning from the stage to rousing cheers from colleagues, his face aglow, his normal doleful expression transformed to that of a child, favorite toy in hand. Sitting in the 'midwest section,' Browne had congratulated him, of course. Firm handshake, broad smile, celebratory pat on the back. Part of him felt proud. Missouri recognized on the media map, usurping the nationals with their big-dollar spend and far-flung arrogance. Good for the whole state, east and west. Would help raise journalism standards, attract more students to local media. Everyone would benefit. He accepted that. But it wasn't easy. Because it wasn't his prize.

Out of collegiate politeness he had been handed the award nestling in an elegant, cherry-wood box with brass hardware. No sooner had he read the inscription, '*Gold Medal Public Service Award*,' than his stomach churned, leaving him as close to being physically sick in a public place as he'd ever felt. Oh, how he'd wished mightily there and then that the newspaper name engraved on it could be magically transformed.

Sitting alone now, these thoughts raced through his mind like wind rushing through a tunnel. But then he remembered the P&L pie charts, the bar graphs, the changing colors when he'd inserted Covington's ad figures, how the red turned sweetly to black.

His fingers drummed a rapid rhythm on the desk. Money or glory? A choice needed to be made. And fast.

Chapter fifty

The house was empty. A quick look and instinctively he knew it. It betrayed a sense of abandonment, of being locked up and left to its own devices. He went through the motions. Knocking, then banging, on back and front doors, peering through windows, shouting out her name. Where could she have gone?

A first thought, dismaying though it was, rushed headlong at him. Home. Had she simply packed her bags and left? In blind panic, headed for the airport? Understandable in the circumstances. She'd been doing it most of her life anyway. Hopping on and off planes, each city, each country a transit point on the way to… where finally? A bit like himself really, searching… but for what? Was he trying to trade the present for the past, to do now what he hadn't been able to do before?

Not for the first time, a feeling of not belonging, of being between places, enveloped him, leaving him hollow. A shadow in a breeze. He shook himself from his reverie. He needed to be in the present, not the past.

Their encounter on the beach earlier hadn't exactly been Cupid's finest hour. They'd been more like unruly children than star-crossed lovers. Still, he couldn't help smiling, remembering how they'd tumbled over each other, then sprawled side-by-side spread-eagled on the sand. Deliciously enticing, if under different circumstances. Then a notion struck him. Did he miss her? How could that be? He'd barely spoken a few words to her and what snatches of conversation they'd managed were more warmongering than peacemaking. Miss her? There was nothing to miss. An angry woman. What's to miss in that?

She'd called Doctor Gray. He'd told him when he called earlier. He hadn't said anything about her leaving. Would he have? Was he completely trustworthy? After all that had happened, yes, he thought so.

Okay, so she's not on a plane. Where then? He had little time. Paparazzi had money aplenty. When they woke up, they'd be doling it out generously for info. And they hunted in packs. More would probably arrive. They'd find her, devour her. Then what? She'd be hurt bad. It'd be too much to take. Feverishly he tried to think of what to do. Only then, did he realize the one thing he hadn't considered. His yearned-for exclusive, his badge of recognition. It'd be one of a million other what-if stories reporters carried to their graves, torn lottery numbers fluttering in the wind. What he'd been dreaming of, what he'd gone to America for, what might have banished the phantoms - would itself be banished. So why hadn't he thought of it first, not Patricia's safety? He tore his mind away from the reason why. He could work that out later. He hadn't much time. Who could help him? Ernie? Ivan? He pulled his cell phone from his pocket, cursed loudly. Of all people, they were the only ones on the entire planet, from Bermuda to Borneo, not connected to the mobile world. Walking anachronisms, they were, one living on an island and the other in the past, his head full of faeries. He thought hard. Bunbeg pier, at the edge of town. Ernie went there a lot, catching herring and sea trout. '*Illegally*'. He'd said the word with pride. '*What the European Union and Bord Iascaigh Mhara don't know, doesn't do 'em any harm. Common EU Fisheries Policy my arse. We only get the tiddlers them Norwegians toss back.*'

Colm was bounced all over the seat as his car raced along the bumpy slice of road, the dark bogs either side threatening to swallow him if he faltered. Seeing them, he shivered, remembering the grim story in the pub the previous night. Being stuck there in the dead of night with ghosts, bog-people, call them what you will, rising out of the dank, bone-sucking earth was not an attractive proposition. After a mile or so, far below him he could make out a clump of miniscule figures near one of the boats. Blurred at first like an image in a faded photograph, he recognized her among them. It wasn't too difficult. She was sitting in the stern wearing a hat with what looked like a feather sticking out of the top. What local would wear a hat, never mind one with a feather in it, in a place like this on such a windy day, on a boat? What's to be expected from a fashionista. A smile escaped his lips.

He pushed down on the accelerator. He didn't know if he could make it before they left harbor. A man in a cap stood on the stone pier, a mooring rope in his hand. Ernie. He was releasing the boat. Another man was walking towards the front cabin. Suddenly a copse of trees blocked Colm's view. He tried driving faster, but couldn't. The bends in the road were too sharp. Then, passing a clearing, he glanced down again. Ernie was throwing the rope into the boat, the man catching it as it spun towards him like a coiled cobra. Colm leaned forward, narrowing his eyes to get a better look. Impatiently, he banged his hand hard on the steering wheel. The thud inadvertently shifted the car's direction. A brick wall appeared out of nowhere. He hit the brake and wrenched desperately at the wheel, but it was too late. Engine screaming, the car twisted this way and that, collided with a sharp edge of stone, careened over the tops of some gorse bushes, threatened to topple over then righted itself, stalling indignantly in the middle of an open muddy field. Fear lighting up their eyes, sheep scattered instantly in all directions. Cursing loudly, Colm tried to re-start. The engine spluttered, coughed, gave out. He waited a few seconds, trying to stay calm, his heart racing. He turned the key again. Again nothing but a grind sound. He cursed loudly, waited a minute, tried again. This time the engine erupted into action. Reversing fast, he screeched out on the narrow road again A few more turns and he'd be at the edge of the pier. Far below him, he heard a spluttering sound like someone with bad lungs, then a soft, rhythmic throbbing.

A few minutes later, turning a last corner on to a makeshift parking lot, he saw Ernie, his arm in the air, waving. Beyond him, leaving a thick line of white foam in its wake, a boat had pulled out of the narrow channel headed for deeper waters. He could make out Patricia's back turned to him. Just then, up ahead, two men stepped out of a Landrover and headed towards Ernie. One of them threw a camera bag hastily over his shoulder. In an instant, Colm realized who they were. Oh, Christ.

* * *

Ernie wondered if he should be worried. It wasn't what Patricia said, more what she didn't. Barely a hello. Just wanted to go to Gola. Fast.

He was in the middle of thinking when he heard footsteps behind him.

"Hello, nice day isn't it? We're sure lucky with the weather."

No-one said 'sure' 'roun here like that. It had to be a Yank.

"Nae bad, nae bad at all, buiochas le Dia," Ernie replied, turning and taking in the two men standing before him. He'd guess late 20s. Dressed in the kind of jackets he remembered seeing on television. Not the kind people dressed in 'round here.' Bright yellow and red. More like a set of traffic lights. A wee multi-colored parachute maybe.

"Gary Kramer," one of the men said, stepping forward and shooting out his hand. Ernie looked at it, not knowing what to do. People didn't do much of that roun' here either. No need. Everyone knew each other. And their cousin's cousin. The Sweeneys, the Gallaghers, the Dohertys, all inter-related. Seeing his hesitation, the man withdrew his hand, embarrassed. Just as Ernie stretched out his. A bit of fumbling ensued. Hands going backward and forward, 'a rusty saw biting through a length of wood' was how Ernie put it later in the pub.

"Wonder if you could help us," he asked. "Will sure make it worth your while." He waited for a response to his offer, but getting none, continued.

"We're looking for a lady by the name of Patricia," he said. "Were told she might be over on one of the islands." He paused. Still no response. Ernie was thinking.

"We need to find her as quick as possible. Could you bring us there?"

"Will sure make it worth your while," the other added.

Ernie found it peculiar the man repeated exactly what his friend had just said. Did they think he couldn't understand English? Or the American version of it at least. Sure hadn't he a brother in New York this past forty years. He understood the lingo right well. Movie theatre. Parking lot. Potato chip. Or was it that the offer was so extraordinary - a rocket ride to the moon perhaps – that it needed to be said twice?

"I have a boat alright," he replied. Slow as it goes, he thought, give the brain space to work.

"That's great, we'll sure make it worth your…"

Not wishing to hear it again, Ernie interrupted. "Ahve a boat, but ah don't have oars." It was the best excuse he could come up with on such short notice. The two men stared at him. He thought they'd burst out laughing. He nearly did. Because they didn't. But he kept it in.

"Do you think you could get some?" one of them said.

"Aye, I suppose so."

"Like right now."

"Aye."

He pretended to look around. That's when he noticed Colm's car and he inside, his puzzled eyes watching him. "Ahll just go have a look," he said and sauntered off. This is turning into quite a day, he thought, mischief writ all over his face.

"Don't help those guys," Colm burst out in a low tone sticking his head out of the car window as he approached. "I know what they're up to. They're bad news."

Ernie held up his hand. "Easy now me boyo. You'll crack a vein in yer head."

"You don't understand. They're working for a..."

"Now no need ta get yoursel' in a twist. They jus' wanna go ta the islands. And they've asked me ta bring 'em there. Said it'll be well worth ma while."

"Jesus, Ernie, they're paparazzi chasing Patricia. You wouldn't sell yourself for a few miserable pennies, would you?"

"More than just a few pennies, ahm thinkin,' a chara. I'd say a fat bundle o' crisp dollar notes. The ones with a photo of ye're man Grant across the front."

An incongruous thought leaped into Colm's head: How on earth did Ernie know what was on the front of a fifty-dollar bill? Ignoring the urge to ask, he said between clenched teeth.

"Do that, Ernie, and you'll be judged a Judas to your dying day."

Ernie put his hand on the roof of the car and leaned over. "All ahm sayin' is that these men asked if ah could take 'em to the islands, an' sure wouldn't that be the proper Christian thing ta do. What harm can they do? Sure won't I be watching them?"

Colm began to protest more but Ernie had turned on his heels and was on his way back up the pier. He felt like jumping out of the car and running after him, but the two men were peering towards him up along the pier. They could have been given a photo of him and might recognize him. Then what? Try to talk them out of it? Say he was here first? They'd laugh in his face. What could he do?

***

"Old friend?" one of the men asked as Ernie approached.

"More an old idiot," was the terse reply.

Ernie pointed to a small boat nearby with a narrow, chimney-like cabin, the words 'Cara na Mara' painted in bright letters along its bow. And 'Friend of the Sea,' she's about to be, he thought, hiding a smile.

"You have an engine," one of the men said seeing the outboard motor.

"Aye."

"I thought you hadn't."

"No, ah said ah'd no oars."

The man stood nonplussed. "But if you have an engine, do you need oars?"

"Not anymore."

241

The two men shot confused glances at each other. Then shrugged their shoulders and stepped on board.

Chapter fifty-one

What the hell was going on out there? The question reverberated through Colm's head as he stared out to sea.

'*Cara na Mara*' was certainly not living up to her name, zigzagging in long, lazy loops back and forth across the bay, rushing headlong, recklessly even, tossing up great swathes of frothy foam either side of her as she swerved this way and that. Hardly the sort of smooth sailing that entitled her to be called '*Friend of the Sea.*'

Colm had no idea what was happening but it looked serious. The boat seemed completely out of control. Had Ernie lost his marbles? In their rush to get to Patricia, had the two on board taken over? Hardly. They'd probably never been in a boat in their lives and certainly not in waters like these. If they hit a rock at full speed they'd be dead. Plenty of them out there, all with strange sounding names. Tor an Ui Arragain. Tor na Sceardain. Tor na gColpach. Tor being Irish for rock. He'd seen them marked on the framed ordinance survey map on the wall of his hotel. Veritable underwater, stepping-stones across Gaoth Dobhair Bay, and far beyond. Several thousand miles beyond. In launching its 'Wild Atlantic Way,' a marketing program to tempt more Americans to spend their hard-earned dollars here, the Irish tourism board had announced they were the undersea remnants of the same mountain range as the Appalachians. The rocks had also been the ruin of the Spanish Armada, a fleeing flotilla of 130 galleons sent by Philip II to help Irish chieftains against their English overlords five hundred years before. Among them, the San Juan de Sicilia, splintered on these very rocks, with two hundred sailors drowned. That's how Robert Louis Stevenson came to write 'Treasure Island,' Ernie had told him. After a summer visit, hearing Gola Island was mispronounced by English soldiers as 'Gold Island' because chests of gold doubloons on the galleons had fallen to the ocean floor, his writer's imagination went into overdrive. If those rocks could sink an Armada, they could certainly sink Ernie and his two hapless photographers, making them literally, 'friends of the sea.'

Standing on the pier, Colm was at a loss what to do. Then he remembered. The coastguard station, it was at the other end of the pier. The large white paneled building, with steel sliding doors in front. Turning on his heels, he rushed there. He twisted on the door handle. It was locked. He peered inside through the glass. There was a large rescue boat there but no people. He ran around to the rear searching for other ways in. There was none. Out of breath, he ran back along the pier.

Just then, he heard a spluttering sound near him. He glanced sideways, seeing a mop of curly hair bobbing up and down in a wooden boat over the edge of the seawall. Something about it was familiar. He took a step closer. The thin angular back, the wiry arms and legs. The lugubrious expression that turned instantly into a childlike grin when the man gazed up at him in recognition from the stern of his boat.

"Jesus, Seamus, am I glad to see you. I need your help, quickly."

Chapter fifty-two

"So, do you come here often?"

Ernie remembered the line from a TV program. He liked it. Smooth as creamy porridge it was. Came sliding off the tongue buttery-like. Once thought of saying it to the pretty widow McCreavy when he spied her in the shop buying milk and sugar near Magheroarty Pier one Wednesday afternoon but decided not to. The priest might hear and be after more money for a good word-in.

They'd been on his boat fifteen minutes and he'd used his best mis-steering skills to frazzle them, but if he didn't say something they might suspect what he was up to and give him what for. He was one and they were two and they were younger, more muscular lads. Time to see if his plan was working.

"Are ye alright back there?" he ventured.

For all the response he got, he might as well have said he was the King of Africa. He stole a glance back from the wheelhouse. The two men were both bent over, heads between their knees, lost in their own world, a rather frightening one by the looks of it, their faces when they lifted them slowly to him as white as bottles of milk. Their eyes were closed, tight as crab shells. He could see the gargantuan efforts they were making to keep 'em that way. Gritting their teeth like they were munching cinders, their cheeks round and bloated like goldfish, their hands grasping the side rail for dear life. He spun the steering wheel again for good luck, first one way, then the other.

Moments later, he remembered, and got worried. The cleaning and repainting job had cost him twenty-two euro, including sandpaper, varnish and a new set of screws. The side-rail was a shiny shade of blue that matched the sea on a fine day. He'd just finished it the day before. He wondered if they'd have the decency to turn their heads, gentleman like, and do their business over the side. Maybe he'd overdone it. Didn't want a thick rainbow coating all over the beam. Would take ages to get off, the smell even longer. Better slow down. He eased back on the accelerator. Too late. He heard groaning, then a series of hollow thuds. He cursed inwardly, the sound all too familiar from city folk up on fishing trips from Derry and Dublin with no sea legs. The kind that didn't know a grub from a grasshopper, a cod from a catfish. He didn't bother turning round. Nothing he could do now. Just the hose, a wet rag and a big dose o' elbow grease when he'd get back. Hopefully, it'd not need a second paint job.

"Amadan," he spat out the Irish word for 'fool.' Aimed both at himself and his annoying guests.

For good measure, he did a few more loop de loops round the bay. He smiled, beginning to enjoy the ride. In fact, the more they didn't, the more he did.

Chapter fifty-three

Driftwood. That's what she was. Floating gently along a meandering river, melodic bird calls the only sounds interrupting the tranquility around her. Worries wheeled away like seagulls in an endless sky. Lulled into a trance she didn't ever want to end. But yet it seemed as if it was. She could feel herself rising from the depths of sleep to which she had slipped, emerging from the soft cocoon that had enwrapped her so comfortingly. Webs of frustration curled around her like wisps of smoke as her senses slowly awakened, signaling a return to harsh reality. The soothing warmth on her back and shoulders and neck, the rhythmic sound of the sea somewhere beyond where she lay, they seemed to be fading like a passing dream.

"You certainly enjoyed yourself," a quiet voice said nearby. "Sorry it had to end. Returning to the world of the real is never easy."

Slowly, with immense effort, Patricia blinked.

"I've made a nourishing herbal infusion for you, lots of natural goodies in it, from land and sea," the voice continued, encouragingly. "Should help you recover."

"It was wonderful, Ivan," she mumbled sleepily, recognizing the voice.

"Who'd have thought a slab of slimy bog mud could be so delectable, eh?" he replied jovially. "Pure Peruvian chocolate isn't half as satisfying."

Pulling the sheet that covered her ever more tightly around her, Patricia swung her legs over the edge of the bed and sat up, dizzy from the effort.

"I met an old farmer here once who told me when he was a child he slipped and scalded his hand on a hot pan," Ivan said. "Described his skin as looking like burned feathers. His mother scooped him up, ran out the door and put him on the handlebars of her bicycle. He thought she was rushing him off to the local doctor. Instead, she rushed to the bog where she wrapped his hand in thick layers of mud. Kept his hand that way for four days. When unwrapped he said you could hardly tell it had been damaged at all."

"So that's the kind of miracle I can expect?" she asked, more fully awake.

"Expect? Have you not had a close look in the mirror recently? Your scars will look like a few specks of sugar compared to what they were."

"In my business even a pimple is life-threatening."

"Time and patience," Ivan replied, encouragingly. "I'll not say you'll be rushing back to New York tomorrow to model the latest skincare cream under the glare of the spotlight. But a few more treatments and you'll have to look real close to see anything wrong. And what the turf and its precious sphagnum and humic acids don't fix, my insect skin creams will." He leaned forward examining her face and neck closely.

Satisfied with his examination, he leaned back in his chair. "You came in here a bit frantic, but you'd tell me nothing. Are you okay now?"

Patricia glanced over at the burly, bearded man, his eyes filled with concern. She wondered, and not for the first time, if she deserved the kind of devoted attention he'd bestowed upon her.

"Have you ever known me not to be okay?" Said in jest, it was a joke well shared. When she'd first arrived in Donegal, she'd been the delicate leaf, quivering and frail and ready to fall. Ivan, the sturdy oak tree. She'd needed no encouragement to shelter under his broad sweeping branches.

"C'mon, young lady, out with it," he said. "That's an order."

"I met with that journalist, Colm Heaney," she said, matter-of-factly.

"Aha, I see," he said, rolling his eyes melodramatically. "And romance blossomed between the bog and the beach."

"More a battle between the bog and the beach," she said joining him at the nearby table where he'd set a pot of tea and cups.

"And?"

"We parted fast, moving in opposite directions."

"Not a meeting of hearts and minds then?"

"Not quite."

"So how did you get into such a mighty showdown?"

"He was trying to tell me he could help."

"Oh my, who writes his lines? That's the worst thing anyone could ever have said to you. How dare he?" He scrunched up his face in mockery.

"Funny funny ha ha."

"I hope you put him in his place."

"What do you think?"

"My best guess is he's nursing a broken ego, if not a broken nose."

"You think that little of me after all we've been through together?" She gave him a playful slap on the shoulder.

"So now you're feeling guilty, is that it?"

"Don't you start."

"Start? I'm just warming up."

Patricia knew what he was thinking. She'd heard it before. *'It's been quite some time and while I've certainly enjoyed seeing the healing benefits of my bog potions and creams on your scars, I can't do much to heal the other wounds... the internal ones... so'...* And she'd always reacted in the same way, making a fast exit. Now, much to her own surprise, her reaction was different. "I don't know. I simply don't know." She stared hard at the wood floor at her feet as if the answer lay there somewhere, trapped between the cracks.

"Doctor Gray trusts this reporter," Ivan said encouragingly. "And we both trust Gray. So perhaps, well, perhaps you should give him a chance. You've been emotionally paralyzed for far too long. Time to shake yourself out of it. Take a step forward, a leap even."

"You mean give him the precious interview he wants?"

"Would that be so bad?" he continued. "People seem to have heard every version of the story except yours. Maybe now's the time to tell it."

"I don't want to be paraded in front of people like some pathetic wounded animal."

"Whether you want to or not, my dear, the truth is that it's already been done. And not as a wounded animal either but a wounding one." His heart sank seeing the grimace on her face as he said that. He knew what he was saying hurt but he pushed on through her pain.

"Look, I understand it isn't easy," he said. "I know how hard it's been for you. But you've got to break out. Maybe this is the way. I don't think this Colm fellow wants to do you any harm. Yes, he's interested in your story but that's only natural. He's a reporter after all. And a pretty damn good one according to Gray and the articles I've read. But he also seems sympathetic."

"Maybe, but it doesn't matter anymore. The situation's all changed."

"Changed?" Ivan said, surprised. "How?"

"Paparazzi arrived. From *'Celebrity News'* in New York."

Ivan's mouth fell open. "You're kidding." Seeing from her expression that she wasn't, he added, "Oh boy, now that is a problem."

"Tell me."

"So that's why you're here. On a non-treatment day."

"I needed to hide somewhere. And this seemed the best place. It is an island after all. They'll hardly find me here. But I didn't want to worry you by telling you earlier."

"Well, thank you, but still... what are we going to do?"

"You aren't going to do anything. I'm not mixing you up in all this."

"My dear lady, I already am, whether you like it or not."

Patricia looked across at him, realizing for the umpteenth time how lucky she was to have people like him and Gray and Ernie rooting for her. Ivan didn't notice her smile of gratitude. He was too busy deep in thought.

"I'd say you've no alternative," he said finally." You've got to speak to this reporter.... "

"See what I mean. It's all about the story."

"My dear, when all's said and done that's what life is – a series of stories. At least this time it's your story." He hesitated then, as if judging the moment. "Maybe you should also speak at the hearing."

Patricia went silent for a moment. "Look, I'm not a speaker, I'm a model. For clothes, for face creams. I'm a poser. A catnip for glossy magazine editors and gossip columnists everywhere. That's what I've done all my life, I'm good at it and I'm not ashamed to say so."

"No-one's saying you should be. But what if you're more than that. You'll never know till you've tried."

Ivan folded his hands under his chin as if deciding something, then continued, a subtle change in his tone. "Look, I'm going to tell you something. Something nobody around here knows. Except for Gray over there cos under that austere exterior he's a rebel at heart." He hesitated, as if deciding how best to begin. "I was in prison once."

She looked at him in astonishment. "You? In prison? I can't imagine it."

"And I don't mean overnight in the drunk tank either. For quite a long time. Two years to be exact. I can almost remember every minute of it. Not too difficult. There's nothing much else to do in a gulag but remember."

Seeing Patricia's eyes widen in shock, he added quickly, "Not gulag as in Aleksandr Solzhenitsyn and his archipelago. I wasn't worked to death, obviously, as I'm still here. But I almost died – of sheer boredom. A fate worse than death in many ways."

"Why were you sent there?"

"Crimes against the state. At least, that's how the charges read."

"Crimes against the state? What does that mean?

"Anything an upstanding member of Soviet internal security wants it to be."

"And in your case?"

"I believed my scientific colleagues and I in the research center where I worked should be spending more of our time on pursuing what I called constructive applied biomedical research. Finding cures for certain cancers, for example. Instead of developing deadly biological weapons, a less-than-worthy vocation at the best of times, but even less so when you know they're never going to be used."

"So? It's not a crime to hold an opinion."

"Oh how I used to envy people like you," Ivan said, shaking his head. "People who take their freedoms for granted. People who don't have to worry about speaking out against something they thought was wrong. You guys have it good. And some of you, maybe most of you, still don't seem to appreciate it."

Patricia's lips puckered in a frown.

"Don't get me wrong," Ivan said soothingly. "I don't mean it as an insult. I just mean we should cherish the precious freedoms we have. People, probably some of them our very own ancestors, fought and died for them. It's an insult to their memories if we simply sit back lackadaisically and take what they did for granted."

"It seems you didn't."

"I tried, but failed miserably. Trapped by my own naivety, and my own ego. Over lunches, over dinners, in the labs, over weekend vodka marathons, I tried to spread the gospel, my gospel, the gospel according to Saint Ivan." The big bearded bear of a man beside her began chuckling, "The secret police, their informants in the research center, their bellies must have been sore from laughing. I went around telling anyone who'd listen that we should go on strike. Even wrote out a specific set of demands. I spent hours telling my colleagues my carefully laid plans. And the informers among them – without as much as a simple thank you – passed it on to their masters. And were well-rewarded for their efforts, I'm sure. Why, if I remember well, some of them were even taking notes as I rambled on. How's that for revolutionary stealth and cunning, eh?"

Patricia felt a surge of sentiment for this gentle grizzly giant sitting across from her. "You did your best. No-one can fault you for that."

"I suppose so," he answered, his face reddening.

A few seconds of silence passed between them, then Patricia spoke up. "So you're telling me I should stand up." It was a statement, but meant as a question.

"I'm not telling you to do anything. All I'm saying is that some things are worth fighting for. That it's important to stand up for what you believe in....sometimes. Did I say sometimes? I mean always," Ivan seemed to hesitate, then continued with a half-smile "Well, actually, *always* is a very long time. Best to start with sometimes and take it from there." His gaze fixed upon her. "But only you can decide if this is one of those times." A mischievous expression appeared on his face, "But I would ask one thing from you. If you do decide to take action, no matter what it is, please, please don't do it the way I did. I couldn't survive another such disaster."

Patricia leaned over and gave him a peck on the cheek. She knew he only wanted the best for her, but ...

"How do you know when it is the right time?" she asked finally.

"Believe me, you'll know. Your soul will tell you."

Just then, a loud continuous banging on the front door startled them, sending droplets of hot tea bouncing on to the table over the rim of their cups. Eyes wide, they stared at each other unblinking, the unfamiliar urgency of the sound echoing in their ears.

Chapter fifty-four

The door burst open before they could reach it, ushering in a blast of cool salty air. Colm stumbled forward, out of breath and agitated, his feet clattering on the bare stone hallway.

"Where are they? Did you see them?" he gasped.

"See who?" Ivan answered puzzled.

"The reporter, the photographer."

"How would we know?" Patricia snapped back automatically, annoyance in her voice. "They're your colleagues. You're the one who should know."

Colm stared at her dumbfounded.

"Didn't you say reporters run in packs?" she reminded him. The words were out before she realized how unfair they were. Deep down she knew. Colm had come to help, not hurt her. And here she was, throwing harsh words in his face as if he was guilty of some heinous crime. She stayed silent, looking at him steadfastly. For a split second, something passed between them, something real yet intangible.

"Would you care to join us for a nice cup of tea," Ivan said, attempting to calm the situation. "Guaranteed to raise your spirits. Leaves picked by my very own hands - on an herbaceous excursion along the Amazon."

Colm's gaze switched from the woman whose face had uncharacteristically softened, to the bearded man with the childlike grin.

"Would love to but these guys... they're on their way. In fact, I thought they'd be here already and I'd not be able to warn you in time....so maybe...," he glanced over at Patricia, half-expecting a caustic comment. None came, surprising him greatly.

"Maybe what?" Ivan asked.

"Maybe we should get out of here. Pronto. Before they get here."

"Mmmm," Ivan murmured turning to Patricia. "It's your call. They're chasing you not me and my precious insects."

Colm's gaze followed his. Patricia felt the intensity of their stares. Events were rushing past too fast for her to keep up, leaving no time to think. She felt cornered like a wild animal. That's why she had gone to the island and Ivan and not to the nearest airport. It was the only safe place she knew.

"I suppose," she said finally, unsure.

"Suppose?" ventured Ivan.

"I mean…," she hesitated. "I don't want to bring trouble on you."

"After what I've just told you about me, do you really think these milk-sucking, latte-loving guys could cause me much trouble? I'm Ivan the Invincible. Remember?"

Patricia's face became a smile. She flung her arms around him. Taken completely by surprise, the big man's mouth dropped, but he accepted her embrace warmly.

Somewhat embarrassed, Colm turned away, puzzled by this beautiful woman's abrupt change of behavior, her erstwhile rigidity and severe self-control giving way to this spontaneous display of sentiment.

"Seamus is at the pier in the boat, keeping an eye out," he ventured finally. "He's ready to take us back to the mainland."

Ivan nodded, disengaging himself from Patricia. "Look, guys, the best plan is that I stay here and you both go on. That way, if they do come, I can stall them."

"How?" Patricia asked concerned.

"Don't worry, I'll think of something. I'll serve them up roasted millipedes on a plate if I have to. Better still, I'll have my little termites feed on them. That should stop them in their tracks."

The other two looked at him strangely.

"Just joking," he said. "My poor critters would only get indigestion."

They moved to the open doorway and bid their goodbyes. "Sorry you can't stay for a cuppa and a wee chat," said Ivan. "Another time."

Colm acknowledged the invite with a handshake. Then he and Patricia made their way quickly along the gently sloping stone path to the rickety pier and the small blue and white boat bobbing in the water.

As he walked along a thought struck him. 'Another time? Would there be one for any of them?' A sense of emptiness rode over Colm. He tried to set it aside, but failed.

Chapter fifty-five

"Is this really a story?" Patricia asked, sitting next to Colm on Seamus's boat, heading back to the mainland.

"Of course it is. And an important one too."

"Who says? You? Your editor?"

Colm was silent, sensing he was stepping on egg-shells.

"In fact, what makes a story important?" she continued, seeing his hesitation. "Much of what I see in newspapers is senseless. Silly stories about the love lives of celebrities, their bizarre antics, what toothpaste they use. Whether they're still sleeping together. And a little paragraph in the corner telling us thousands of children die of hunger every day in Africa. Is that what journalism is all about nowadays?"

"Look, I agree celebrity culture has taken over media to some extent but this is more than a celebrity story...." Colm began but again was cut off.

"To some extent? Who cares whether Gerard Depardieu relieved himself in a bottle in first-class seating? Yet it's breaking news worldwide. You'd think Iran had just launched a first strike."

"You're right. But people want to read that kind of stuff. They play along with the game. They suspend their better judgment." He was trying to sound wiser than he felt. He didn't want to be an apologist for that kind of media.

"Is that true? Or are they simply force-fed until they finally accept this junk as a normal diet of information. Are they ever given a choice? Is it not simply that there are empty pages to fill, deadlines to meet and papers to sell, so editors say, 'let's just go the easy way and titillate' rather than work to give people something interesting to read that's important, that affects their daily lives. Depardieu and his overactive bladder hardly qualifies, does it? No matter what his urologist might say."

Colm couldn't help but smile at the cartoonish image of the corpulent star of 'Cyrano de Bergerac' explaining in court how he pissed into the bottle as discreetly as possible and apologizing for spilling some of it on the plane's carpet. His smile almost erupted into a burst of laughter at the sheer incongruity of his present situation, discussing the complexity of media ethics with a beautiful model on a tiny wooden boat rocking to and fro in the middle of the Atlantic and the sheer stone-faced expression on Patricia's face in the midst of her ferocious rant of righteous indignation. Not to mention that toilet talk together with the swaying movement of the sea made him realize that he himself needed to go to the bathroom – and quickly. By doing so right there and then, he thought, could he thus also achieve celebrity status? Based on recent experience, he couldn't have imagined anything this woman said could have made him laugh but in thinking about doing so he felt himself relax, realizing how his body had been an elastic band ready to snap. Their tumble-over beach encounter still fresh in his mind, he'd subconsciously been bracing himself for another onslaught. With relief, he realized Patricia's remarks weren't a prelude to launching another full-scale attack on him personally. She was simply airing her views, rather abrasively granted, and seeking a response, albeit without giving him too much time to give it.

"Do these editors ever consider readers might think the emperor has no clothes?" She was on a roll, not seeming to notice the smile that Colm hurried to disguise. "That people might be offended by the sheer idiocy of stories in their papers? And the celebrities? Do they ever stop to consider that the antics they get up to in public – things they should be embarrassed doing even in private – are just tedious, ludicrous?"

Colm looked at the woman before him as if seeing her for the first time. He had already faced the brunt of her anger, the coldness of her comments. Now he was delighted to see those same attributes directed elsewhere. And to elements of the media he felt fully deserved them. He was about to answer her when he noticed a movement out of the corner of his eye. Seamus had stepped out of the wheelhouse and was staring out to sea. Colm followed his gaze, his apprehension rising. Was it the paparazzi in Ernie's boat approaching fast? He looked around but there was no other vessel in sight. Instead, Seamus was staring at a raggedy knot of inky black clouds that had gathered on the horizon.

"Sea's getting lumpy, a storm's comin,' " he said, glancing down at them, then turning back into the wheelhouse. "We better get ta shore quick."

Colm began to worry. Where was Ernie? What had happened? Though Seamus had told him on the way to the island everything would be okay, that Ernie knew these waters like the back of his hand, he still felt a rising sense of concern. Why did he take them anyway? The paparazzi could be ruthless. What might they do? To Ivan, not to mention Ernie, to get their way. Especially if they were in the pocket of somebody else other than the magazine.

"There's something I don't understand," he said finally, turning to Patricia, not wanting to create even more stress for her by talking about his concern. They were seated in the stern of the boat, tight against each other on a narrow, wooden bench, the sensation of their bodies touching sending a vicarious thrill running through him. A strong breeze ruffled her hair, brushing it back off her face, accentuating her high, sculpted cheekbones. A scarf prevented him seeing the soft curve of her neck up close. He wondered what was beneath.

"What's that?" she responded.

"I don't understand how you of all people don't understand the media."

She titled her head, her eyes narrowing. With suspicion? With puzzlement? Both? He wasn't sure.

"You more than anyone should know exactly what forces are at work. You've created them."

"I don't know what you mean."

"It's your lifeblood. You and your industry depend on them."

"On what?"

"Carefully constructed publicity campaigns in cahoots with the media. It's a massive cottage industry created by people just like you, celebs of all kinds - fashion models, actresses, actors, soap stars - and around you all a tightly-knit cadre of others, press agents, photographers, advertisers, merchandisers. All metamorphosing people like you into saleable products. Let's face it, that's how you became famous…"

Seeing her eyes narrow even further, a spark within, he sensed he'd gone too far. But he'd taken a lot of heat from her, now it was his turn. The journalist inside him felt her attacks were too one-sided. He knew he was dancing on the edge, but out here floating among the lobsters and the crabs, it didn't seem to matter much anymore. A chasm separated them and he needed to bridge it. If that meant tough talk, so be it. At least on a boat she couldn't run away. He felt free, freer than he'd felt in a long time. His publisher was pulling the rug on the story anyway so what had he got to lose? If there was to be mutual respect, both sides had to have their say, he reasoned. Out of respect might come something else, something more lasting, he hoped.

"You mean I'm merely a product of consumerism and popular culture..." Her interjection stopped him momentarily.

"In a nutshell, yes," he replied. "So why get all upset about it now? I mean you've benefited well from the dog-and-pony show. You're rich, famous, have a fancy pad in New York. Your image is splashed across the front covers of Vogue and Vanity Fair in glorious color."

"That's exactly what it is." Her tacit agreement shocked him. He'd expected a hefty, harsh denial. He was left speechless.

"What?" he said finally.

"Imagery. Nothing more, nothing less. It's not real. It's not me."

The answer was more than he had hoped for. At last, she was talking about herself. Like the hungry Eskimo over the fishing hole in the ice, he added more bait to his line.

"The glamor, the glitz, the parties, the luxury. Bright lights. World travel. Adoring eyes. All canapés and caviar. Surely you're not telling me you didn't enjoy all that schmoozing and razzmatazz?"

For a second he could have sworn her eyes went shiny and cat-like. If all the lights in the world had gone out, he'd swear there'd still be these two bright, laser-like spots left, both fixed immutably on him. The skin on her face tightened as if someone behind her was pulling on it. Having been vilified by her over the last few days for deigning to be a member of that lowliest of clubs known collectively as the media, Colm had to admit to a certain nefarious pleasure. Revenge was sweet. But there was something else he longed for that would taste even sweeter. Plain blunt honesty.

"You think I'm spoiled, don't you?" she shot back. "You think it's all been an easy downhill ride. That I've milked the media for all its worth and now have no time for it."

Colm didn't answer. Fire had taken hold between them and was beginning to burn brightly.

"Let me tell you, it hasn't been easy." Patricia swung round on the wooden bench to face him head-on, her thigh touching his, sending tiny shock waves of pleasure through him like little scurrying mice.

"And glamorous? You've no idea about the hours of preparation every single day. Endless facial exercises first thing in the morning, then a shower, then skin cleansing and temporary moisturizer. Then tweezing eyebrows and massaging cuticles and touching up chips on toenails, then feet exfoliation, a pedicure, a face pack. Then hair, wash and blow-dry, over and over and over again. Then serum followed by moisturizer and sunscreen, then the make-up. Then a meal that's not a meal, of thin tomato and apple slices. Skinless of course."

She stopped to take in breath.

"Does that sound glamorous to you?"

"Not really," he acknowledged, trying to holding back a comical quip about skinless apples.

"And my routine is considered normal," she continued. "You should see what other models do. Pay a few hundred dollars to a spa in Manhattan to have the excrement of a nightingale spread all over their skin. On stopovers in Dubai, have facials of human placentas gleaned from Russian maternity wards. In London, have bull semen wiped all over their hair to keep it fresh and feathery. And not just any old semen either, it must be organic and Aberdeen Angus. 'Viagra for hair,' they call it. Oh, and then, of course, there's the number one."

"Number one?" Colm asked, confused, still trying to come to terms with the shit of nightingales, not to mention bull semen and human placenta.

"Yes, number one. As in urine."

"Urine?" The thought crossed his mind this was all a joke and that any minute she'd burst out laughing, point at him and shout, 'Gotcha!' But she didn't. She just continued. In expository mode.

"Yes, the HCG diet. Human chorionic gonadotropin. Produced by the placenta and excreted in pregnant women's urine. Suppresses appetite, stops you from feeling weak or hungry on daily low calorie intake. Has been around since the fifties but sales went through the roof when rumors went out that Britney Spears used it after giving birth."

Excrement? Semen? Human placenta? Urine? Colm felt his stomach begin to churn. If there was a sudden lurch he might be sick over the side. And then he'd piss in his pants. There was no stopping her.

"Wearing fine clothes, strutting the boards, that's the easy part. Then there's the hanging around with absolutely nothing to do because the make-up girls might be free any minute so you can't leave your chair. The going-to-parties routine, simply to meet the right people, invariably men in the throes of middle-aged crisis in Milan, lecherous Lotharios in London, roaming Romeos in Rome. Men who inevitably try to touch you up and tumble you into the nearest closet."

"Is this just some kind of existentialist response to your bad luck, your fall from grace?" he ventured, to stop the storm of words rushing at him

"It certainly sounds like it."

He expected a sharp slap to the face and suffered a twinge of guilt when none came, more so upon seeing a sudden vulnerability etched in her eyes, a vacant sense of loss.

"Maybe… I was only seven when I started modeling." Her tone had changed completely, her voice quiet. "As a teen I failed nearly every exam at school, was thrown out of several for poor attendance, had few friends yet earned more money than anyone I knew. A few weeks ago I was to be the public image of a multi-million dollar cosmetic campaign. Now I'm 'a loose party girl, drug addict, binge drinker.' You're right, I've turned into what I am because of my industry's incestuous relationship with the media. But I've fallen far enough, I can't fall any farther. There's nowhere else to fall. I'm just a face. There's nothing more to me."

She stopped speaking, her eyes welling-up as she fought back tears. Seeing her so broken, Colm felt an urge to put his arms around her, hug her close, tell her everything would be alright, that there was nothing to be afraid of, that she was the most beautiful, intriguing woman he had ever met and probably would ever meet. But he didn't do any of those things. The words stuck in his throat and wouldn't come out and his arms were suddenly made of concrete.

Finally, he placed his hand gently on top of hers. She didn't pull away, simply looking at it as if with infant's eyes, wondering what it was, what it was doing there.

"You're not just a face, you're much more. But if you truly want to find out who you are, hiding away here is probably not the best way," he said finally. She was studying him hard as he spoke, a subtle expression in her face as if she was seeing something there she hadn't seen before.

"Look, I'm probably not the best person to give you advice?" he added. " I came here to write a story about you participating in an experimental skin procedure. And I got that information by tricking your mother into telling me some things."

Colm held his breath, fearing a ferocious reaction, with him maybe him ending up in the water below. But a smile formed slowly on her lips, breaking up the clouds that veiled her face.

"Not to put cold water on your powers of persuasion," she said, her face brightening. "But say hello to my mother and she'll tell you her life story."

Colm returned her smile, relieved. It emboldened him. "Doctor Gray told me about Washington, I didn't know anything about that until you mentioned it on the beach. He cares deeply about you, and after what happened to his daughter, his concern goes far beyond that of a doctor for a patient. I don't think he'd ever ask you to do something that would cause you harm."

She was listening, her eyes now fixed on a point beyond him. He took the plunge. No better time. Land was approaching fast. Even if she tried to toss him out of the boat, he'd only be waist-deep in water not fathoms below.

"Why not speak at the committee hearing?"

The change in her features was dramatic. From contemplative to agitated.

"No, I can't. A room crowded with photographers and journalists elbowing each other for space. A flood of questions about my life."

"But if you spoke up, then you'd be more than just a face. Isn't that what you want?"

"Yes, but…," she replied. "Not that. Anyhow, I've still got a job to do here."

"A job? I thought you came here for treatment."

"Yes, but for something else also."

"Something else?"

"I can't talk about it, you'll understand soon enough."

***

Intrigued but realizing he'd get nowhere plying her with questions, he backed off. He didn't want to jeopardize the personal bond he'd achieved in just a few short minutes on a simple boat ride. He was confident he'd be told, eventually. But when? And would there be enough time? And for what exactly? At the outset it had been clear. Reporter in search of an exclusive combining rare coupling of staid science with sexy celebrity. But things had changed. And not just because the paparazzi had arrived. He sensed a blurring of roles. He was breaking rule number one. Becoming involved in the story rather than standing back from it. He felt the gap between the professional and the personal nudging ever closer. Even more worrying, it didn't seem wrong.

"There's only one way to persuade you to speak to that committee," he said breaking his train of thought.

"Which is?"

"To remind you whom you'll have to speak to if you don't speak there."

"Who?"

"Our two resident paparazzi."

Her expression turned grim.

"You'll have to tell them you're a fraudster, a fake," he cut in quickly.

She started up quickly from the wooden bench, a wicked look on her face. For a second, he thought they were both about to end up in the water. Not an entirely undesirable scenario, he had to admit.

"That you're not even an American citizen," he continued, remaining poker-faced. "Nor an Irish one for that matter." She looked at him wide-eyed as if he'd gone mad.

"That you're actually an alien from the planet Pluto on a scouting mission here to study the cultural habits of ancient Celts."

A tiny vein began to throb in her temple.

"That your Mother Ship is due to dock here within the next few days to pick you up and bring you home."

He watched her closely, thrilled by the interplay of emotions dancing in her eyes, dancing like a multi-colored array of dots. An ever-changing aurora borealis. He continued, enjoying the moment.

"And further, that you're a downright cheat. That your legendary beauty has absolutely nothing to do with lotions, potions or motions. That it's not even skin deep. That it's nothing but a sophisticated human bodysuit made from a unique intergalactic material created through advanced Otherworld technology. That, in truth, you care sweet nothing for beauty or make-up and all the claptrap that goes with it. That it's an alien concept to you, literally. For you and your kind, green and squiggly like little baby toads, come from a planet where your kind never grows old anyway so no worries on that score."

What began as a bout of nervous giggling turned quickly into laughter so hearty her cheeks began to turn a shade of crimson. To Colm, it was as if a bright light had illuminated a very dark place. His stomach felt light as if he'd just driven over a bump in a road at high speed. Patricia bent over double, becoming giddier by the second, unable to catch her breath, was irresistibly contagious. He too began laughing, feeling something inside break free from its moorings. Next minute they were like children sharing a funny story, teasing and jostling each other playfully. Finally, Patricia caught her breath.

"An interesting theory…' she blurted out. "but there's just one… teeny-weeny problem,"

"What's that?"

"Pluto … it isn't a planet anymore."

Just then the boat hit an errant wave and they lurched side-ways.

Caught off-balance, they toppled off the bench and rolled helplessly along the wooden floor like a couple of floundering fish.

Back inside the cabin, Seamus heard a thud. Remembering it wasn't the first time a silly landlubber had fallen over the side, he swung round, pole in hand, ready for action. As his eyes swept around the boat, his face - a mask of anxiety - melted into a question mark. The sight of four legs flailing in the air left him baffled. What the hell was going on? How on earth did two intelligent human beings become entangled inside his brand-new, nylon, mildew-resistant fishing net? Reluctantly, he stepped out of the cabin to begin the unenviable task of unraveling them. Then he heard laughter. Letting out a heavy grunt, he went back into the wheelhouse shaking his head vigorously. No matter how long he lived, even if it was to be a hundred and ten, he'd never be able to understand city folk. It was right what he and the boys said down the pub. These people live in a world of their own.

Chapter fifty-six

"We'll have to stop meeting like this, Gorgeous George will get jealous," he said, pointing to the Nespresso machine.

She turned and smiled. He wished he'd studied smiles more closely, then he'd know if there was more to this one than just her appreciation of his irresistible wit.

He was seated in the living room of her white-walled cottage on the hill. Dusk was beginning to settle, the dying light making the islands resemble the metallic remains of sunken warships, as well they might be for he'd learned this part of the Atlantic had been a watery graveyard for them during World War Two and they still lurked motionless far below the surface. After Seamus had dropped them at the pier, they'd taken the road between the dark rolling bogs making small talk about the pristine beauty of the landscape and how it was a haven for artists of all kinds.

"Who knows?" he said, gazing dreamily out of the window at the sea beyond. "Maybe I'll stay here. Live off Mother Nature. Eat fresh fish and organic vegetables. Drink wine and black beer and listen to fiddles and flutes playing in the local pub every night. Yeah, a bohemian lifestyle sounds attractive. Maybe even write a best-seller."

Her smile broadened. He liked that.

"What about you?"

"I'd make cosmetics." Her reply came with enthusiasm and without hesitation, as if she'd already been considering the idea. "Natural ones, no toxic chemicals. Made from the abundance of sweet-smelling flora around here."

Seeing his interest piqued, she continued excitedly. "There's a treasure trove of colors and smells to choose from. Do you know there are more than three hundred different types of plants in the bog alone? And not just heather, mosses and lichens. Tormentil, with bright yellow flowers and woody roots. And asphodel with yellow, star-shaped flowers and six-pointed petals. Their leaves are shaped like a sword, bright green in spring before turning orange at the end of summer. And I'd give my creations romantic Gaeilge names. Like *Tír Na nÓg*. No more suitable title for a cosmetic line, don't you think? '*Land of the Ever-Young.*'"

Mention of the fabled Celtic land took Colm back to the afternoon in the Kansas City hospital gift store, a time and place worlds away from where they were now. Hearing the name now, he glanced across expecting to see a mocking smile on Patricia's lips indicating she knew very well she'd 'stolen' the music CD with the mysterious cover from right under his nose back then. But there was none.

"What is it about this legend?" he said finally.

She looked at him puzzled.

Not sure her expression was merely a charade and she was really teasing him about the gift store episode, he said instead, "I was in the pub with Ernie and Seamus the other evening and they both talked about it, about Oisín and Niamh." He watched her closely, no sign of smirk or smile. He decided to go on. "I came across it back in Kansas City, too. With you."

It was obviously not a set-up for she gazed at him with even greater puzzlement. "Us, together, in Kansas City?"

"Well, no, not exactly together. It was in a store in a hospital lobby, the place where I first saw you. I wanted to buy a music CD I saw there, one with two ghostly figures on the cover, in a swirling fog…"

She walked over to a nearby bookcase and lifted something from it, then turned, holding it high in the air.

"Yes, that's the one," he said, recognizing the CD immediately. "You beat me to it. The young store assistant told me I should use it as an excuse to chat you up."

"Wouldn't have worked."

"I gathered that much when you drove off so fast."

The silence was thick.

"So you did see me?"

"Waving your arms like a windmill." She smiled mischievously, her eyes lightening up. "You were hard to miss."

"But why did you ignore…"

"Please, let's not go there now. It's history now."

He was about to say something but let it drop. She was right. It was in the past. And he being from Ireland should know better than most how staying in the past causes much damage. He'd already stayed there far too long. In his case, as in Patricia's he sensed, it was knowing just how to move on. And where.

But the CD cover, his conversation with Ernie and Seamus and now Patricia mentioning it. Tír Na nÓg? He remembered reading of persons who, unknown to themselves, act as message carriers in life, passing on snippets of information that change other peoples' lives dramatically. A shiver passed through him. Was Patricia such a carrier? Was he? Was it just coincidence, or did Oisín and Niamh, their tragic love story, have a deeper significance? His reason battled with his imagination. He couldn't see how but was open to the possibility.

As Patricia brought their empty coffee cups to the kitchen sink, he took the opportunity to look around him. The cottage was simply furnished. An open-style kitchen with wall-to-wall cupboards bordered by a refrigerator and small, flat-topped stove, an adjoining living room where he sat, with a bare, pinewood table in the center, four chairs around it, a soft, lime-green sofa, and a reading lamp.

"I'm sorry if I said some things I shouldn't have said in the boat coming over," he began quickly, feeling an urgent need to set things right. "The success you've had you've earned through hard work. You don't deserve the trouble you're having."

She lowered her eyes, suddenly coy, a change of expression that made her beauty all the more appealing. "I'm sure you've wondered yourself how you managed to get through it all over there and then have to come here of all places without going completely mad," he continued.

"Yes I have, often," she replied, sitting down on the sofa. "But then again, what's the definition of madness? Living in a tiny box on the twentieth-fifth floor in the middle of a noisy, whacky, polluted city of twenty million people, a box that costs what most people around here never earn in a lifetime? And paying for it by ping-ponging back and forth around the world in the sky, then prancing up and down on stage like a painted peacock."

She shook her head. "Isn't it mad to think people here enjoy the cleanest of air, the most breathtaking of scenery, utter tranquility, safety and security, all for a tiny fraction of what others pay for a room not much bigger than a box, in a concrete high-rise, with gas fumes, robbery, murder and road rage all around? I'm not sure which of my lives is madder. This one, or the one I left behind?"

"Makes it hard to leave, eh" he ventured. "But where from here?"

She was silent for a moment, deep shadows in her eyes reflecting her uncertainty. "That's the problem. I don't know."

"I'm sure you'll still find plenty of modelling work, though I can understand, after all that's happened, if you don't want to. There must be many other things to go back for." He hesitated, fearful of the answer to the question he needed to ask. "What I mean is …you must have left a broken heart behind. Is it not time to go back and… repair it?"

He stopped. The phrasing was all wrong. It was as if he was talking about a wristwatch. She cocked her head at him with curiosity.

"Tell me Colm. Do you investigative journalists even know what broken hearts are? Because considering the work you do, you all must have the hardest of shells to protect against that kind of thing." She hesitated for a second. "I'd bet you've never loved anyone in your life." She was testing him, not expecting an answer, he could see that in her eyes. But the words 'never loved anyone in your life' tore at him. His mind rushed back through time, pumping out flashbacks, re-interring images that seared his insides. He breathed deep, tried to change his focus but that all too familiar serpent rose up from the depths, repugnant in its ugliness. Sensing his weakness, it began to wrap itself around him, coil-like, its grip becoming ever tighter. His vision blurred. He shut his eyes hard, tried to push the monster away, back into the dark cave from which it came. The moment passed. When he opened them again, her attention was riveted on him.

"Colm? Are you okay? You look ill. Can I get you something?"

"No… no… I'm fine." She was watching him, concern written deep on her face.

"I did love someone once," he said finally. "But… she went away."

His voice sounded suddenly weary, his throat dry, a smarting pain stabbed at his eyes. Heavy droplets of rain started beating against the window.

"Look, I didn't mean to…" she started, but he didn't let her finish. He didn't want sympathy. That was the last thing he deserved.

"It was a long time ago," he said as if in saying it the image might fade from memory. But he knew it wouldn't. He had tried before, many times. "We loved each other, probably longer than we'd realized. But what was happening then in Belfast made what we had impossible."

He heard a bitter sadness flutter its wings, flickering embers of fire inside him.

"Colm, I'm really sorry. I… sometimes time stays still when we least want it to."

The words were addressed to him but he sensed they applied to her also.

"What happened?" she asked softly.

He didn't want to talk about it but she sat staring at him, her hands resting on her lap. He stood up and started walking around the room, hoping the simple movement would ease the emotion rolling around in his head.

"It was near the end of the fighting in Belfast, before the ceasefire. I was a beginning journalist on a local paper. After her brother was shot dead by British soldiers at a civil rights march, Maria had joined Cumann na mBan, the female wing of the Irish Republican Army."

He glanced over. The skin on Patricia's face was taut with interest.

"There was a lot of trouble then. Buses and cars hijacked. Street barricades going up. Maria's job was to bring weapons to a designated meeting place under cover of darkness. But there must have been an informer. Or they were just unlucky. They turned a corner and walked right bang into a British army foot patrol. There was a chase. Shots were fired. Two bullets went through her neck. She was probably dead before she hit the ground."

Hearing a gasp, he glanced up from the floor where his eyes had rested. Patricia's hand covered her mouth as if trying to stop further sound escaping.

"Oh my God," she muttered under her breath.

He stopped speaking. He couldn't go on. He needed to change the subject, fast. Otherwise…

Only the rhythmic thud of rain outside could be heard. Thunder echoed in the distance, a storm was brewing.

"There are times you've got to stand up for what you believe in," he said finally. "Maria did. And paid the price. I miss her. It's hard to say goodbye."

A veil of silence fell across the room. Their breathing shallow, Colm and Patricia lingered in their own thoughts. A shrill sound startled them. Their eyes darted around the room, momentarily confused. Then Colm pulled out his cell phone. It was McCarthy. He stood up, speaking in a hushed tone. A few minutes later he sat down again, his expression dark.

"Patricia, I'm really sorry…" he began, struggling for words, grappling with how best to say what he had to. Not thinking of an easy way, he spurted it out. "Christine's dead."

At first, she didn't react, remaining motionless where she sat. For a second, he thought she hadn't heard him. But then he saw them. Tears, glistening and shiny, welling up. They slipped over the lids of her eyes. He had a sudden urge to brush them away. He walked towards her and bent down to comfort her. But she pulled away sharply.

"I'm sure Doctor Gray was trying to reach you earlier when we were on the island," he whispered. His words didn't seem to register. She sat staring into space, tears rolling snail-like down her cheeks.

"Please go," she whispered. Her words had a strange guttural sound to them.

"Sorry?"

"Go, please. Now."

"But…"

"Leave. I just want to be alone."

"I can't leave you now. I want to help."

"Your story? Your precious story is that what it is?"

"No, I…"

"Can't you see? It's not here, it's gone. You're wasting your time. Don't you get it? I'm not the story. I never was. I'm just the decoy. That was the plan. Not just the treatment, but to keep attention on me, keep the paparazzi away from her. I was to protect her… so that she'd get well… that's what we'd hoped for. But I couldn't protect her, could I? She's dead and it's all my fault. So just go. Write your story. I don't give a damn." She stood up, her eyes blazing.

Confused and fearful, a part of him wanted to hold her close to him, the other to grab her and shake her violently. He watched helplessly, an avalanche of emotions rising up in him, a flood of questions waiting to be answered but if he wanted answers, he'd have to stay, and she didn't want him to. Frustration batted its wings and he let loose.

"I'm not the monster of your warped imagination, Patricia, nor are you," he called desperately after her as she suddenly rushed towards the bedroom. "And I'll not be target practice for your devil-haunted conscience. I've my own devils to deal with. I'm simply a journalist doing my best, making mistakes, getting things wrong. But at least I get up each time and try again. Maybe you should also. If not for yourself, then for Christine, especially now."

The words, barely out of his mouth, filled him with regret, but it was too late. The look in her eyes told him he must leave. If he didn't, there'd be just another argument. He'd had more than enough. Patricia. The story. The newspaper. Screw them all. He was finished. It wasn't worth it. A publisher who didn't want to publish. A source who didn't want to talk. A woman dead and a culprit getting off scot-free. He'd better things to do with his time.

Yanking open the door, he strode purposefully outside, the sudden chill making him shiver.

The storm had gotten worse, matching his mood. Clouds as black as ink. Rain pelting down as if heavens' drains had opened. Fog as thick as cement draped the coastline, blotting out buildings, fields, islands. He could scarcely see his car standing in the driveway. A blustery wind howled around him, plastering his hair in a wet mess against his forehead. Impatient to put miles between him and this brooding place, he twisted the ignition key sharply, stamping down hard on the pedal. The tires squealed, tossing up gravel. He didn't care. There wasn't too much he cared for anymore. Past memories, present frustrations, they made for a potent cocktail. He careened out of the driveway, the car slipping and sliding on the muddy ground. Then he was on the steep slope leading down between the bogs, Patricia fading into his past with each passing second.

Chapter fifty-seven

"My goodness, they look a proper mess," Ivan said, keeping his voice low.

"It's no' my fault they've no sea legs," Ernie replied, feigning innocence.

"What did you do to them?"

"Just took 'em for a wee spin 'roun the islands," said Ernie, a mischievous grin on his face.

"The islands? All ten of them? In fifteen minutes?"

"O' course, on Ernie's exclusive sightseein' tours ya see e'rything in wan go?" he said deadpan. "Anyway, they may not get a chance to come back again."

"Back again? By the looks of them, I'd say they can't wait to be out of here never mind come back again."

"Even brought 'em out beyond Tory ta the Three Sisters."

"What, you're in the matchmaking business now? Another Irish language grant I suppose. Is there anything around here there isn't public funding for? Anyway, there's only two of these guys and they're not pretty. At least they don't look so now."

"You've a head like a sieve, Ivan. I tol' ye before. The Three Sisters, the farthest rocks offshore. The three Druid priestesses who transformed themselves into beautiful swans and flew outa Tory Island when Christianity came, then turned themselves into rocks saying they'd stay there until Paganism returned."

Ivan shook his head nonplussed. Then turning, he gazed intently into a side room through a square of glass in the door. Two bedraggled men sat there on chairs, bent over, heads in their hands, staring fixedly at the floor, their eyes shut tight. They were barefoot, dressed only in underwear and vests. Their wet clothes hung over a nearby heater.

"So what shall we do with them now?" Ivan whispered.

271

"Dunno," Ernie replied softly. "Thought you'd have an idea or two."

"Me? Why me?"

"Well, you're the smart one. You wear a white coat."

"Oh, for goodness sake Ernie. You drive me nuts sometimes."

"Well, at leas' tis only sometimes. Not all the time."

Ivan ignored the quip. "At least we've time to think. That door locks automatically, so they can't get out unless we let them. Anyway, they're in no fit state to go anywhere. And their cell phones are here on the table."

"That's grand, sure," Ernie said. "We canny let 'em out anyways or they'll go chasing after Patricia again."

"Are you sure they're paparazzi?"

"Tol' me themselves on the way over."

"How did they know Patricia was even here?"

"That Maggie woman back at Teach Jack's, she's got the mouth 'o a hungry whale on her. Canny keep it shut, for love nor money."

"Well, it does us no good fretting about it now…"

Just then, a strangled sound rose from behind the door. They jumped to their feet. One of the men was still seated, a look of astonishment on his face. The other man was nowhere to be seen. Ernie and Ivan pressed their faces to the window, jostling each other for a better view. That's when they saw him. The other man. He was backed up tight against a wall, staring wildly at something immediately ahead. His eyes seemed ready to pop out of their sockets. He let out a loud groan. Everyone, Ernie, Ivan, the man seated, stared at him, dumbfounded. The poor man seemed to be having an apoplectic fit. Suddenly, the frozen expression on Ivan's melted. His eyes lit up.

"Aha," was all he said, walking away from the window, caressing his chin, deep in thought.

"Wha's happenin'?" Ernie said, his mind racing.

"I think I have a plan," Ivan replied, smiling.

Ernie shot him a quizzical look.

"Who'd have thought my forced vacation on Vozrozhdeniye Island working for Russian intelligence all those years ago would pay dividends now, here of all places?"

"I havna clue what ye're on 'bout," said Ernie, utterly confused. "Ye're abou' as clear as a bowl of my mammy's pea soup."

"Back in the dark days of the Cold War," Ivan began. "Back when members of our sensitive, visionary Communist apparatchik felt the need to uphold the glory and independence of our fine nation, they required intelligence, and lots of it. In order to obtain it, they'd use whatever creative methods they could come up with, regardless whether it was on a captured foreign agent or a pesky political prisoner. So for a few years, some of my hapless fellow researchers were ordered to focus their efforts on finding out as much as possible about one of the most vulnerable aspects of human psychosis."

Ernie stared at him as if he had fallen from space.

"For the love o' Jesus, is it an 'cyclopedia ya swallowed? Will ya hurry up and get ta the point. We dunno ha' time for an entire histry o' modern civilization."

"Okay, okay," said Ivan, indignant. "For a nation that's supposed to have no notion of time and an incurable predilection for story-telling, you display an uncharacteristic lack of patriotism. It's not as if our two friends in there are going anywhere. At least, not without our say so."

Ernie was hopping from one foot to the other with impatience. "If ah'd a lobster pot, I'd wrap your head up in it."

"Entomophobia."

"Wha' ...?"

"Inadvertently one of our captives has revealed to us that he's deathly afraid of insects."

Ernie had a puzzled look.

"Are ye sure, cos it sounds real daft ta me?"

"Believe me, I'm sure. I had the misfortune many years ago to hear some of the screams and shouts as I passed room B137 on East wing on my way to the lunchroom. I'm familiar with the symptoms. It's unmistakable. I don't mean to be cruel, but I'd say we've just struck gold. This unfortunate fellow's at our mercy."

Ernie stood up quickly, making a beeline for the front door.

"What are you doing?" Ivan asked, shocked. "Where are you going?"

"Chickens," Ernie replied, a solemn expression on his face. "Avhe got ta get to ma chickens."

Ivan was dumb struck, lost for words.

"If ah don' get there soon, that pesky fox will get 'em for sure."

"But you can't leave now," Ivan demanded. "What am I supposed to do with these two?"

"Well, seems ya have lottsa 'xperience in these matters. And as ya say, you've got 'em at your mercy."

Without another word, Ernie disappeared out the door, closing it quickly behind him. Ivan rushed out after him and began shouting, but his words fell on deaf ears. For a man so lacking in stature, Ernie could certainly move fast on his feet.

"Well, I'll be," Ivan murmured to himself in amazement. "The wee pipsqueak. Would you believe it? Who says the Irish don't take their responsibilities seriously?"

A noise behind him grabbed his attention. He swung back round. One of the men was pulling frantically on the door handle, his face red with exertion.

"What the hells' going on?" he screamed. "This bloody door's locked. Let us out of here."

Ivan hesitated. If he did, they might catch up with Ernie and make him bring them back to the mainland, maybe even force him to take them to Patricia. He needed to play for time. The banging got louder, the other man having joined the first. One pulling on the handle, the other beating on the door panel itself.

"Look, it's no good going on like that, you'll exhaust yourselves," Ivan said, attempting to sound conciliatory.

"What the hell are you locking us up for?" one of the men demanded.

Ivan tried to think fast, then an idea came to him out of the blue. "Stopping you from stealing my secrets, that's what."

The two men turned to each other confused, then shouted.

"Secrets? What secrets?"

" Is that why these disgusting creepy crawly things are in here?" one of them added.

"They're not disgusting," Ivan replied, insulted. "They're part of a highly sensitive experiment. They're..." He was interrupted before he could go on.

"We don't care. We want out," the other man cried out.

"Yeah, all I care about is whether they're dangerous?" the phobic one added. "And can they get out of these boxes? They don't look too sturdy to me."

Ivan sensed his opening and took advantage.

"They sometimes escape. I don't know how. Maybe holes in the boxes they squeeze through."

Suddenly both men were staring intently at their feet.

Ivan pushed on. "But nothing to worry about. They usually don't bite. Well, not unless someone unfamiliar enters their territory. Then they're known to clump together... a little army of sorts... and ...well... subdue the situation."

"Subdue the situation?" The phobic one's voice had risen a decibel or two. "What the hell does that mean? Is it what I think it means?"

Recalling the various stages of interrogatory technique, Ivan didn't answer.

"Mister, you've got to let us out of here." The phobic man's voice was tremulous.

"I will, but first you've got to answer some questions," Ivan said confidently.

"Go ahead, ask. We got nothing to hide."

"Why are you here?"

"Mister," the phobic one pleaded, ignoring the question. "Will you just let us outa here before these things start crawling across the floor?"

Ivan pressed home his advantage. "Who sent you?"

"Our magazine, of course."

"But how did you know Patricia was here?"

"A guy called Larry. He's with a cosmetic company."

"Which company?"

"Hi guy, who do you think you are? Homeland Security?" the other man said. Ivan didn't answer. His silence was his trump card.

"Okay, okay," the phobic one blurted out. "It's a company called Bellus and our guy had been in touch with someone on a newspaper in Kansas City. A fella called Pratt."

"And no-one is out to steal your secrets," the other chimed in. "We had no idea you existed until that idiot brought us here in his boat. Now let us out."

Ivan glanced at his watch. Ernie would be back on the water by now and there wasn't another boat until tomorrow. By persuading them this was one big miscommunication, he was confident his captives wouldn't strangle him with a length of his own fishing line. If that failed, he had a bottle of Seamus's homemade poitín in the cupboard. It wasn't nicknamed *uisce beatha*, 'the water of life,' for nothing. A few sips of that and they'd be pacified until morning, giving Patricia and Colm more than enough time to skidaddle. He slowly unlocked the door.

Chapter fifty-eight

Ernie was in the stern of the boat caressing and tickling the largest trout he had ever seen. A feisty one - its belly shimmering speckled shades of silver in the sunlight. Smooth and shiny as a brand new penny, it twisted this way and that in his hands trying to escape – a real beauty, one that was sure to land him the county's top angling award for the season.

A noise broke loudly behind him. Startled, he spun round quickly, too quickly, for in an agonizing instant he felt the soft, slippery body slide away from his fingers. He spun back again, trying desperately to catch it but instead it fell through the air, shattering into a thousand tiny pieces.

A thousand tiny pieces? A fresh trout? Ernie's muddled mind began to grapple with the incongruity of it, but before it could do so, he felt warm liquid splash across his knees. His eyes shot open. Bright coals blazed before him. A flicker of flames warmed his face. His boat on fire? How was that possible? He didn't even smoke. Feeling a burning sensation between his legs, he looked down bewildered. A dark stain had spread around his crotch. At first he thought it blood, then, with a twinge of shame, something else.

"Ah Mother of Sweet Jaysus," he muttered.

Then he noticed white shards scattered around his feet and on the tiled floor in front of him. Tiled floor on a boat? Utterly confused, he shifted uneasily in his armchair. Armchair? What armchair? His boat didn't have an armchair. What the fuck? He gazed around with a frantic look. At the poker, the neat pile of cut turf, the framed pictures on the wall, the hanging mirror. What the hell? This was his house. How did he get here? With a sudden realization, he cursed loudly, recognizing the delft fragments from the mug he'd been sipping his tea from when he'd fallen asleep by the fire.

Out of the depths of his mind, he remembered. The sound that had entered his subconscious as he'd dozed off. The faraway revving of a car engine. The screeching of brakes. He remained motionless listening for a few seconds, then stood up quickly. Was Patricia okay? He grabbed a pair of binoculars and made his way to the window. Rain lashed down and a thick fog hovered in an eerie latticework of patches around the tree line. He could barely see the little white house at the top of the hill. Lights were on in the front room. Colm was probably with her. That eased his concerns. She was safe at home at least. But still, something bothered him. He'd handled the two Americans pretty well – in fact, was chuffed at his simple plan of action - but now he wasn't so sure. They'd be stuck on the island until tomorrow. But what if they became desperate and forced Ivan to call the mainland for another boat?

He ran his fingers nervously through his hair. What to do? He didn't want to be a nuisance. But then again. If something happened to Patricia and he just lying around here like a mackerel caught in a net? Unsure, he lifted the binoculars again, took another long look. The inside light of her house was still on, illuminating part of the garden. At first, he could see no movement. But then? Out of the corner of his eye. What was that? There seemed to be something right outside. A vague outline, vibrating, changing shape. Was it lingering wisps of fog? Strange shadows cast by the light and the shifting branches of trees? No, it seemed more solid. Something with more substance.

He adjusted the lens to get better focus. Whatever it was, it was moving closer to the house, making mischief among the red and yellow chrysanthemums by the front door. Teasing their slender stems backwards and forwards, shaking their silky heads from side to side, making them flutter like butterflies. Seemed to be taking on a more distinct shape. Circular, the size of a Gortahork cabbage, and as transparent as chiffon, reminding him of the scarf his mother used to wear. The strange object was suspended now in mid-air, revolving slowly. Ernie could make out a rainbow of colors as it spun. Then, nothing. In an instant, it seemed to just vanish from view.

Stunned, Ernie stood by the window, binoculars at his side. Was there something in the tea he'd just drank? It was the herbal stuff Patricia made him take. It might as well have been brewed from grass. She'd said it'd be good for his stomach, but she'd said nothing about his eyesight. Or was it that he wasn't properly awake? Maybe bringing those two rascals for a wild spin on the boat around the islands had taken more out of him than he reckoned. Of course, it might be just the fog and light playing tricks on him. Or the aurora borealis, maybe it was something to do with that.

He stood still, thinking. He'd call just to make sure she was fine. That'd do it. Should he tell her what he thought he saw? Better not. If she was fine and dandy, he'd leave it at that. She'd probably think he'd gone nuts and start worrying about him. That'd do nobody any good. He walked across the room and lifted the phone from the wall. His face clouded over in an instant. All he could hear was a constant clicking sound. He pressed the reset button. No tone. He cursed the weather and shoved the phone back in its cradle, sighing deeply. Now what to do? He walked back to the window, lifted the binoculars. Thick fog had returned. Bloody Foreland was infamous for it. One minute clear as daylight, the next dark as night. He couldn't see anything anymore. It'd take him a while to walk there, especially in the fog, but he'd better go, just to make sure. Better change his trousers first though. Seeing him in that state, thinking he'd wet himself, she'd probably serve him up another batch of that awful, foul-smelling tea.

Chapter fifty-nine

Patricia sat in the hollow of the bed, her back to the window. Behind her, a wan moon rested upon her shoulder. Bent over, she held her face flat in the palms of her hands. Her cries came softly. She pressed the tips of her fingers hard against her eyelids, squeezing them hard until slivers of pain shot through her, but it was in vain. The tears flowed ever stronger, stinging her eyes, wave after wave in an outpouring of long-held grief walled up inside for so many lonely days and nights. Jerking spasms swept through her making her arms shake uncontrollably.

How long she remained there lost in a world of despair, she couldn't tell. Time meant nothing as her anguish spilled out into the cobwebbed shadows of the room. Then, without any conscious effort on her part, she became aware of an eerie silence around her, imbuing her with the strong sense that an unseen presence was near. A silence so all-pervading it seemed, on a single command, all movement had stopped instantly. The wind had died, scurrying leaves had stopped rustling and the rain had ceased battering against the window pane.

Slowly she uncovered her face. Her hands trembled. Fearful what might be lurking in front of her, she kept her eyes closed, then opened them quickly, wide. In the gloom she could barely make out anything at all. Everything seemed out of focus and disjointed. Staring straight ahead, she rubbed her tired eyes, blinking rapidly to release pent-up tension. Then she gazed around her tentatively. Nothing strange. Just the curtains, the carpet, books piled on the bedside table, a radio. And herself, alone, in an empty room, in the dark. She relaxed, and started to ease herself off the bed. That's when she saw it. Wisps of mist, feathery and light, rising almost imperceptibly from under the door leading to the garden. It seemed like curling fingers of fog slipping into the room from the outside. She sat spellbound, surprised by her own reaction, not one of dread and incredulity but calm, controlled. It was as if in some way, she had expected something unusual to happen and now, her curiosity roused, she wanted to know what it was. Within seconds, the feathery shapeless wisps had begun re-aligning themselves, weaving together, becoming denser, more substantial, reshaping themselves into more recognizable forms. Where had she seen that image before? Unable to move, she watched mesmerized as out of this nebulous mass, a hazy outline emerged, a figure, a man, stocky, muscular, his angular face framed by waves of thick hair.

The apparition now loomed above her, floating in mid-air as the last wisps coalesced. Broad, wide shoulders, cloaked in a vivid garment of purple and green, decorated with a spiral motive – a design vaguely familiar to her - that replicated itself along the line of the sleeve. Penetrating eyes, the color of the sea, almost translucent, looked down upon her, not in a threatening way, but with compassion. As she watched, it spread its hands and reached forward. She let out a gasp and scrambled backwards, but the apparition remained where it was, motionless, holding her in a fixed gaze. Then it spoke, a soft voice, almost a whisper, that seemed to echo across the room.

"Take warning. Do not get lost in the mists of the past. Look deep within. Move into the light, for there it is clear what you must do."

Patricia remained transfixed, her mind a whirl of colliding thoughts. A wave of warmth spread over her bringing with it an immense sense of comfort and wellbeing she had never felt before. It was as if threads of incandescent light had entered every fiber of her body. And as she bathed in its utter loveliness, the apparition began to turn, moving slowly toward the window, its hands still outstretched, an index finger pointing out into the night. Then it was gone. That's when she remembered. That mist, that face. The CD Colm and she had spoken about earlier.

Chapter sixty

Impatient to get away, Colm slammed down on the accelerator and jerked on the gear lever, causing the car to veer wildly from side to side on the narrow strip of road. Screeching around sharp S bends with a high-pitched squeal of rubber, it barreled down the steep slope towards the bog. Heavy raindrops pounded on the windscreen as if demanding entry while all around ethereal-like fog encased him in a sheet of cellophane.

He stared fixedly ahead, but focused on nothing in particular. He wasn't interested in seeing anything, hearing anything. He had seen and heard enough. Her words echoed over and over in his head, tearing into the very fabric of his being. '... *just go. Write your story. I don't give a damn.*' Drained of emotion, man and machine rushed further into the depths of the black void ahead.

A line of hefty oak trees bordered the road, a battalion of soldiers keeping intruders out of the ancient turf bogs beyond, but these gradually gave way in the glare of the headlights to straggly bushes like war-weary remnants of a bedraggled army in retreat, then to stunted patches of grass and reed. Sturdy drywalls that had defied a thousand storms and the bone-chilling winds sweeping across the Atlantic seemed to retreat now in the glare of his headlight, leaving behind a sullen emptiness, a bitter, forlorn landscape that matched his mood.

Questions rushed at him, tormenting him, reminding him of feelings he thought he'd buried deep inside. It was as if his heart had been ripped from his chest and tossed raw and bleeding into the cold, wetlands around him where it lay inert and shapeless. The mask of hope he'd dared to wear upon entering her home had been torn asunder and cast into the billowing waves below. And the awful, gut-wrenching truth that whatever he'd tried, whatever efforts he'd made, he'd failed, rushed at him, drowning him, sucking his emotions in a downward spiral. Then a sudden realization dawned. It wasn't Patricia he was hearing. It was the ghost of Maria. Taunting him, blaming him, accusing him of not caring enough to believe in anything. Or was it just himself, refusing to forgive himself for not being there for her? And now, here he was. Running away yet again.

Such were his thoughts, he didn't notice that the rhythmic drumming of raindrops on the car window had grown louder, clouding the windscreen in a torrent of water, threatening to shatter the glass itself. Nor did he see the pothole until the left front wheel skidded down into it with a metallic screech, the tire exploding in a deafening noise that shook the silence. His mind still lost in a wave of conflicting thoughts, he was unable to react when he was lurched violently sideways and the engine screamed its protest as the car swerved in a half circle, rushing out of control, wheels grinding, seeking desperately to hold on to ground that was no longer there.

He felt a sharp pain as his head snapped back. Then his world started spinning, over and over, as if caught in the eye of a tornado. Then nothing.

Chapter sixty-one

Patricia sat on the edge of the bed stunned. Had it been a waking dream? A hallucination? An aberration of her mind brought on by stress? Yet it had seemed so tangible. Now, however, there was no sign anything strange had happened. The room was empty. Whatever it had been was gone, vanished into thin air. Confused, she didn't even know how much time had passed. An hour, a day, a week? Outside, all was velvet as heavy raindrops quarreled at the windowpane.

Such had been the apparition's effect on her she stumbled into the living room half-expecting to find everything around her changed – unfamiliar rooms, different furniture, complete strangers turning to stare quizzically at her. Her gaze flitted from chair to table to sofa. Everything was as it had been. Then, with a painful jolt, she remembered. She tried to push it away, but the news lurched at her, scratching at her mercilessly with its sharp talons. Christine was dead. The words reverberated in her head, her mind unable to accept their meaning. Those innocent eyes closed forever? The kid who'd hooked on to her as the older sister she didn't have. Waifish, vulnerable, her childlike exuberance a breath of fresh air, a foil to Patricia's worn cynicism. That's the only reason she'd gone to that party. She hadn't wanted to, would much rather have gone to bed. *'Please, please, just for an hour,'* Christine had pleaded, beaming that big round smile of hers. Then the drive back, the quiet road, the dancing lights, the dizziness, the blackout.

She'd been warned but she never lost hope. With her bubbly energy, she believed Christine would pull through. With today's technology, doctors could do anything, right? She'd learned the jargon. *'Vegetative state,' 'acquired brain injury,' 'minimally conscious state,' 'deep brain stimulation.'* She'd read the stories. About people waking up, being okay. A dark abyss appeared before her and she felt herself slide helplessly into it. There are no miracles. No fairytale endings. Panic gripped her. She needed to talk to Doctor Gray. She rushed across the room and grabbed the phone off the wall. But all she heard was a buzzing sound. Frantically, she stabbed at the buttons. Nothing. The line was dead. She turned and looked outside. A seething storm had erupted. Swirling clouds, wind pummeling the trees, tearing branches off like they were mere strips of wallpaper.

She flopped down on the sofa feeling miserable, and so alone. Trying to shift her legs under her, her feet tangled on something. Irritated, she tried kicking it away but couldn't. Finally, bending over, she pulled at it, snatching it up. It was a leather satchel with a long shoulder strap. She hesitated, wondering what it was. Then she remembered. Colm had brought it from the car, saying he wanted to show her something. A metal clasp held it closed. She fingered it for a few seconds, then gave in to temptation. The clasp opened easily. She spilled the contents on to the coffee table beside her. Pens, pencils, colored markers. A reporter's notebook was open at a page with writing on it. She glanced at it. Her name scrawled in capital letters across the top. Below it, a story with a headline.

Tragedy turns to triumph
Her heart began to race.

Hers is not a Cinderella story – in fact, quite the reverse. But it's one that is every bit as inspirational, its ramifications of redemption and resurrection touching even those places in our hearts tainted by the cycle of cynicism that swirls savagely around us every day in modern life. Once a social pariah – unjustly accused of drug abuse and injury to a friend, toppled from her coveted position as America's queen of the catwalk, hounded by the paparazzi until she was stripped of common decency - Patricia Roberts has emerged an unlikely heroine.

In a world exclusive, The Kansas City Guardian reveals the story of this young woman's enduring battle against the worst excesses of corporate America to become a leading voice for the protection of consumer rights. Not only has the 27-year-old fought her battle with dignity but has also bravely taken part in sensitive research that officials say illustrates categorically the benefits of many natural treatments and the inherent dangers of chemicals in everyday cosmetics.

That was it. There was no more. She flipped through the rest of the pages. They were filled with notes in shorthand she didn't understand. She sat motionless, thinking over what had happened earlier. When she'd heard the terrible news, Colm said he wanted to help but she'd accused him of wanting only his precious story. She'd attacked him, ordered him to go away. Why? When would she ever learn? No wonder she was alone. The word was invented for her. She imagined ending up like her mother. In a Midwest suburb, a TV in the corner her only companion, a bottle on the table her only relief. The image made her shudder. Why couldn't men realize her bark was bigger than her bite? Or just bite back.

She had to do something. For once, she regretted not having a car, but driving would bring back too many bad memories.

Within seconds, she'd grabbed a coat and was rushing across the room, tearing savagely at the handle of the old wooden door, her eyes mad with desperation as if a blazing fire raged behind her ready to engulf her. Tightened by the constant stream of rain and wind, the wooden door creaked in defiance. Planting her feet apart, she arched her back, pulled with all her might. Grunting, her breath coming in short, heavy bursts, she felt animal-like, almost brutal, with a strength she didn't know she possessed. With a sigh of resignation, the door sprung open, catching her off-balance, sending her stumbling backwards into the room. A wave of frigid air engulfed her. For a few seconds, she stood glassy-eyed staring out into pitch darkness, a maelstrom of emotions swirling within her like a basket of writhing snakes. Then she rushed headlong into the storm, dragging the door shut.

Only halfway along the pebbly driveway with rivulets of rain cascading down her face did reality hit. She didn't know where she was going or what she was going to do whenever she got there, wherever there was. She'd shed so many tears she thought she'd none left to give but now she could feel them welling up in her again. She was too weary to stop them. Let the rain wash them away. She rushed on, head down, not knowing where her legs were taking her but glad to be away from the house where she'd felt trapped and helpless. She thought again of what she'd experienced in the bedroom. Whatever it was – a waking dream, a hallucination, a force far greater than herself yet she part of it – it had unlocked something deep within her. The doubts, the fears that had haunted her for so long seemed to dissipate. A balloon loosened from a string, she felt a buoyant sense of release. And while she had no fixed plan, she knew with immutable certainty what she had to do. Find Colm. She'd lost Christine. She couldn't lose him. If she did, she knew. She'd lose herself.

Below, a band of mist stretched across her vision etched with tiny lights blinking like stars indicating the whereabouts of scattered homes among the hills. The silhouetted slopes of Errigal and Muckish mountains loomed around her, their respective pyramid and bread-loaf shapes barely recognizable in the gloom. Beyond lay the endless sea, its constant ebb and flow the sound of a slumbering giant snoring softly, each rhythmic breath, she imagined, blowing a ripple of surf along the surface of the water. The dark humps of Gabhla, Inis Oirthir and Inis Meain islands lay in a disheveled cluster, mismatched jigsaw pieces, their jagged edges like fingers reaching valiantly out to each other.

Trees swayed beside her, their branches waving to and fro maniacally as if delivering a dire warning, 'Stop, go no further, go back, go back…before…' She felt goose pimples form on her arms and started to shiver, the damp seeming to enter her very bones. She felt a sudden urge to rush back to the house but when she turned the house had melted into the fog, which had grown denser and was billowing all around her. It seemed as if she had stepped into a limbo, a non-man's land between the living and the dead. She stopped nervously in her tracks listening, sensing a presence nearby. But there was only the groan of the wind, the smack of raindrops splashing against leaves. She started walking again but felt ever more disoriented in the fog and was forced to stop every few minutes to avoid sliding into the deep ditch that ran along the side of the road. As time passed she began to tire, her breath coming in heavy gulps. Her clothes clung to her, hanging heavy like a blanket. She began to worry. It was because of her stupidity that Colm had left angry. She remembered hearing the screech of tires. Where could he have gone? Teach Jack? Hiudai Beag's? Was he okay? She had to know. If something happened to him, she'd never forgive herself. She needed help. The only person she could think of was Ernie. His house lay somewhere below, isolated, at the edge of the sea. In fact, so close to the water, it seemed to float there. She recalled asking him why he lived there.

'The wind and sea keep me company, they lullaby me to sleep every night,' he'd said ironically. 'I don't like the world to be too quiet. It'd be lonesome then.'

But could she make it? Rather than abating, the storm seemed to be getting worse by the minute. Worries whispered in her ears like village gossips. She'd made a mistake. She should have waited for it to blow over. As she leaned into the wind and rain, her bedraggled hair and clothes making her feel like an old witch, she thought about taking a shortcut through the bog. But she'd been warned. About its slippery, striated surface, its sheer mud walls. How a wrong step in a soft spot and she'd be sucked in, forever.

"Step on a landmine and you'd be dead instantly," Ivan had told her morbidly. "But the bogs, they're cruel, they bide their time, taking a person down slowly."

After what seemed like hours of walking, she reached a rise in the road and peered down into the darkness. A few scattered houses stood solemn and sturdy up ahead, their eerie shapelessness making her think of decomposed corpses. Only the half-hearted cry of a dog lost in the drama of dreaming marked her passing. Turning a sharp corner, she saw the skeletal outline of Ernie's beloved fishing boat in Bun na Inbhir harbor. The words 'An Draiocht,' were painted large on her stern. On a night like this, the meaning 'Druid's Magic' somehow seemed appropriate. Like an infant seeking comfort at its mother's breast, it hugged the shelter of the small stone pier. Then his whitewashed house emerged. A dim light inside raised her spirits. She moved faster, fearful it might go out any minute, leaving her directionless. Reaching it, she tapped lightly on the front door. Nothing, no sound, no movement. Just the wind leaping out of the sea as if trying to wrap its arms around everything. Perhaps he was asleep. In bed or on the seat by the fire, that old lime-green throw-over faded with age across his knees. The warmth helped his rheumatism, he'd told her.

She leaned on the windowsill and peered inside through a chink in the curtains. A smoldering fire burned in the hearth, flames licking hungrily around lumps of brown turf. But the seat beside it was empty. She could see an unwashed dinner plate on a table. Her spirits began to sink. He might have gone to Teach Jack's for some company. A wave of tiredness rushed over her. Standing there, unsure what to do, she heard a soft muffling sound behind her. Swinging around sharply, something hard bumped against her shoulder. Startled, she fell back against the wall in the dark but without warning her arm was seized tight as if in a clamp. She screamed, tried to swipe it away, but she felt too weak to resist. Her legs lost power, her head began to spin. Everything became a blur. Then the ground rushed up to meet her. In an instant, her world went a shade darker than the night around her.

Chapter sixty-two

A thick arm stretched across her vision. Out of glazed eyes, she noticed it was streaked with mud and dirt.

"You scared the Bejasus outa me," a voice said. "Thinking ye were that cunning old fox after me chickens again, I coulda shot ye where ye stood."

Groggy and confused, she struggled to understand. Slowly, a bearded face came into focus. Weather-beaten, mere inches away. The eyes, filled with concern, studied her closely.

"Are ye able ta sit up a wee bit?"

Suddenly fearful, remembering the apparition in her bedroom, she jerked her head away.

"'azy does it, now, slowly, no quick movements," the voice cut in, gentle, reassuring, somehow familiar. An arm was at her back, supporting her. "Grand, that's the way. Now, try sipping on this. It'll put some heat inta ya."

She recognized the voice now, saw the face clearly. It was Ernie. He was holding a cup out to her. She pushed herself up on her elbows, feeling welcome waves of heat from a fire in front of her stacked high with wood. Dry-mouthed, unable to speak, she took the cup and started to sip slowly from it. But the pungent liquid within sent her into a paroxysm of coughing.

"Sin é, maithu, that's it, good," Ernie said encouragingly. "The poitín's working. Nothing quite like it for revivin' a body. Seamus makes good stuff, ahll give the sly ol' bugger that much. Now drink up."

More awake now, Patricia looked down dubiously at the clear liquid in the cup, then glanced up at Ernie. "I'd rather die," she mumbled, handing it back.

"You almost did," Ernie rejoined quickly. "When ye collapsed outside like a heap a' turf piled all wrong ah thought ye'd gone surely."

Patricia began to shiver, recalling the walk, the lashing rain, the numb cold as if inside the very marrow of her bones. She took a deep breath to calm herself. Then remembered.

"I need your help," she gasped quickly. "But we've got to hurry."

Ernie stared at her confused. "Where? What?"

"Colm and I had a fight," she began in hurried explanation, feeling awkward talking about it.

Ernie blinked, a hint of mischief in his eyes. "Is this the one you tol' me about before on ta beach when yez both went flying like a pair o' drunk geese?"

"No, another one."

"Jaysus, you've only known each other a cupla days and you're already havin' lovers' tiffs."

She blushed. For what, she wasn't sure. "No, it's not like that," she blurted out, not quite knowing what 'that' was.

"What was it then?"

"I'm not sure, but...." she hesitated, lost for words. The rush of feelings for Colm uplifted her spirits but left her emotionally confused, their unfamiliarity leaving her ill-equipped to acknowledge them, never mind accept them. Ernie was staring at her, a smile poorly hidden in the corners of his mouth.

"Never mind." She sighed, unwilling to enter such treacherous territory. A topic that had eluded her most of her life could hardly be dealt with over a blazing fire and a cup of poteen in the middle of nowhere. Sentiment had never come easy but she had a strange sensation something powerful was burrowing its way through her shell. "Will you help me?" she said.

"O' course," he said, his response immediate. "How?"

Ten minutes and a few phone calls later and she was hopped up in one of Ernie's thick, rainproof fishing jackets, a woollen balaclava pulled down low over her ears. Ernie handed her a pair of sturdy rubber boots.

"As he's not at Teach Jack's nor in Hiudai's pub and he's not answering his phone and it isna exactly the weather for a leisurely stroll, there's only wan thing to do," he said, his tone decisive. "That series of wee roads crisscrossing the bog, just down a bit from yer house - the shortcut to Jack's - he might ha taken one ah them. The daft idiot. Ah warned him. When tis wet, it's a mud trap. If ye start slidin' God only knows where ye end up. Anyhow, we'll try to go through 'em slowly and keep an eye out."

"Keep an eye out?" she repeated, realizing the implication. The fear she'd kept under wraps leapt out. "Do you think something bad's happened?"

"Well, ya did say ya had a big fight," Ernie said matter-of-factly. This simple truth made Patricia's spirits sink further. There must have been a placard across her face saying so for Ernie held her shoulders in a fatherly way.

"Don't worry, ahm just a morose old jackeen," he said. "He's probably just decided he dunno wanna see either o' us right now and he's hoisting pints o' porter in some shebeen a ways from 'ere."

He winked knowingly and guided her gently towards the door. "C'mon let's hurry or ah'll be tempted to hoist a few cold wans meself."

Outside in the pitch darkness, the wind sent up a wailing howl, as if in protest at their sudden intrusion. They kept their heads down, shielding their eyes. Ernie's car was small, so small Patricia's head was pressed close to her knees in the front seat. By American standards, it probably wouldn't have been allowed on the road, she thought, probably not even on a child's go-kart track but it was perfect for the narrow twisted byways around here. Before starting the engine, Ernie pulled something out of the glove compartment. "We'll be needing this," he said handing her a torch.

After a few miles, they turned on to what was little more than a pathway, all covered in mud and gravel and peppered with potholes and bits of broken branches tossed nonchalantly there by the wind. Raindrops splattered off the window and rolling fog made it hard to see. Putting her face close to the side window and peering out, Patricia could make out a precipitous drop below into a deep ditch. She feared the car would slide off into it any minute.

"Tight as a duck's arse, eh," said Ernie. "Built afore cars were invented. Fer ponies and carts. Dinna worry, Shumaker's the name, drivins' ma game." He chuckled softly.

She smiled, but didn't feel much better for it. Worries loomed larger by the minute. An avalanche of 'what-ifs' poured through her head. What if she hadn't invited Colm up to the house? What if she hadn't been so damn contrary? What if she'd just stayed in America? Then none of this would ever have happened.

The car shuddered to a stop, shunting her out of her reverie. She turned to see Ernie's eyes narrow, his attention riveted by something up ahead. She followed his line of sight but couldn't make out anything. He pointed ahead, not saying a word as if afraid of frightening off a wild animal. She still couldn't see anything. He pointed again. After a few seconds, she noticed triangular-shaped mounds of black sods, stacked bricks of turf. Then a series of darker shadows beyond, deep channels from which the turf had been sliced clean from the earth like meat cleaved from a bone. Her eyes opened wide. There was something else out there, something incongruous in this barren landscape. Too smooth for turf, its shiny surface gleamed in the rain. It looked vaguely mechanical, but its shape seemed all wrong, though she couldn't understand why. A tractor maybe? Just then strands of fog parted and for a split second, she saw it clearly. It was a car, but upside down, its roof firmly lodged in the wet bog, its wheels pointing into the air. A recurring image from a lonely road rushed to her mind, one she had tried hard to forget. Her heart began palpitating, she felt light-headed.

Ernie was halfway out the door. "Hand me that torch," he said gravely. But it was as if he was speaking from the end of a long tunnel. His words echoed in her ears, losing their meaning in a cacophony of sound that assaulted her eardrums. Her vision began to blur. She could barely see the window in front of her. She started trembling, the tremors growing stronger, coming in waves. She bent over, putting her head in her hands and closed her eyes. Her heart pounded so hard she felt it might burst right through her chest.

"Patricia, are ye okay?" The voice seemed far away.

She tried to answer but couldn't. It was as if her vocal cords had been cut. "Christine's dead. And so is Colm. And it's all my fault." The words erupted like phantoms soaring from the dark stillness of her mind. She pounded her hands on the dashboard. She felt jolts of pain rise through her palms into her shoulders, but she couldn't stop. Next instant her door was flung open. "Patricia, Patricia. Settle down now. Everything'll be alright. Stay calm fer Chrissakes."

Hands eased her back against the seat. She couldn't resist. The time for resistance was long past.

"Breathe deep," Ernie said, nervous but soothing. "Nice 'n aisy now."

The trembling subsided, but her body felt as if it was bruised all over.

"C'mon now. Pull yourself together, girl, we've got work to do, and fast."

The grave tone of his voice made Patricia struggle upright. She opened her eyes.

"Gie' me the torch."

Momentarily confused, she looked down. It had fallen off her lap on to the floor at her feet. She bent down and handed it to him. He took it quickly without a word and turned to go. Seeing him walk away, she took a deep breath, swallowed hard and pushed open her door. Swinging her feet slowly out on to the path, she stood up, almost fell, but recovering her balance, started walking, keeping Ernie within sight up ahead. As they drew nearer to the overturned car, she expected it to be battered and broken, to see fragments of glass and metal everywhere, but to her surprise it seemed untouched. It was as if some Alien Force had simply picked it off the road, turned it over and placed it back down again in the bog.

Ernie indicated for her to move closer. The torchlight swung in a slow arc towards the bog. They edged forward gently, the slippery surface sliding beneath their feet. Glancing down, the ditch's sheer drop reminded her of the legends about bog people. As if reading her thoughts, Ernie took her arm, "Be careful. Ah may not be able ta pull ye out."

They were now barely twenty feet from the car, its rear end facing them, smeared with mud. Ernie directed the beam of light towards it, sweeping it back and forth in the darkness. Then he stopped. Something was poking out from behind the open car door. Patricia tried to make out what it was but it was small and partially hidden behind tufts of grass and difficult to distinguish. Taking a few steps closer, staring hard, Patricia let out a gasp, her heart skipping a beat. It was a human hand. A tiny spur of broken white bone partially congealed in blood sprung out from the flesh of the index finger like a sharp flint arrowhead.

Chapter sixty-three

The low moaning, constant in its cadence, sounded like that of a small animal in pain. It was strangely familiar but Colm couldn't work out why. With an effort that seemed to send shards of glass shooting through his body like pointed needles, he prized his eyes open. That's when the moaning ceased. That's when he realized what it was. That's when the first shockwaves of knowing shook him into full awakening. He had no idea how long he had lain here giving voice to his pain. Or even where 'here' was.

Rain beat down on him yet his tongue felt thick and dry. Something was draped across his cheek, its unfamiliar dampness tight against his skin. Thinking it a tiny lizard, he tried to toss it off but when he tried to move he couldn't. It was as if his entire body, muscle, bone and sinew, had fallen into a deep slumber and refused to waken from its hibernation. His eyes seemed the only part of him that worked. Blind panic rose, a monster from the deep, forcing him to harness whatever mental energy he possessed to calm the seething waters of distress. Slowly, moving one finger at a time, he began making tiny circular movements, feeling a rush of childlike joy at accomplishing such a seemingly impossible task.

He raised his hand slowly to the thing stretched across his cheek. It felt spongy, string-like. He brushed it off then tried moving his other hand but jolts of excruciating pain shot through him almost making him black out. With sheer willpower he remained conscious staring into the gloom. Within minutes, his eyes began to decipher vague shapes and forms. Stones, rocks, weeds. A desolate terrain bereft of bushes or trees. To his fevered mind, it seemed a futuristic, post-Armageddon world. His eyes fell upon the spongy substance, recognizing it for what it was – a clump of sphagnum moss. Then realization dawned: he was lying in the middle of a bog. He could feel it under him, soft as if alive, clasping him closer. Thinking back as to how he had got here his mind conjured up a series of fast-moving images as if on a film spool. A woman's sad face; raised voices; a slammed door; heavy rain; tendrils of fog; screeching brakes; the world turning upside down; pain. Then nothing. Feelings rushed at him snarling like rabid dogs foaming at the mouth - guilt, fear, loneliness, an abject sense of failure.

Feeling a tugging sensation from behind, he turned his head slightly. A thick swathe of mud had encased itself around his legs, just below his waist. It clung to him tenaciously like wet cement. Then he felt the tug again. Was there a reptile below the surface pulling at the cloth of his pants?. The sinking sensation made him stiffen but he couldn't muster the strength to pull himself out. The more movement he made, the more pain he endured, the more he was being sucked in. The viscous mud itself was dragging him slowly downwards into it

Hopelessness weighed heavy on him as he lay there not knowing what to do. Around him howling wind and heavy rain screamed their warnings. Realizing that staying conscious was vital, he tried to stay awake but tiredness overwhelmed him and his eyes slowly closed and he returned to the darkness from which he had come.

When he opened them again there was a light but not the kind signifying the approach of dawn. Strangely, it illuminated only a small area immediately around him. It seemed to emerge from a shapeless cloud of mist advancing slowly across the undulating terrain. As he watched, confused, the mist began to swirl and billow as if whipped up by an errant breeze. It became thicker, its finger-like tentacles entwining themselves around clumps of rocks, swallowing them whole. Still disoriented, Colm's eyes flickered nervously, struggling to make visual sense out of what was happening before him.

Then he heard it. A soft sound, the merest whispering echo. To his astonishment, it seemed to come from somewhere deep within the mist but he couldn't make out any shape, man, beast or bird, within. Nor could he hear any movement. Not the rustle of grass or the scraping of footfall against stone and earth. He held his breath, thinking if it was a predator, it might pass without seeing or smelling him.

In an instant, as if controlled by an unseen hand, the mist's swirling movement ceased abruptly. A distinct feathery pattern began to form, a pattern strangely familiar, one he had seen somewhere before. He tried desperately to remember but failed. Its outline was so fuzzy he thought it might be simply a figment of his imagination. Then the feathery wisps began to slowly coalesce and form a more defined shape. Within seconds it emerged, clear and unmistakable, a spectral figure that seemed to float mid-air. Colm's heart thumped madly against his chest, a lunatic banging on a cell door. The sudden rush of blood made him feel light-headed and nauseous. He could feel the bitter taste of bile rising up through his throat.

'*A hallucination, nothing more, a simple optical illusion,*' a voice inside his head told him. Another, more menacing, screamed at him: '*You're among the cursed dead now, in…*' Hell? It must be, for it certainly wasn't heaven. A shiver ran through him. His breath came in short, shallow draughts. He shut his eyes tight, thinking maybe if…. but when he opened them again it was still there, the image moving in and out of focus, blurred one minute, clear the next, making it seem both real and unreal at the same time. Though it seemed he was peering through opaque glass, he could make out certain features. A woman - tall, slender, long locks of blonde hair billowing in the breeze. Her clothes strangely out of place, making him think of a time long gone. A flowing cloak tossed back over her shoulder, falling down below her knees. Beneath, a muslin tunic. Boots, hardy, functional, not elegant and refined.

Utter fear at the sight of such a ghostly apparition suddenly turned to bewilderment and perplexity. For now he remembered. The hospital gift shop. The music CD on the rack. He could see clearly the title scrawled in a peculiar font - *Niamh's Lament for Tír Na nÓg*. But how could the woman on that cover appear in front of him now? What was happening? Was he awake? Was he dreaming?

A slender leather pouch hung from a rudimentary belt of twisted strands of rope that looped around her waist. She seemed to hover in the air, her gazed fixed directly on him. The expression on the woman's face was serene, comforting even, a hint of hope in her eyes, like someone on a long quest having found what they were searching for.

Suddenly, the specter started speaking. "You know me, you know my story. Looking back was our undoing. I have come to warn you. Let it not be yours. Let the past remain where it lies. Open your eyes, see only the present and look to the future."

As he watched, a sense of dread descending upon him, the features of the woman's face began to change, slowly dissolving, imperceptibly realigning themselves. How could this be possible? The eyes, once round like pennies, became oval, their color changing from brown to green. The nose, upturned, became straight and smooth. Then he saw her. The flowing ringlets of black hair. The knowing smile. It had been so long.

Why now? Why here? In what illusory place was he, was she?

"Maria?" His voice thick with emotion, he could barely say her name but as he did so, tendrils of mist coiled around him, raising him off the ground. Effortlessly, weightless as if in outer space, he was drawn closer to where she was. She stretched out her hand. Slowly, as if mesmerized, he reached out too. Their fingers touched, curled around each other. Their foreheads almost touching, eyes mirroring eyes. It was as if they shared a secret they dared not say, a dilemma they dared not face. Then, without warning, the mist whorled around them, separating them. She let out a sigh and began drifting backwards as if drawn by some invisible force. He tried to grasp her, her hands, her arms, but they were insubstantial. She was turning slowly from him.

"Don't go, please don't go," he heard himself cry out, pleading. "I need you. I don't want to lose you. Not again."

She seemed to hear his cry for she turned her face again, tears in her eyes. "You haven't lost me, Colm. I'm here. Beside you. I always will be. Open your eyes, you will find me wherever you go."

Agonizing pain ripped through his chest as if a burning spear had been thrust right through him. His heart broke, shattering into a thousand pieces, mingling with the rocks and stones scattered around this forbidden landscape. As the thick, glutinous mass of mud gripped him ever tighter, dragging him slowly downwards, his eyes grew heavy and he felt his last ounce of strength ebb away.

Chapter sixty-four

"Glioblastoma? At least we have a name for it."

"I realize it must be difficult for you."

"So how long?"

"It's hard to say," Doctor Tompkins replied.

"Give me an idea at least. Surely you can do that."

"I wish I could, I really do, but with favorable response to treatment…"

"Be honest, give me your best guess."

Doctor Tompkins hesitated. "A study has reported that some patients could live five years or longer."

"Some? What is some? Five per cent or ninety-five?"

"On the lower end I'm afraid. But median survival is between one and two years."

The Senator stared blankly in front, his mouth falling open. He swayed slightly on his feet seeming as if about to faint, then leaned back against the wall and closed his eyes.

"So… little… time," he stammered. "I thought… I read…"

"They can be quite different. It all depends, on location, cell type, other factors like…" The voice trailed off, then stopped. Medical jargon would only make matters worse. Plenty of time for a fuller explanation later. Better silence to absorb what had already been said.

The two men faced each other, the hum of an air-conditioner providing a faint backdrop of sound. Then the Senator started pacing slowly back and forth across the room. The doctor, hooded eyes under dark, unruly thick brows, the lazy brushstrokes of a bored artist, watched closely, a stethoscope hanging from his neck.

"You've looked over the materials I sent you, haven't you?" asked the Senator, his tone firm.

"Yes, of course. And as much else as I could find on the subject. It's called precision medicine and it's a growing field. I was aware of it, but I've learned even more since."

"Does it have the potential they speak of?"

"Yes, it could have."

"Could?"

"Early tests show encouraging results. Nano applications is a fast-developing field in medicine. In this case, they've developed mini-syringes that can infiltrate tumors with drug-packed nanoparticles that are not toxic to normal neurons and other non-cancerous brain cells. It's complex but if I were the researchers, the clinicians, I'd be satisfied with results so far, but..."

"But... ?"

The doctor hunched his shoulders in a 'don't know' gesture, adjusting the thick glasses on the bridge of his nose as if doing so might let in the greater light of understanding.

"I know this is not easy but ..." he began.

"Please, spare me the sentiments, doctor," the other cut in. "We both know I don't have time for them. What I need to know is, can it work?"

"Perhaps, but as you know, it's still in an experimental stage. And the way regulations are nowadays, passing through the various stages could take quite some time... rigorous procedures are in place. For good reasons."

"That's the problem in a nutshell isn't it? Regulations."

"I know how you must be feeling... but..."

"But?

"Well..."

"This is a desperate situation. And desperate situations require desperate measures."

"I wouldn't use that term. I mean we have developed treatment modalities. They can have strong ameliorating effects."

"Ameliorating isn't enough, it doesn't cure. The question remains. Is this procedure worth trying?"

A heavy silence lay between the two men for a few moments.

"What can I say? I don't have a crystal ball, I wish I had. I can't see into the future. I do as I've been trained to do using the latest techniques and treatments at my disposal. I can't do more than that. Like the rest of my colleagues in this building, I have to be optimistic. But I'm also realistic. We have to be. We've got little choice."

"But I do have a choice. That's the root of the problem."

The doctor looked puzzled. "Choice?"

"Regulations on use of nanoparticles – whether to strengthen them. Or reduce them."

"Not knowing the circumstances you speak of, I cannot say," the doctor replied. "In the end, the decision is yours. I can give you my best opinion, but I can't put a finger on time. You'll have to do what you think best, for you, for others. That's why you do what you do. That's why I do what I do. We're no different. We make tough decisions every day."

"Yes, and this is the toughest decision I've ever had to make."

The Senator let out a heavy sigh, equal parts resignation, frustration, indecision. Not being sure which path to take had led to mental paralysis over the last few days, a most unusual state for him, but then again this whole situation was most unusual. Grotesquely so. He'd managed to keep his condition hidden, but couldn't keep up the pretense indefinitely. Headaches came more often, lasted longer. He thought, hoped, coming here might help provide some answers, some stepping stones upon which he could move forward. Instead, they added ever more questions to the increasing pile already facing him. Personal? Professional? Where did one end and the other begin? Since hearing the news, since reading the materials, the differences between the two had become blurred. And sleepless nights and withering pain had not accommodated clarity. Talk about conflicts of interest. Even he had to admit, this one topped them all. Push a regulatory agenda and he'd be pushing himself into a coffin.

Chapter sixty-five

Traffic was snarled along Purchase Street, a snake of steel that curled tightly around itself, motionless, almost languorous in its lethargy. The midmorning gridlock along Pearl, Broad, Oliver and Summer only added to Larry's growing consternation. Running late for a meeting with Covington, he glanced impatiently from the long line of stationery vehicles in front of him to the passenger seat, his eyes resting on the still-flashing light. The phone had been calling for his attention for the last half hour but he'd resisted the urge to answer. It was not someone he was keen to talk to. Talk to? Hardly the right term. More like the scene in front of him, all one-way traffic, he failing to get a word in edgeways, then ending up taking orders like a silly messenger boy. Unwanted memories flooded back. A cold, damp basement – a place of punishment, mistakes made, consequences to pay.

But the way things were now, perhaps he should answer. Could be important. He mulled over his options. Not that there were many. Covington was on his back, demanding results from Ireland. He'd none to offer yet. The light flashed on and off again. He took a deep breath. He'd be brusque.

"Hello," he said, a hint of irritation in his voice.

"What took you so long to answer?" his father demanded impatiently.

"A meeting. What's up?" He kept his tone even, controlled.

"Delay the product launch."

Here we go again. Another order.

"Why?" he asked trying not to sound skeptical.

"Clarke's up to no good."

"Whatya mean no good?"

"He and his people are trawling the corridors. Knocking on doors. Doing deals. Too cocky for my liking."

"Cocky? About what?"

"Dunno. That's the problem. But something tells me he's got something up his sleeve, something big. It'll take me a while to find out so better to delay the launch."

Larry tried to be diplomatic. "I can't just go to Covington with a hunch and tell him to call off a well-planned product launch."

"Yes, you can, and you will. Anyway, who said anything about calling it off? Is there wax in your ears? I said delay."

Larry felt bile rise. He breathed deep, resisting the urge to snap shut the phone.

"He won't be convinced," he said, maintaining his calm. "I need something tangible."

"No you don't. Listen to me, I could call him directly and he'd jump as high as a kangaroo. He knows I won't go down over this. I've other political backers. I don't need him."

Larry didn't reply. He'd heard the same line before. Often wondered how his father had the audacity to keep saying it when it was blatantly untrue. There were no other big backers out there waiting in line. Bellus, the biggest, and richest, employer in the state, was the Granddaddy of the PAC. Maybe that was the reason for his short temper now. He might just have to swallow his words. The voice on the other end started again.

"And I'd like to hear a bit more thanks out of you. Why do you think I'm telling you first, huh? So you'll look good when my hunch turns out true and you get them off the hook, that's why."

"But…"

"No buts, just do it."

Larry heard a click.

The dead phone in his hand brought the past home again, left him dealing with the same feelings he'd become accustomed to down through the years – awe, fear and something much darker, something he was reluctant to give a name to. He had a good mind to spill the beans. It'd be sweet revenge.

***

"That's it. That's all I know. That's all he knows right now."

All eyes were directed at Larry as he spoke.

"But he was damn sure we should delay the release date," he added quickly.

"That's gonna be difficult…" Covington said, shifting uneasily in his seat.

"Difficult?" Cathy leaned across the table at the three men, incredulous. "More like impossible. It'll could kill us. If we lose momentum now, it'll be hard to get it back. It can't be done."

Covington spun in his deep leather chair to face her, annoyance writ large on his face. "Don't tell me what can or can't be done," he snapped.

Cathy hesitated for a second, then pressed on, her tone more conciliatory.

"What I mean is we've already spent tens of millions on developing the product and launch preparation…Everything's a go. POS. PLVs. Advance media spend, including a half page in The New York Times on launch day, and big market regionals. We've a dozen sound-bites packaged for the networks and cable. Specifics on the product. General on nano and the battle against ageing. My guys have been working full out for the last two months. Stopping now would be a disaster, both to our image and staff morale."

"We can and we will – if I decide so." Covington's terse rebuff left her deflated. There was a cold finality to it she hadn't expected, his words so cutting they left her wondering whether there would still be a job for her tomorrow. Their relationship had never been warm and cordial but while she hadn't expected a daily round of pleasantries when she'd taken the job, she hadn't expected this either. And Larry's joining the company had just made things worse. Yes, influence on the Hill had to be purchased but the company was already footing a hefty chunk of Barden's campaign expenses so Covington's hiring the Senator's son was an unnecessary expense.

As these thoughts flashed through her mind, Covington turned to Larry.

"What's your view?"

"We'd lose some money but we could lose a lot more if the hunch is right."

Cathy couldn't believe what she was hearing, that these men were considering delaying a major launch on an innovative product with the potential loss of millions. It just didn't make sense. Not for the first time, Cathy wondered what it was she wasn't privy to. The wheels of her mind started spinning furiously.

Just then Larry's phone beeped. He pulled it out of his pocket and glanced down at the message. A shadow fell across his face. He turned to Covington, a mix of anxiety and apology there, "I need to make an urgent call." Something passed between the two men, almost indiscernible, but

Cathy noticed it. Eyes don't lie. Covington nodded and Larry stepped out of the room.

She felt both foolish and angry. It was a ridiculous situation. She was the marketing director and she didn't know what was going on. She'd have to confront Covington no matter the price. She couldn't go on like this. In the meantime, there were others outside this room she could check with.

Larry's quick return interrupted her reverie. The self-confidence he'd exuded earlier had vanished. In its place, worry. And plenty of it. As clear as daylight.

"We need to talk," he said, addressing Covington.

"Okay, we'll adjourn this meeting until later," Covington said peremptorily, seeing the look on his face.

Cathy swept up her briefcase and scurried down the corridor. Something had gone badly wrong. And if Chris was right, someone would be made a scapegoat. As sure as hell it wasn't going to be her.

***

"What's this all about, Larry?" Dick Covington's voice was etched with worry.

"We've been chasing the wrong person."

"What the hell does that mean. Chasing the wrong person?"

"We've been duped."

"What on earth are you talking about?"

"We've been thinking all along that Patricia was the big threat, that if we dealt with her everything'd be hunky-dory, that we'd be home and dry. Well she's not, perhaps never was. It's the other model, Christine, the one who was with her when the crash happened."

"Nonsense. That woman's not even on our books. Ongoing discussions with her agency, yes, but we haven't signed a single modeling contract, not even a prelim. And we certainly haven't given her the concealer to use so how could she be a threat? Anyway, she's in a bloody coma, for Chrissakes."

"Not anymore."

Covington stared at Larry uncomprehending.

"She'd dead. And Gray's conducted a post-mortem on her."

"A post-mortem? Why?"

"Searching."

"For what?

"Cause of death."

"What's to search for? The reason's obvious. A bump on the head. The woman should have followed the rules of the road. Worn a seatbelt, like the rest of us."

Covington scrutinized the younger man's face. The crumpled look he saw frightened him. His heart skipped a beat. Without thinking, he stretched out for the glass of water in front of him. That God-awful acid had started to gather in his stomach again. He had the distinct sense things were slipping from his grasp but he had no idea why or how. He needed to calm down.

"Okay, okay," he said with an effort of self-control. "What's this all about?"

"Seemingly Patricia may not have been the only person suffering vision problems," Larry continued, his voice faltering. "From what I know, the two of them got pretty close over the last year, shared a room on assignments. Shared other things as well."

"Like what?"

"Cosmetics"

Covington's mouth fell open.

"The committee's just been informed Senator Clarke will present the post-mortem results tomorrow."

Chapter sixty-six

"We're not there yet."

"Not there, sir? I don't mean to be crude but we've got both a dead victim and a potential live witness. Surely that's enough."

"My dear Chris, you've been reading too many detective novels."

Chris looked at Senator Clarke the way a scolded dog looks at its master.

"Don't be upset," the gray-haired politician said, seeing the injured look on his young assistant's face. "Your enthusiasm is an endearing trait. Sometimes, I wish I could be that way but I've been too long in the game. Too long wheeling and dealing. Too long listening to nonsense when truth is obvious. It wears you out sometimes."

Something in his voice, a kind of resignation that bordered on fatigue, made Chris feel uneasy. Could he be having second thoughts about this campaign? Now he thought about it, he had noticed an awkward shuffle come into the Senator's gait over the last few weeks. Sometimes he seemed out of breath on their routine walks to the committee chamber. Maybe it was just his imagination toying with him, maybe it was he who was tired not the Senator. After all, hadn't they'd been working flat-out on this campaign leading up to tomorrow, the crucial day, the last day of committee hearings? What with Patricia's flying in on the red-eye from Dublin to JFK then to Dulles and Doctor Gray already settled on the third floor of the Watergate Hotel, preparations over the last twenty-four hours had been nothing less than frenetic.

The concern on his face must have been obvious, for the Senator continued in a more upbeat manner, "Don't get me wrong now Chris. I'm not saying we haven't got anything. Gray's evidence from the post-mortem on Christine is strong and if we get him to put it across in clear, simple language and avoid complicated jargon, it'll be even stronger. As for Patricia, her beauty alone will win over some committee members."

"So I don't see what the problem is then."

"The whole point Chris is not only to show these nano products could be dangerous – our friends across the aisle will point to hundreds of other products on supermarket shelves that could be dangerous. They'll say what happened to the two women is the exception, not the rule."

Chris listened intently.

"Ultimately, we need to show that these kinds of cosmetics should be monitored more closely, to convince committee members that self-regulation is simply not working, that it's anachronistic policy when compared to how other industries are treated, and that it must be replaced. And that's a helluva task. Maybe an impossible one. Our Republican friends don't like government interference, it's anathema to them, and unless it's a voting-winning measure like immigration reform, or at least not a vote-losing one, they'll stick to that line."

Chris had to admit. What the Senator said was true. Some Republicans on the committee were painting the Democrats as anti-patriotic, '*Downright anti-entrepreneurial*,' was the way Senator Barden had put it during yesterday's hearing, a sound-bite good enough for CNN, never mind Fox News. '*More in favor of ever fatter bureaucracies – in this case the FDA - than in the indomitable spirit of free enterprise and individual achievement that has made this great country of ours the leading nation in the world*,' he'd added, driving home his point.

"But what about the documents from Cathy?" Chris said, a blush warming his face at mention of her name. "Okay, she didn't do it for entirely altruistic reasons, but still. I don't think she knew anything about Bellus's deception. And she had a right to ask us to keep her name out of all this. A small price to pay for what she brought us."

Chris stopped. Was his personal feelings taking over from his professional ones? Not wishing his words to be interpreted as him simply protecting the woman he'd come to like - a lot - he changed tack. "The lab results clearly show Bellus was aware the product was dangerous yet they ignored the findings and went ahead without conducting further research."

"Went ahead with what Chris?" the Senator asked. "They haven't even launched their product on the market yet. Something that isn't on the shelves can hardly be defined as a public health hazard."

"But these two women, one almost blinded, the other dead, they…"

"The fact remains they both chose to use the product, they weren't tied hand and foot and forced to do so," the Senator interjected. "And they were to get big money for putting their faces to it. Or at least Patricia was. It's unfortunate she gave it to Christine. A case of kindness turning to tragedy. Bellus and its lawyers, if it comes to legal proceedings will no doubt say she volunteered to use the product."

"But now Christine's dead," said Chris, his frustration rising upon hearing the unfamiliar sense of defeat in the Senator's voice. "And Patricia's brave enough to speak out. Surely that'll impress committee members."

"And Bellus will say her evidence is just sour grapes, pure and simple," the Senator replied. "They'll say they were already in discussions about cancelling her contract. That her disfigurement, the scar from the car accident, had ruined her good looks, forcing them to find other models to advertise the concealer product. That this automatically made the personal services contract between them null and void."

The Senator's arguments, said with such conviction, sounded as if he was supporting the other side not his own. It made Chris think the unthinkable. Were political favors being exchanged that he didn't know about?

"So where do we go from here?" he asked, seeking an urgent dose of reassurance.

"Well, wear out more shoe leather. Cast our pride and dignity aside, walk the halls, stick our heads through doors and beg, borrow and steal as many votes as we can, and then wait for the final roll call. What else can we do?"

Chris couldn't remember the last time the Senator ended with a question. It just wasn't his style. He was confidence personified, the man with the answers, Chris the one with the questions. And anyhow, his tone was all wrong. It wasn't the battle cry he was used to hearing, the one that had fired his blood and filled him with endless possibilities. Something was amiss. Chris couldn't resist, the feeling overwhelming him with an urgent need to know. Without thinking, his words came out in a mad torrent.

"Senator, is something wrong? I mean not wrong in the wrong sense, not in the sense that we may not win this but wrong in the sense of wrong, real wrong, wrong like..." he found himself floundering, a fish out of water, unable to find the words to express what he meant.

The Senator smiled at the childlike sincerity of the question.

His eyes narrowed, his gaze shifting to a point on the wall above Chris' head. Then it reverted back to his face, unblinking.

"Yes, I guess you could say there's something wrong... I'm dying."

***

Chris's mouth dropped open. A malignant brain tumor, a glioblastoma, the most aggressive kind. The Senator's only hope – precision medicine - nano-size cocktails of chemotherapy drugs implanted directly into the cancer cells. His mind was a whir, his thoughts in a tailspin, the avalanche of information was too much to process.

Chris stared wide-eyed, the Senator still talking, tossing out technical details that overwhelmed him. About nanomedicine researchers at the Methodist Neurological Institute and Rice University; about something called a hydrophilic carbon cluster - an antibody drug enhancement system called HADES, named after the Greek god of the underworld; about a carrier with protective properties and a high kill rate of cancer cells. Chris heard the words but their meaning eluded him. His mind was riveted by something else. All this time, this man seated before him had been haunted by demons, battling two terrible choices. To save others? Or to save himself? With no in-between. Strengthening the FDA's powers, imposing stronger regulatory control of use of nano-materials would inevitably mean slower progress of experimental nano products on to the market, not just cosmetics, but all kinds, including cancer drugs. Though stated unemotionally, the phrase the Senator had used was all too ominous, '*median survival time, one to two years.*' The logical conclusion was unavoidable. If a bill came out of committee now and far-reaching legislation limiting nano use was adopted, the Senator's life would be over.

Was this why he had seemed less than enthusiastic recently about the campaign? Why he had poured cold water on Chris's growing confidence? Had he decided not to pursue the issue to give himself a chance to live? If so, could he blame him? If it were Chris, would he not do the same? Wouldn't everyone? After all he'd accomplished in his life, especially in healthcare, innumerable bills he'd penned that helped so many people, saved so many lives, did the Senator himself not now deserve help to save his own life? Desperately trying to reconcile himself to this new reality, Chris didn't register the urgent knocking on the door, the woman's voice on the other side.

"Yes, come in," said the Senator in calm, even tones.

"Excuse me, sir." Mary, the Senator's long-time assistant, looked visibly nervous, creases of stress obvious on her 60-year-old mottled

308

skin. "I'm really sorry for disturbing you but your phone must be off the hook. I've been trying to call you for the last ten minutes."

"Apologies Mary, we needed a little uninterrupted time to discuss a delicate matter," the Senator explained. "What can I do for you?"

"It's a bit unusual, sir, or I wouldn't have…" Mary's apology was waved away congenially by the Senator.

"It's fine, Mary, perfectly fine," he said, affection in his voice. "Do you think I kept you on here just for your delectable good looks? Without you, I'd be licking stamps in the basement mailroom. So tell me, what has put you into such a flutter?"

Mary eyes sparkled at the praise but her voice still had a ring of uncertainty to it. "Well, sir, someone has just arrived to see you."

Senator Clarke's eyes narrowed disconcertingly.

"But I have no appointments this afternoon. With the last day of committee hearings tomorrow, I cleared the schedule. We talked about this. Remember?"

"Yes, sir, of course I remember. Distinctly. That's why this …"

Her voice trailed off.

"Yes?" the Senator said encouragingly, noting her reluctance to continue.

"I told him that, sir, but he said the matter was too urgent to wait. That it was related to the hearings. That he had to talk to you right now and that he wasn't going to leave until he did so. I tried to dissuade him but he simply wouldn't leave. He's sitting in the outer office right now…"

She hesitated momentarily as the Senator continued to stare at her non-comprehendingly.

"…I've never seen him so flustered," she added, as an afterthought.

"Who, Mary? Who are you talking about?"

"Senator Barden, sir. It's Senator Barden."

Silence filled the room as if an invisible force had stripped all three of the faculties of movement and speech. The Senator stroked his nose lightly.

"Mmmm, I see."

Chris watched him closely. He could have sworn he was hiding a smile.

"Okay, Mary, please tell the esteemed Senator I'll be finished in a moment," he said finally.

Mary left, closing the door quietly behind her. The Senator turned to Chris.

"Well, well, I see FEDEX really does live up to its reputation." He rubbed his hands together gleefully. "I guessed he'd be interested in reading the documents but I didn't think he'd get through them this fast."

Chris's head was spinning. Too much information, too many surprises.

"As you said yourself, Chris," the Senator continued, his tone playful. "It was a very admirable thing Cathy did, bringing us those documents. Invaluable, I suspect, is the most appropriate word. So the very least we owe her is a nice, long lunch. And, as you've just heard, I'll probably be somewhat busy for the next hour or so... if you would be so kind ..."

Chris's face was a question mark.

"I'd already booked a table at 1789, a fine eating establishment, a good distance from the Capitol to avoid pesky eavesdroppers. I thought I'd have Senator Barden bring me there to iron things over, but under the circumstances, I don't think that's necessary. I'd hate to lose the table and anyway, such good food would be wasted on him. He's a basic burger and BLT man. Though now it seems the vulture has come to chew on whatever pickings we deign to offer. As one shouldn't keep a lady waiting, make sure you go into Virginia, then cross back into DC on the Key Bridge, it's faster that way."

Chris smiled, the beginnings of understanding dawning on him.

"Oh, and before you go. You might just want to read up on the Consumer Product Safety Improvement Act, Public Law 110-314. A fine piece of whistle-blowing legislation, one I helped pass myself. A few years back, one gentleman, John Kopchinski, a sales rep, was paid fifty million dollars for blowing the lid on erroneous marketing by Pfizer of one of its big-selling painkillers."

Seeing confusion on his assistant's face, he continued, "I know it's outside your realm of research, Chris – at least for now – but there's one important thing you should know from the outset. Weddings cost a lot of money these days. I know from experience."

Then he turned to the papers on his desk and began chuckling to himself.

Chapter sixty-seven

"Intriguing piece," said Browne, leaning back from the computer and turning to McCarthy.

"Best kind, Richard."

"Cosmetics create beauty, but when that turns ugly, it's lethal. Talk about evolution of story-line, eh."

"One-person celebrity feature becomes big issue, front-page news splash."

"Wonderful. That's what I love about this business, Kevin. Finding a great story. No amount of money matches it. I've missed this journalistic thrill over the years."

McCarthy glanced at Browne as he spoke, feeling slightly uncomfortable. He still hadn't got used to sitting so close, and certainly not this way, side-by-side editing together. The last time he was with his boss was a more formal occasion, being offered the editor's position, in the top-floor executive suite of a downtown Manhattan brownstone overlooking Central Park that made the Kansas City newsroom seem like an enlarged cubbyhole. Then the man wore Berluti shoes and an impeccable Giorgio Armani double-breasted suit, probably bought at Brooks Brothers on Madison Avenue. And a two-hundred dollar silk tie to match. Now he was open-collar, no coat, his sleeves rolled up to the elbows as if he was a plumber fixing a leak.

"Age," Browne continued interrupting his thoughts. "Mark my words, it does something to you, especially if you've a particularly endearing and nagging wife as I have. But you've no need to worry, its way, way off for you. For me, it's here and now. You start to yearn for what you might have missed." Then turning back to the computer, "What do you think of the lead?"

"Certainly grabs your attention," McCarthy said encouragingly.

"And focuses on the one thing we can be absolutely sure about -

Patricia. Right?"

"Yep, slated to give evidence later this week. And a press conference to follow. That should be a real humdinger."

"Can't miss that. Fancy going together?"

McCarthy turned, startled. Was he serious? The expression on his face told him he was.

"Yeah, why not," he replied collegiately.

Not for the first time in the last twenty-four hours, McCarthy sat in disbelief. Browne, the publisher, his boss, everyone's boss, bubbly and effervescent, sounding like a student just out of journalism school in his first job. He'd even proudly showed him a nice-looking pen he'd been given years before while editor of the university paper. Seemed he hadn't stopped rattling on excitedly since he got off the plane at KCI the previous day and they'd dined together at Chaz restaurant in the Raphael.

"Brilliant quotes from Patricia and Christine's parents," Browne said, his eyes fixed on the screen. "Very touching. Readers will weep when they read them. Colm did a great reporting job."

"Yes, he did," McCarthy replied, a part of him wanting to remind the man beside him that just a few days before he'd wanted to drag Colm back on the next plane and abandon the story altogether. He wisely decided against it. His shrewd idea had worked. That's all that mattered. "Their sentiments complement Doctor Gray's impressive scientific analysis of nano particles and their hidden dangers," he said instead.

"And the doctor's not overly technical or convoluted," Browne replied. "Some medical types can lose you in a maze of multi-syllables. All Latin and Greek. What he says is simple, straightforward. I failed high school biology and I understand it. Let's hope those in that committee room do also."

McCarthy smiled, feeling more at ease. He was getting to like this guy a lot. If he'd stayed in the writing side of the business, he'd have made a helluva good journalist. He was tempted to offer him a job. The thought tickled him no end.

"The visuals showing the lab test results on the two women are impressive," Browne continued. "Your graphics guys are spot on. That bar graph showing the amount of botulin and other chemicals in the samples is dramatic."

"Nowadays you gotta look like television on a page," McCarthy replied. "Plenty of color photos and charts. It's the only hope for newspaper survival."

"Tell me about it," Browne said rolling his eyes. "And Covington? Has he commented yet on the record?"

"Declined at first, then called back saying he needed some time. Told him we'd put 'no comment' in if he didn't get back to us before deadline."

"Don't worry, he'll get back," Browne said confidently. "Would look bad if he didn't. His lawyers' fingerprints will be all over the statement. How the company's past record stands for itself, how it has produced hundreds of products, all safe to use, lah-di-dah. Better for us to have something, than nothing. Shows we're being fair and helps avoid potential litigation down the road."

"A record that's hard to check all the same," McCarthy added. "With the industry regulating itself for so long now, information on bad products was kept well under wraps."

"Well, that may all change now," McCarthy replied, pride in his voice. "Our Washington correspondent tells me there's movement afoot in the corridors of power. Senator Clarke, a lone voice in the wilderness on this issue for so long, is on to a winner. No lawmaker wants to be tagged anti-consumer."

"Tomorrow's hearings are pivotal and our timing on this story couldn't be more perfect," Browne said, his voice filled with barely-contained excitement. "We'll lead the nation on it. I'd like to see the expressions on the faces of our colleagues on the Post and Times. Even the networks will go big on this."

"That's why we're thinking of running a double-decker headline with a 48 font across the cover," McCarthy said. "What do you think?"

"Perfect, the bigger the better." Browne's reply came brimming with enthusiasm. "What about pictures? Got good ones to go?"

"Think so. One of Doctor Gray in a white coat among vials and test tubes in a lab, looks suitably erudite. Another of Christine, doe-eyed, pretty as a peach, at her high-school prom."

Browne smiled, delighted.

"And a most bizarre one of Patricia with three strange-looking characters on a tiny boat in the middle of the ocean. Peculiar words 'Cara na Mara' emblazoned on the side. Feisty-looking fellas. Big toothy grins on their faces. Looks like they've been on the liquor, homemade Irish poitín most likely. Colm is keen we use it, says they're Patricia's best buddies over there, that we wouldn't have the story if it wasn't for them. Maybe he's gone native."

"Who took the pic?" Browne asked.

"We lucked out. Coupla freelance paparazzi had been sent over courtesy of Covington and a sleazy sidekick called Larry to do a hatchet job on Patricia. But Colm told me they were 'dissuaded' by two old fishermen and a Romanian scientist, the same characters who're in the boat. Don't know what he meant exactly. Was rambling on about three sisters, seasickness and strange insects."

"Sounds like potent poitín doing its work."

"Maybe. Though he did warn us to expect a hefty bill from the photographers."

"Worth every cent. Speaking of sleazy, did you take care of Pratt?" Browne shot a conspiratorial glance over his shoulder.

"Sure did, yesterday before you arrived. Screamed and kicked when I told him he was history. Cursed Colm to the high heavens, called him all kinds of names. Threatened to bring us to court. But went quiet when I showed him his telephone records, and the calls to Bellus."

"A case of hanging him with his own telephone cord, eh? So I don't need to punish him further then?"

"You not talking to him is punishment enough. He'll be gone by the end of the week anyhow."

"By the way, what about the source of this whole controversy?" Browne asked. "That little cosmetic thing. The revealer. I mean concealer."

"Either word is good enough. In the end, it worked both ways."

"Indeed it did, but where is it now?"

"Well-concealed," quipped McCarthy, smiling at his own pun. "It'll be used as evidence in the hearings tomorrow. 'As well protected as Alien bodies in Roswell.' Gray's exact words. But he did let us take pictures of it. Under strict conditions, of course. I'm thinking of using it as a logo on our stories."

"Great idea. Considering what's about to hit the fan it'll be a long-running series..." Browne's eyes brightened like shiny buttons. "Did I tell you my wife bought me a brand new monkey suit?"

McCarthy looked at his boss askance, his worse fears filtering into his mind again. That the stress of endless falling ad revenues had put him over the edge. In light of this, "Really!" was the only reply he could muster.

"Yep. Brioni. An Italian fashion house. Established in '45, right after World War Two. Specializes in handmade suits. Mine's a pinstripe. Made from the expensive wool of the vicuna, a rare South American animal. Stitching is made of white gold."

McCarthy was stumped. He hadn't read the handbook, the one that told you what to do if you're boss suddenly went mad. Biding for time to devise a proper strategy, he made the same limp reply, "Really!"

"Cost forty-eight thousand dollars."

Though now doubly shocked, McCarthy felt it incumbent to keep his tone even and avoid repetition, so said simply, swallowing hard, "Oh, and what's the occasion?"

"Why, that glittering event you promised me, of course. Between the Doric columns of my old alma mater at Columbia. Accepting the Pulitzer Public Service Award."

Chapter sixty-eight

"Are you sure you want to go through with this? It'll be a mad scramble. Lots of meddlesome reporters, just like me."

"I don't think they could possibly be like you," Patricia smiled, adding mischievously. "They couldn't be that bad surely."

"Ha ha." Colm made a face, then turned serious.

"It's very brave of you to speak out publicly," he said, looking deep into her eyes. "I just want to make sure it's what you really want."

"I appreciate your concern," she said, returning his gaze. "But I have to do this. I couldn't live with myself if I didn't, especially if it turned out to be a close vote against us. For the first time in my life maybe I can accomplish something more than winning a beauty pageant and modeling a face cream." Suddenly, tears welled up in her eyes. She swallowed hard. "It's the very least I can do for Christine."

"Stop thinking like that," Colm said seeing her face begin to crumble. "It's not your fault. You had no idea there was anything wrong with the product. Those bastards at Bellus, they're to blame... and now, hopefully, they'll pay for it. And you fooled Bellus and the entire cosmetic industry, didn't you? You coming here, taking the focus away from Christine and her family. I'm sure that helped a lot."

"I hope so," she said, dabbing at her eyes.

"And now, by going over there, saying what you've got to say, you can accomplish even more. For Christine, for Doctor Gray. And for so many others who could have faced these same problems in the future."

They stayed silent for a while, each in their own world.

"What about your own situation?"

Patricia looked at him as if confused by the question.

"The tests you had back at the hospital last time. Were they okay? I mean did they show... did they show....?" He faltered.

"So far so good," she replied, understanding. "The scars on my neck have probably put an end to my modelling career but I was getting tired of it anyway, and not getting any younger. As for the concealer, I wasn't using it for a long period of time so the botulin doesn't seem to have caused a lot of harm inside this head of mine. They say my brain seems to be working normally."

She stopped and fixed him with a wicked smile. "So I guess I'm not as mad as you thought I was after all."

Surprised, but not slow, he shot back. "Really? Well, I've got a straight-jacket here in my bag just in case." Seeing a twinkle in her eye, he continued, "Seriously though. That's great news. You'll be okay over there then?"

"I'll be just fine," Patricia said, touching his hand, finding pleasure in the simple gesture. "Anyways me laddie sure haven' ah faced plenty o' cameras afore?"

Her spontaneous imitation of their two favorite Irishmen made him laugh. They glanced to the stern of the boat where Ernie sat between Seamus and Ivan. Fishing rod in hand, he was animatedly explaining the merits of mackerel head over maggots as bait for black bream.

"Anyway, I'll have plenty of protection," Patricia continued. "There'll be no shortage of Secret agents there. I'll be like Whitney Houston in that movie."

She hesitated a few seconds. "Will you be my Kevin Costner?" She felt her cheeks glow saying it.

Colm's beamed. "Where's the sign-up sheet?"

They looked at each other for a long time without speaking.

"Anyway, I'm one to talk about protection," she said finally. "It's you who needs it. That was a nasty bang you got. When I first saw you lying there, sliding down into that mud, I thought ...." Her voice trailed off.

"You'd be so lucky," he said, seeing her difficulty. "Anyway, no need to worry, I'm well protected." He raised his arm. "This plaster of Paris weighs a ton. One swipe and you'd be bowled over."

She stretched over suddenly and kissed him softly on the cheek. "I already am." He felt a soothing warmth rush through him. Patricia leaned back, inhaling deep.

"Look, I have to tell you something but don't think I'm crazy," she said finally.

"Aha, so I was right to bring a straight-jacket after all."

"Maybe, especially when you hear what I've got to say."

Seeing her hesitate, he urged her on. "C'mon let's have it. I promise

I'll not tie the jacket on too tight."

"Something strange happened to me after you rushed out of the house in the storm and crashed in that bog."

"Strange?"

"Yes, and I just wondered if anything peculiar happened to you that night also?"

"To be honest, finding myself upside down in a car that was itself upside down in a bog in the middle of nowhere in the middle of a storm - that was peculiar enough for me," Colm replied.

She nudged him in mock annoyance, then continued. "I had a dream. A dream related to you."

"Me? In your dream? I'm honored."

"Sorry to disappoint you," she said, sticking out her tongue. "But you weren't in it. But I think the dream was about you."

"Is that like saying. 'I had a dream about my house, but it wasn't actually my house in the dream?' "

"Something like that. I say dream as that seems the only rational way to explain it. But at the time it seemed very real. Scary, but comforting at the same time." She glanced at Colm, his eyes narrowing with interest. "I know I'm not making sense, but...

"Go on. Let me be the judge of that."

"Well, after you told me the terrible news about Christine, I went to my bedroom. I lay down. I just wanted to forget about the world. That's when I saw an apparition, a ghost-like image. And it looked just like the mysterious image on that music CD at the medical center. The only difference being instead of two figures in a swirling fog, it was one, the man. I wondered, did you happen to see anything unusual out there in the bog that night cos it was about the same time?"

Colm stared at her, saying nothing. Feeling idiotic for bringing it up, Patricia looked down at her feet, embarrassed, but a sudden movement made her glance back up again. He had leaned closer, his eyes wide, his gaze fixed on her. "Colm?" she said, worry in her voice. "Are you okay?"

"I saw the same thing ...in the bog...in the mist," he said, excitement rising in his voice. "Not two figures, but one. Except what I saw was the woman. I thought I was hallucinating."

They looked at each other confounded.

"What do you think?" Patricia asked finally.

"I've no idea, it's bizarre." Then he thought of something. "Well, if you consider the legend of Niamh and Oisín and the Land of the Ever Young. Seems they were following their dream, going to a place where they could start a new life together, free of everyday stress and worry."

"Except he gave up the dream by going back," she added.

"Yes, but I don't intend making the same mistake."

"What do you mean?"

He didn't answer at first.

"You are going back to America, aren't you?"

"I'm not sure."

"About what?"

"About where I'm going." He stopped and gazed around him. "With the newspaper world collapsing, perhaps this isn't such a bad place to make a new beginning."

"As what?"

"A novelist."

She looked at him, incredulous. "You're serious?"

"Well, can you think of anywhere better than this achingly beautiful place to start afresh? Anyway, didn't you say living in a tiny box on the twentieth-fifth floor in the middle of a noisy, whacky, polluted city was crazy?"

She slowly nodded her head, remembering her words.

"And didn't you also say you wanted to start afresh and create a line of natural cosmetics with authentic Irish names, to help people stay young?" She glanced sideways at him, cocking one eyebrow. "I'd say there's no better scientist or skin specialist than Ivan to assist with that."

They turned and gazed out to sea in silence, deep in contemplation. Then a loud voice rang in their ears.

"Hey you two over there, wha' are ye both gawkin' at?" Ernie's singsong voice mingled with the swishing sound of the waves. "You look as if you've just seen Tír Na nÓg."

They swung around startled as if he'd read their minds.

"It's out there somewhere ye know," he said, seeing astonishment in their eyes, "but ye've got to believe in it afore ye can see it."

Colm and Patricia smiled at each other. It was as if his words had scattered stardust in the air and they were both holding their breath at the beauty of it all and the promises it offered.

The question was: Would it be there tomorrow?

ABOUT THE AUTHOR

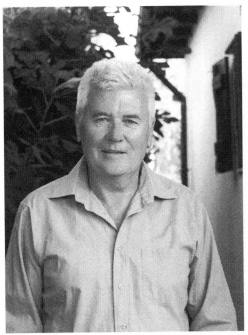

During a 40-year media career, Sean Hillen has been war correspondent, medical reporter, arts reviewer, travel writer, editor, publisher and author, as well as media trainer and creative writing coach with Ireland Writing Retreat.

Born in Belfast, northern Ireland, he wrote for Belfast Telegraph newspapers and The Irish Times before emigrating to the United States to work at the United Nations Media Center in New York. From there he moved to the Midwest with Scripps Howard Broadcasting, now an NBC-affiliate, and then The Kansas City Times, becoming the daily newspaper's health and science correspondent.

Sean's writings have also appeared in other newspapers including Time magazine, The Wall Street Journal, the Daily Mail, The Sunday Times, The Sunday Business Post, as well as specialized publications such as American Medical News, the national newspaper of the American Medical Association, American Nurse, national magazine of the American Nurses Association, and Nursing Times in England.

After winning regional and national journalism awards, Sean left the US for Eastern Europe immediately after the fall of the Berlin Wall in 1989 as a volunteer with the Human Rights League to establish the first post-Communist journalism schools in Romania. This led to him working with international aid agencies such as the British Council, United Nations Development Fund, Soros Foundation, Rockefeller Foundation and the US Agency for International Development (USAID). He was a foreign correspondent for The Times and The Daily Telegraph, London, before establishing his own national publishing and events company based in Bucharest for 15 years.

Reflecting his achievements in academics – including two postgraduate degrees in economics and journalism – Sean was elected chairperson of the US Fulbright Commission in Romania, a position he held for four years. He was also honored by the President of Romania for launching the nation's first-ever Corporate Citizen, Civic Journalism and Community Service Awards.

Sean's other books include a guide to media training and a light-hearted, intra-country travelogue entitled 'Digging for Dracula.' His travel writings can be found at Worlditineraries.co and JustLuxe.com

Sean shares his life with his Transylvanian wife, Columbia, and two enchanting collies, Siog ('fairy' in Irish) and Lugh (the Celtic Sun God) in the 'Forgotten County' of Donegal, a northwestern region boasting the most awe-inspiring landscapes on Ireland's 'Wild Atlantic Way.'

Author's Note

I welcome, indeed yearn, for your comments, good or bad, extraordinarily generous in your praise or downright critical (constructively so, preferably). Either way, please get in touch. It's always gratifying for any writer to receive feedback.

'Pretty Ugly' is intended as the first in a series of novels focusing on Colm Heaney and his particular, some might say peculiar, journalistic penchant for uncovering intriguing truths that matter, even in the most remotest of places on the planet.

seanhillenauthor.com

Made in the USA
Columbia, SC
24 May 2017